Soft Tissue Sarcomas:
Present Achievements and Future Prospects

Cancer Treatment and Research

Steven T. Rosen, MD., *Series Editor*

Hansen HH (ed): Basic and Clinical Concepts of Lung Cancer. 1989. ISBN 0-7923-0153-6
Lepor H, Ratliff TL (eds): Urologic Oncology. 1989. ISBN 0-7923-0161-7
Benz C, Liu E (eds): Oncogenes. 1989. ISBN 0-7923-0237-0
Ozols RF (ed): Drug Resistance in Cancer Therapy. 1989. ISBN 0-7923-0244-3
Surwit EA, Alberts DS (eds): Endometrial Cancer. 1989. ISBN 0-7923-0286-9
Champlin R (ed): Bone Marrow Transplantation. 1990. ISBN 0-7923-0612-0
Goldenberg D (ed): Cancer Imaging with Radiolabeled Antibodies. 1990. ISBN 0-7923-0631-7
Jacobs C (ed): Carcinomas of the Head and Neck. 1990. ISBN 0-7923-0668-6
Lippman ME, Dickson R (eds): Regulatory Mechanisms in Breast Cancer: Advances in Cellular and Molecular Biology of Breast Cancer. 1990. ISBN 0-7923-0868-9
Nathanson L (ed): Malignant Melanoma: Genetics, Growth Factors, Metastases, and Antigens. 1991. ISBN 0-7923-0895-6
Sugarbaker PH (ed): Management of Gastric Cancer. 1991. ISBN 0-7923-1102-7
Pinedo HM, Verweij J, Suit HD (eds): Soft Tissue Sarcomas: New Developments in the Multidisciplinary Approach to Treatment. 1991. ISBN 0-7923-1139-6
Ozols RF (ed): Molecular and Clinical Advances in Anticancer Drug Resistance. 1991. ISBN 0-7923-1212-0
Muggia FM (ed): New Drugs, Concepts and Results in Cancer Chemotherapy 1991. ISBN 0-7923-1253-8
Dickson RB, Lippman ME (eds): Genes, Oncogenes and Hormones: Advances in Cellular and Molecular Biology of Breast Cancer. 1992. ISBN 0-7923-1748-3
Humphrey G Bennett, Schraffordt Koops H, Molenaar WM, Postma A (eds): Osteosarcoma in Adolescents and Young Adults: New Developments and Controversies. 1993. ISBN 0-7923-1905-2
Benz CC, Liu ET (eds): Oncogenes and Tumor Suppressor Genes in Human Malignancies. 1993. ISBN 0-7923-1960-5
Freireich EJ, Kantarjian H (eds): Leukemia: Advances in Research and Treatment. 1993. ISBN 0-7923-1967-2
Dana BW (ed): Malignant Lymphomas, Including Hodgkin's Disease: Diagnosis, Management, and Special Problems. 1993. ISBN 0-7923-2171-5
Nathanson L (ed): Current Research and Clinical Management of Melanoma. 1993. ISBN 0-7923-2152-9
Verweij J, Pinedo HM, Suit HD (eds): Multidisciplinary Treatment of Soft Tissue Sarcomas. 1993. ISBN 0-7923-2183-9
Rosen ST, Kuzel TM (eds): Immunoconjugate Therapy of Hematologic Malignancies. 1993. ISBN 0-7923-2270-3
Sugarbaker PH (ed): Hepatobiliary Cancer. 1994. ISBN 0-7923-2501-X
Rothenberg ML (ed): Gynecologic Oncology: Controversies and New Developments. 1994. ISBN 0-7923-2634-2
Dickson RB, Lippman ME (eds): Mammary Tumorigenesis and Malignant Progression. 1994. ISBN 0-7923-2647-4
Hansen HH (ed): Lung Cancer. Advances in Basic and Clinical Research. 1994. ISBN 0-7923-2835-3
Goldstein LJ, Ozols RF (eds): Anticancer Drug Resistance. Advances in Molecular and Clinical Research. 1994. ISBN 0-7923-2836-1
Hong WK, Weber RS (eds): Head and Neck Cancer. Basic and Clinical Aspects. 1994. ISBN 0-7923-3015-3
Thall PF (ed): Recent Advances in Clinical Trial Design and Analysis. 1995. ISBN 0-7923-3235-0
Buckner CD (ed): Technical and Biological Components of Marrow Transplantation. 1995. ISBN 0-7923-3394-2
Muggia FM (ed): Concepts, Mechanisms, and New Targets for Chemotherapy. 1995. ISBN 0-7923-3525-2
Klastersky J (ed): Infectious Complications of Cancer. 1995. ISBN 0-7923-3598-8
Kurzrock R, Talpaz M (eds): Cytokines: Interleukins and Their Receptors. 1995. ISBN 0-7923-3636-4
Sugarbaker P (ed): Peritoneal Carcinomatosis: Drugs and Diseases. 1995. ISBN 0-7923-3726-3
Sugarbaker P (ed): Peritoneal Carcinomatosis: Principles of Management. 1995. ISBN 0-7923-3727-1
Dickson RB, Lippman ME (eds): Mammary Tumor Cell Cycle, Differentiation and Metastasis. 1995. ISBN 0-7923-3905-3
Freireich EJ, Kantarjian H (eds): Molecular Genetics and Therapy of Leukemia. 1995. ISBN 0-7923-3912-6
Cabanillas F, Rodriguez MA (eds): Advances in Lymphoma Research. 1996. ISBN 0-7923-3929-0
Miller AB (ed): Advances in Cancer Screening. 1996. ISBN 0-7923-4019-1
Hait WN (ed): Drug Resistance. 1996. ISBN 0-7923-4022-1
Pienta KJ (ed): Diagnosis and Treatment of Genitourinary Malignancies. 1996. 0-7923-4164-3

Soft Tissue Sarcomas: Present Achievements and Future Prospects

edited by

J. VERWEIJ
Department of Medical Oncology
Rotterdam Cancer Institute
Rotterdam, The Netherlands

H.M. PINEDO
Department of Medical Oncology
Free University Hospital
Amsterdam, The Netherlands

H.D. SUIT
Department of Radiation Medicine
Massachusetts General Hospital
Harvard Medical School
Boston, Massachusetts, USA

KLUWER ACADEMIC PUBLISHERS
BOSTON/DORDRECHT/LONDON

Distributors for North America:
Kluwer Academic Publishers
101 Philip Drive
Assinippi Park
Norwell, Massachusetts 02061 USA

Distributors for all other countries:
Kluwer Academic Publishers Group
Distribution Centre
Post Office Box 322
3300 AH Dordrecht, THE NETHERLANDS

Library of Congress Cataloging-in-Publication Data

Soft tissue sarcomas : present achievements and future prospects / edited by J. Verweij, H. M. Pinedo, H. D. Suit.
p. cm. – (Cancer treatment and research; 91)
Includes bibliographical references and index.
ISBN 0-7923-9913-7 (alk. paper)
1. Soft tissue tumors. 2. Sarcoma. I. Verweij, J. (Jaap)
II. Pinedo, H. M. III. Suit, Herman D. (Herman Day), 1929–
IV. Series.
[DNLM: 1. Sarcoma-diagnosis. 2. Sarcoma–therapy. W1 CA693
v. 91 1997 / QZ 345 S681 1997]
RC280.S66S65 1997
616.99′4–dc21
DNLM/DLC
for Library of Congress 97-9988
CIP

Printed on acid-free paper.

PRINTED IN THE UNITED STATES OF AMERICA

Contents

Contributing authors

ADLER, Lee P., Division of Nuclear Medicine, University Hospitals of Cleveland, 11100 Euclid Avenue, Cleveland, OH 44106

BEN-ARI, G., Department of Surgery, Chaim Sheba Medical Center, Tel-Hashomer, Israel

BIDMEAD, Margaret, Department of Physics, The Royal Marsden NHS Trust, Fulham Road, London SW3 6JJ, United Kingdom

COOPER, Colin S., Section Chairman, Molecular Carcinogenesis Section, The Haddow Laboratories, Institute of Cancer Research, 15 Cotswold Road, Belmont, Sutton, Surrey SM2 5NG, United Kingdom

CORNES, Paul, Molecular Carcinogenesis Section, The Haddow Laboratories, Institute of Cancer Research, 15 Cotswold Road, Belmont, Sutton, Surrey SM2 5NG, United Kingdom

DEVLIN, Phillip M., Joint Center for Radiation Therapy; Harvard Medical School; 330 Brookline Avenue, Boston, MA 02215, USA

EGGERMONT, A.M.M., Department of Surgery, Rotterdam Cancer Institute (Dr. Daniel den Hoed Kliniek) and University Hospital, Groene Hilledijk 301, 3075 EA Rotterdam, The Netherlands

FAULHABER, Peter F., Division of Nuclear Medicine, University Hospitals of Cleveland, 11100 Euclid Avenue, Cleveland, OH 44106

FLETCHER, Jonathan A., Department of Pathology, Brigham and Women's Hospital, 75 Francis Street, Boston, MA 02115, USA

HARMER, Clive, Head of Radiotherapy Services, Department of Radiotherapy, The Royal Marsden NHS Trust, Fulham Road, London SW3 6JJ, United Kingdom

HARRIS, Martin, Consultant Histopathologist/Honorary Reader in Pathology, Department of Pathology, Christie Hospital, Wilmslow Road, Withington, Manchester M20 4BX, United Kingdom

HARRISON, Louis B., Brachytherapy Service, Department of Radiation Oncology, Memorial Sloan-Kettering Cancer Center, 1275 York Avenue, NY 10021, USA

HARTLEY, Ann L., CRC Paediatic and Familial Cancer Research Group, Royal Manchester Children's Hospital, Pendlebury, Manchester M27 4HA, United Kingdom

KLAUSNER, J.M., Department of Surgery, Ichilov Hospital, Tel-Aviv Medical Center, Tel-Aviv, Israel
KROON, B.B.R., Department of Surgery, Netherlands Cancer Institute, Amsterdam, The Netherlands
LEJEUNE, F.J., Department of Surgery, Centre Pluridisciplinaire d'Oncologie, CHUV Lausanne, Switzerland
MIRALDI, Floro, Professor of Radiology and Engineering, Director, Division of Nuclear Medicine, Division of Nuclear Medicine, University Hospitals of Cleveland, 11100 Euclid Avenue, Cleveland, OH 4416-5000, USA
PAPPO, Alberto S., St. Jude Children's Research Hospital, 332 North Lauderdale, Memphis, TN 38105-2794, USA
PASTORINO, Ugo, Department of Thoracic Surgery, Royal Brompton Hospital, Sydney Street, London SW3 6NP, United Kingdom
PINEDO, Herbert M., Department of Medical Oncology, Free University Hospital and Netherlands Cancer Institute, De Boelelaan 1117, 1081 HV Amsterdam, The Netherlands
PRATT, Charles B., St. Jude Children's Research Hospital, 332 North Lauderdale Memphis, TN 38105-2794, USA
ROBINSON, Martin H., YCRC Department of Clinical Oncology, Weston Park Hospital NHS Trust, The University of Sheffield, Whitham Road, Sheffield S10 2SJ, United Kingdom
SCHLAG, P.M., Department of Surgery, Robert Rössle Hospital, Umboldt University, Berlin, Germany
SCHRAFFORDT KOOPS, H., Department of Surgery, University of Groningen, Hanzeplein 1, PO Box 30001, 9700 RG Groningen, The Netherlands
SPEAR, Matthew, Department of Radiation Medicine, Massachussetts General Hospital Harvard Medical School, Boston, MA 02114, USA
SPIRO, Ira J., Department of Radiation Medicine, Massachussetts General Hospital, Harvard Medical School, Boston, MA 02114, USA
STEWARD, William P., Co-Director, Investigational New Drug Program NCIC Clinical Trials Group, Queen's University, 82–84 Barrie Street, Kingston, Ontario K7L 3N6, Canada
SUIT, Herman D., Department of Radiation Medicine, Massachussetts General Hospital, Harvard Medical School, Boston, MA 02114, USA
VERWEIJ, Jaap, Department of Medical Oncology, Rotterdam Cancer Institute (Dr. Daniel den Hoed Kliniek) and University Hospital, Groene Hilledijk 301, 3075 EA Rotterdam, The Netherlands

Preface

The previous volumes in this series on soft tissue sarcomas highlighted the importance of the multidisciplinary approach to treatment, and this focus is continued in the present volume. Proper diagnosis and staging remain the cornerstone of the treatment strategy. Sophisticated histopathology techniques and growing consensus on grading systems have further increased the importance of the histopathologist in providing estimates of patient prognosis as well as in providing data for planning the treatment strategy. The use of cytogenetics in this field is rapidly increasing and might enable the distinction of subgroups in specific histological tumor types. Furthermore, molecular biological studies not only help reveal inherited predispositions and details in tumor oncogenesis, but they may also provide additional predictive factors for tumor behavior. Further data on treatment strategy will be provided by diagnostic imaging, and in this volume the value of PET imaging, a relatively new achievement, is highlighted.

As far as the actual treatment is concerned, surgery still provides the major opportunity for cure. The addition of radiotherapy to surgery is of utmost importance in efforts to spare as much tissue as possible. The chapters on the planning of radiotherapy, brachytherapy, and the treatment of benign soft tissue lesions using radiotherapy are new contributions to this book. One of the potential late problems of radiotherapy is the occurrence of secondary soft tissue sarcomas, which is discussed in Chapter 10. The functional outcome of treatment is obviously dependent on the skills of the surgeon and the vicinity of the joints, and is known to be dependent on the expertise of the treatment center. Detailed information on this topic is given in Chapter 6.

Recent reports on metastatic disease have indicated the excellent results achieved with metastatectomy with proper patient selection, as discussed in Chapter 5. There appears to be growing consensus on the role of chemotherapy in metastatic disease, in which only doxorubicin, ifosfamide, and DTIC are known to be active. Although it may differ, for individual subsets, in general, single-agent chemotherapy appears to be as effective as standard doses of combination chemotherapy. The lack of efficacy of adjuvant chemotherapy with standard doses of the drugs presently available has been definitively shown. Like radiotherapy, chemotherapy may have an important role in the preoperative treatment of advanced soft tissue sarcomas. Of great interest for this purpose is the application of isolated limb perfusion using tumor necrosis factor-alpha and melphalan. Finally, clinical behavior, treatment strategy, and the outcome of treatment in childhood soft tissue sarcomas are differ significantly than in adult soft tissue sarcomas, as described in Chapter 14.

We would like to thank all of the contributing authors for their work. Hopefully this book will stimulate further expansion of multidisciplinary approaches to cancer treatment.

J. Verweij, H.M. Pinedo, and H.D. Suit, editors

Soft Tissue Sarcomas:
Present Achievements and Future Prospects

1. Value of peer review of pathology in soft tissue sarcomas

Martin Harris and Ann L. Hartley

Introduction

The level of accuracy of diagnosis in general histopathological practice appears to be high, although the number of published studies is few [1–3]. The clinically significant discrepancy rate between the original and reviewed or audited diagnoses in these studies varies from 0.26% to 1.2%, with the lower figure coming from a North American community hospital [3] and the higher levels from a British University Teaching Hospital [2]. The difference does not appear to reflect variations in case mix at the two institutions because the details given suggest that the errors were often the result of oversights by the reporting pathologist and that the interpretive errors were mainly common, rather than rare, problems.

When tumor pathology is considered, a more substantial problem is found, although published data, excluding studies of specific tumor types or diagnostic techniques, such as intraoperative frozen section, are even more scarce. A recent publication compared 227 selected tumor diagnoses made in a British District General Hospital with those made on review of the same material by specialist oncological pathologists when the patients were referred for treatment to a Regional Oncology Center [4]. A major (i.e., clinically significant) discrepancy rate of 8.4% was found; the most important area of disagreement was in lymph node pathology, but 5 diagnostic errors (one major and four minor) occurred amongst 17 cases of soft tissue tumor, suggesting that this is also an important area of diagnostic difficulty.

Size of the problem in soft tissue tumors

Most studies that have assessed discrepancy rates between the original diagnoses of soft tissue tumors and the diagnoses made by expert reviewers have been based on series of patients referred to specialist centers for entry into therapeutic trials [5–8]. As such, it is likely that they received especially critical histologic scrutiny, even at the stage of making the original diagnosis. The discrepancy levels in these four studies are summarized in Table 1 and show

J. Verweij, H.M. Pinedo, and H.D. Suit (eds). SOFT TISSUE SARCOMAS: PRESENT ACHIEVEMENTS AND FUTURE PROSPECTS.

rather consistent findings, with 5–10% of cases having the original diagnosis of sarcoma revised to nonsarcoma and with 16–32% having a revision of the histologic subtype of sarcoma. Where grade was analyzed, there was disagreement in up to 40% of the cases.

A large study conducted in Manchester, UK took a different approach, which may give a more accurate assessment of the size of the overall problem [9]. Using the North West Regional Cancer Registry, all cases registered as soft tissue, visceral, or bone sarcomas in the 3 years 1982–1984 (inclusive) were traced. An attempt was made to review the pathological material for all of them, thus providing population-based data. The review was conducted by a panel of five consultant histopathologists, some of whom had special experience in sarcoma diagnosis. A pathological review was obtained in 96% of the 468 registered cases, and it was found that the level of disagreement on the basic diagnosis of sarcoma was much higher than in the studies cited earlier, with 22% of cases having a sarcoma diagnosis revised to nonsarcoma. Furthermore, in 39% of tumors the panel disagreed with the original subtype (this figure includes revision of diagnosis from one specific subtype to another; revision from sarcoma, not otherwise specified, to a specific subtype; and revision from a specific subtype to sarcoma, not otherwise specified). The results of the study are also summarized in Table 1.

The revised diagnoses for the cases reclassified as nonsarcomas in the Manchester study are listed in Table 2. It is evident from Table 2 that the most common type of malignancy mistaken for sarcoma was carcinoma, and that borderline or benign connective tissue tumors formed a significant group in

Table 1. Revision of sarcoma diagnoses in five studies

	Cases studied	Diagnosis revised to nonsarcoma	Sarcoma subtype revised	Grade revised
Baker and Benjamin, 1978 [5]	130 cases: soft tissue; therapeutic trials	7%	32%	—
Presant et al. 1986 [6]	216 cases: soft tissue and bone; therapeutic trials	6%	27%	17–28% (varies with grade)
Skiraki et al. 1989 [7]	488 cases: soft tissue, bone, mesothelioma; therapeutic trials	10%	16%	—
Alvegard et al. 1989 [8]	240 high-grade soft tissue sarcomas; therapeutic trials	5%	25%	40%
Harris et al. 1991 [9]	413 cases; population-based study; soft tissue, visceral, and bone sarcomas; 96% ascertainment level	22%	39%	—

Table 2. Final diagnoses for cases diagnosed as nonsarcomas in the study of Harris et al. [9]

Histology	Total (1982–1984)
Malignant tumors	
Carcinomas NOS	11
Squamous cell carcinoma	8
Clear cell adenocarcinoma	2
Hepatocellular carcinoma	1
Renal cell carcinoma	1
Malignant melanoma	4
Mixed Mullerian tumor	8
Yolk sac tumour	1
Astrocytoma	1
Lymphoma	5
Malignant tumor NOS	21
Borderline tumors	
Smooth muscle tumor of uncertain malignant potential	3
Epithelioid leiomyoma	1
Cellular leiomyoma	1
Hemangiopericytoma NOS	3
Benign tumors	
Fibrous histiocytoma	1
Lipoma	2
Leiomyoma	3
Bizarre leiomyoma	2
Capillary hemangioma	1
Juxtacortical chondroma	1
Neurofibroma	2
Benign soft tissue tumor NOS	1
Non-neoplastic conditions	
Proliferative myositis	1
Fibrous dysplasia	1
Fibromatosis NOS	4
Nodular fasciitis	1
Non-neoplastic NOS	1
Normal cellular morphology	1
Total	93

NOS = not otherwise specified.

which malignancy was overdiagnosed. In practice, the classical traps of non-neoplastic reactive fibroblastic proliferations, such as nodular fasciistis, were rarely mistaken for sarcoma.

The reclassification of sarcoma subtypes in the Manchester study is shown in Table 3. It is notable that many of the sarcomas originally labeled as unclassified were allocated to a specific type by the panel and also that there was a very poor level of agreement in the groups originally diagnosed as leiomyosarcoma, malignant fibrous histiocytoma, liposarcoma, fibrosarcoma, and rhabdomyosarcoma.

Table 3. Reclassification of sarcomas in the study of Harris et al. [9]

		Final diagnosis																	
Original diagnosis	Total number reviewed	Sarcoma NOS	Leio	MFH	Lipo	Fibro	RMS	Hemgio	Endo Stro	Synovial	MPNST	Osteo	Chondro	Ewing's	Other specified sarcoma	Other malignant tumor	Malignant tumor NOS	Benign/ border-line	Non-neoplastic
Sarcoma NOS	73	11	10	8	2	2	0	1	2	1	5	4	1	0	5	11	9	1	0
Leiomyosarcoma	66	1	**43**	2	0	0	0	0	1	0	1	0	0	0	0	6	1	10	1
Malignant fibrous histiocytoma	52	6	10	**23**	1	0	1	0	0	0	0	0	0	0	1	4	3	2	1
Liposarcoma	35	1	2	4	**17**	0	0	0	0	0	0	0	0	0	1	6	1	3	0
Fibrosarcoma	28	5	4	5	0	**2**	0	0	0	1	2	1	2	0	1	1	2	1	1
Rhabdomyosarcoma	25	5	1	5	1	0	**9**	0	0	0	0	0	0	0	1	1	2	0	0
Hemangiosarcoma	14	2	0	0	0	0	0	**9**	0	0	0	0	0	0	0	2	0	1	0
Endometrial stromal sarcoma	10	1	0	1	0	0	0	0	**7**	0	0	0	0	0	0	1	0	0	0
Synovial sarcoma	4	1	0	0	0	0	0	0	0	**3**	0	0	0	0	0	0	0	0	0
Neurofibrosarcoma	10	0	1	0	0	0	1	0	0	0	**6**	0	0	0	0	1	0	1	0
Osteosarcoma	28	1	0	0	0	0	0	0	0	0	0	**21**	1	1	0	2	1	0	1
Chondrosarcoma	30	0	0	0	0	0	0	0	0	0	0	2	**24**	0	0	2	0	1	1
Ewing's tumor	9	0	0	0	0	0	0	0	0	0	0	0	0	**9**	0	0	0	0	0

NOS = not otherwise specfied.

Reasons for the high discrepancy rate

It is clear from the data summarized so far that the diagnosis and classification of soft tissue sarcomas is an area of major and difficulty for general histopathologists, and all of the studies cited have concluded that specialist review is desirable. The reasons for the difficulties are well understood by histopathologists but perhaps not by clinicians. Part of the problem arises from the intrinsic difficulties in interpreting the histology of these tumors. This is compounded by their rarity, so that any one histopathologist working in a general hospital is unlikely to encounter enough cases to develop or maintain expertise in the field. For example, in North West England the incidence of soft tissue sarcomas is 18.6 per million person years [10], which equates to 84 new cases per annum amongst a population of approximately 4.5 million people served by 61 consultant histopathologists. If the cases are distributed equally amongst those pathologists, each will see only one to two new examples each year; in practice, the distribution is not even, so that while some see more cases, others see less.

It is possible, however, that the figures quoted in all the studies referred to may exaggerate the problem as it currently exists. In all cases the initial diagnoses were made in the preimmunohistochemistry era, whereas immunohistochemistry was available to the reviewers, giving them an advantage in both the differentiation of pseudosarcomas from true sarcomas and in the accurate subtyping of sarcomas. It may be that the substantial differences between first and reviewed diagnoses would be reduced if, as would be the case nowadays, immunostaining was used in making the primary diagnosis. A study to examine this proposition would be valuable. Nevertheless, immunohistochemistry cannot solve all diagnostic problems, and it is likely that significant diagnostic discrepancies will continue to arise between general histopathologists and specialists.

Why is accurate diagnosis important?

The immediate and obvious reason why accurate tissue diagnosis is important is that it determines clinical management of the individual patient, including the assessment of prognosis and, where appropriate, the determination of validity for entry into clinical trials. However, it is also important in the collection of reliable epidemiological data, which may reveal trends in incidence, and it facilitates assessment of the effectiveness of health care systems in dealing with these rare tumors. Furthermore, it is essential in the analysis of etiological and pathogenetic factors, especially in familial syndromes such as the Li-Fraumeni syndrome, and the analysis of the results of therapeutic studies can only be meaningful when accurate diagnosis is assured.

Review systems in the achievement of accurate diagnosis

The generation of clinically relevant immediate diagnoses and the requirements of data collection for scientific and clinical research operate under different time constraints. The latter are easier to achieve because diagnostic review can be obtained in a planned manner without clinical pressures. All of the studies cited so far have made use of panels of reviewers who saw the pathologic material and clinical data some time after the original diagnosis had been made, although the size and modus operandi of the panels varied. In some cases initial review was conducted by one reviewer only, and if there was agreement the original diagnosis was accepted without involvement of other panel members [6,7]; only where there was disagreement were other panel members asked to see the case.

The European Organization for Research and Treatment of Cancer (EORTC) organizes and coordinates numerous therapeutic studies in the field of oncology with member institutions from a total of 14 countries, creating special problems in the organization of the pathologic review process. Currently the EORTC Soft Tissue Sarcoma studies accrue approximately 300 new case per annum, and the pathological diagnoses for all of these cases are reviewed in a manner similar to that described in the last paragraph. The six members of the Pathology Subcommittee, who come from Holland, Denmark, France, Italy, Spain, and the United Kingdom, take responsibility for cases from their own and, in some instances, other countries.

Contributing hospitals refer representative sections to their EORTC pathologist, who also has access to clinical data recorded on a standard proforma. If the referee agrees with the original diagnosis, the pathology data sheet recording subtype and grade is completed and sent to the EORTC data center without further review. If there is disagreement, the referee consults another pathologist from his own country who is not a member of the EORTC group but who has an interest in sarcoma pathology; if they agree, the agreed, revised diagnosis is recorded. In cases in which these steps do not produce agreement, the sections are discussed at one of the biennial meetings of the full Pathology Subcommittee before the final diagnosis is entered into the database.

Referring clinicians and pathologists, as well as referees, operate on a defined time scale to ensure that there is conformity with the requirements of the trial protocols. This method has been successful in overcoming the difficulties of organizing review of cases when they originate in many countries and when the reference panel is multinational and able to meet only infrequently. In the future alternative schemes employing 'telepathology' may be possible [11–13], but until then this appears to be an acceptable compromise.

However, this panel approach does not offer a solution to the problem of optimizing the immediate working diagnosis for each patient. It is difficult to devise a practical answer to this problem, but a modification of the approach of Safrin and Bark [3] to general surgical pathology sign-out could provide a solution. In this study all surgical pathology sections in the authors' laboratory (excluding those cases for which a second opinion would have been sought anyway) were reviewed by a second pathologist in the same department *before* reports were issued, and any discrepancy was resolved before reports were signed out.

The clinically significant discrepancy rate was very low (0.26%), and the process generated an added cost of US $7 per case or US $2700 per discrepancy. This may not be cost effective in general histopathology, but a similar approach could be routinely applied to selected tumor groups where problems are known to occur frequently, including soft tissue tumors. The number of cases reviewed in this way would thus be limited and the costs/time involved contained. The reviewer might well vary for different tumor types, with the local expert in a given field acting as a referee for his or her own area of interest. Once again, telepathology could have an important role in gaining immediate access to national and/or international expertise.

Conclusions

A consensus exists that expert pathologic review is desirable for soft tissue sarcomas. Review by panels for the analysis of clinical trials and the production of accurate epidemiological and scientific data is an acceptable method and can be adapted to local needs. An example of an adaptation for the EORTC international studies has been described. Panel review is not appropriate for immediate diagnosis to determine clinical management, and an alternative local peer review mechanism has been proposed to overcome the difficulties experienced by general histopathologists in dealing with these rare tumors.

References

1. Whitehead ME, Fitzwater JE, Lindley SK, Kern SB, Ulirsch RC, Winecoff WF. Quality assurance of histopathologic diagnoses; a prospective audit of three thousand cases. Am J Clin Pathol 81:487–491, 1994.
2. Ramsay AD, Gallagher PJ. Local audit of surgical Pathology. 18 months' experience of peer review-based quality assessment in an English teaching hospital. Am J Surg Pathol 16:476–482, 1992.
3. Safrin RE, Bark CJ. Surgical pathology signout. Routine review of every case by a second pathologist. Am J Surg Pathol 17:1190–1192, 1993.
4. Prescott RJ, Wells S, Bisset DL, Banerjee SS, Harris M. Audit of tumour histopathology review by a regional oncology centre. J Clin Pathol 48:245–249, 1995.
5. Baker LH, Benjamin RS. Histologic frequency of disseminated soft tissue sarcomas in adults (abstr). Proc Am Soc Clin Oncol 19:324.
6. Presant CA, Russell WO, Alexander RW, Fu YS. Soft tissue and bone sarcoma histopathology peer review: The frequency of disagreement in diagnosis and the need for second pathology opinions. The South Eastern Cancer Study Group experience. J Clin Oncol 4:1658–1661, 1986.
7. Shiraki M, Enterline HT, Brooks JJ, Cooper NS, Hirsche S, Roth JA, Rao UN, Enzinger FM,

Amato DA, Borden EC. Pathologic analysis fo advanced adult soft tissue sarcomas, bone sarcomas and mesotheliomas. The Eastern Cooperative Oncology Group [ECOG] experience. Cancer 64:484–490, 1989.

8. Alvegard TA, Berg NO. Histopathology peer review of high-grade soft tissue sarcoma: The Scandinavian Sarcoma Group experience. J Clin Oncol 7:1845–1852, 1989.
9. Harris M, Hartley AL, Blair V, Birch JM, Banerjee SS, Freemont AJ, McClure J, McWilliam LJ. Sarcomas in North West England: I Histopathological peer review. Br J Cancer 64:315–320, 1991.
10. Hartley AL, Blair V, Harris M, Birch JM, Banerjee SS, Freemont AJ, McClure J, McWilliam LJ. Sarcomas in North West England: II Incidence. Br J Cancer 64:1145–1150, 1991.
11. Weinstein RS. Telepathology comes of age in Norway. Hum Pathol 22:511–513, 1991.
12. Nordrum I, Engum B, Rinde E, Finseth A, Ericsson H, Kearney M, Stalsberg H, Eide TJ. Remote frozen section service: A telepathology project in Northern Norway. Hum Pathol 22:514–518, 1991.
13. Oberholzer M, Fischer H-R, Christen H, Gerber S, Bruhlmann M, Mihatsch M, Famos M, Winkler C, Fehr P, Bachthold L, Kayser K. Telepathology with an integrated services digital network — a new tool for image transfer in surgical pathology: A preliminary report. Hum Pathol 24:1078–1085, 1993.

2. Cytogenetics of soft tissue tumors

Jonathan A. Fletcher

Introduction

The past decade has witnessed tremendous advances in our understanding of the chromosomal and DNA mutations responsible for soft tissue sarcomas. Many research groups have characterized cytogenetic and molecular genetic mutations in soft tissue sarcomas, and a surprising number of sarcoma mutations have proved to be specific for particular histologies (Tables 1 and 2). Virtually all malignant soft tissue tumors contain clonal cytogenetic aberrations [1–4], and clonal cytogenetic aberrations are also found in many benign soft tissue tumors [2–4]. Sarcoma cytogenetic aberrations arise by diverse physical mechanisms. Common mechanisms include deletions, amplifications, and rearrangements of various chromosomal regions.

There are several reasons why so many research groups have studied sarcoma genetics. Sarcomas are relatively common during childhood, for one thing, accounting for approximately 10% of all pediatric malignant solid tumors. Pediatric tumors are generally viewed as excellent models for defining novel genetic mechanisms. Productive genetic studies of pediatric solid tumors have focused on Ewing's sarcoma, peripheral primitive neuroectodermal tumor, rhabdomyosarcoma, and neuroblastoma, among others. Genetic studies of soft tissue sarcomas have not been restricted to pediatric cases, however. Adult sarcomas have also been subject to intensive research efforts. This is, in part, because sarcomas in adults often contain genetic aberrations that are less complex than those in carcinomas and other common types of adult malignancies. This chapter describes some of the cytogenetic aberrations that have been characterized recently in soft tissue sarcomas (see Tables 1 and 2).

Cytogenetic and related detection strategies

A variety of approaches are used to demonstrate chromosomal aberrations in soft tissue sarcomas. The principal approaches include cytogenetic analysis, chromosomal fluorescence in situ hybridization (FISH), and polymerase chain reaction (PCR). It is understandable that the variety of alternate diagnostic

J. Verweij, H.M. Pinedo, and H.D. Suit (eds). SOFT TISSUE SARCOMAS: PRESENT ACHIEVEMENTS AND FUTURE PROSPECTS.

Table 1. Cytogenetic and molecular aberrations in malignant soft tissue tumors

Histologic findings	Cytogenetic events	Molecular events	Frequency	Diagnostic utility?
Chondrosarcoma, extraskeletal myxoid	t(9;22)(q31;q12)	*CHN-EWS* fusion	?50%	Yes
Clear cell sarcoma	t(12;22)(q13;q12)	*ATF1-EWS* fusion	>75%	Yes
Dermatofibrosarcoma protuberans	Ring form of chromosomes 17 and 22		>75%	Yes
Ewing's sarcoma	t(11;22)(q24;q12)	*FLI1-EWS* fusion	>80%	Yes
	t(21;22)(q12;q22)	*ERG-EWS* fusion	10%	Yes
	t(7;22)(p22;q12)	*ETV1-EWS* fusion	<5%	Yes
Fibrosarcoma, infantile	+8, +11, +17, +20		90%	Yes
Hemangiopericytoma	Translocation at 12q13		>25%	No
Intraabdominal desmoplastic small round cell tumor	t(11;22)(p13;q12)	*WT1-EWS* fusion	>75%	Yes
Leiomyosarcoma	Deletion of 1p		75%	No
Liposarcoma				
Myxoid	t(12;16)(q13;p11)	*CHOP-TLS* fusion	>75%	Yes
Well differentiated	Ring chromosome 12		>75%	Yes
Pleomorphic	Complex		>90%	No
Malignant fibrous histiocytoma				
high grade	Complex		90%	No
Myxoid	Ring chromosomes		>50%	?
Malignant peripheral nerve sheath tumor	Complex		90%	No
		Mutation and/or deletion of *NF1* gene	>25%	?
Mesothelioma	Deletion of 1p, 3p, 6q, 9p and/or 22q		>90%	Yes
		Deletion of *p15 and p16*	75%	Yes
Neuroblastoma				
Good prognosis	Hyperdiploid	No amplification of *MYCN*	90%	Yes
Poor prognosis	Diploid or tetraploid	No amplification of *MYCN*	50%	Yes
	Diploid or tetraploid, with double minute chromosomes	Amplification of *MYCN*	50%	Yes
Primitive neuroectodermal tumor (see Ewing's)				
Rhabdomyosarcoma				
Alveolar	t(2;13)(q35;q14)	*PAX3-FKHR* fusion	>75%	Yes
	t(1;13)(p36;q14)	*PAX7-FKHR* fusion	10–20%	Yes
Embryonal	+2q, +8, +20		80%	?
		Deletion at 11p15	>80%	Yes
Synovial sarcoma	t(X;18)(p11;q11)	*SSXT-SSX* fusion	>90%	Yes

approaches has engendered a great deal of confusion amongst clinicians. Even those specializing in cytogenetic and/or molecular diagnostics are often uncertain as to which method is best suited to demonstrating a particular cytogenetic aberration. A comprehensive discussion of the pros and cons of

Table 2. Cytogenetic and molecular aberrations in benign soft tissue tumors

Histologic findings	Cytogenetic events	Molecular events	Frequency	Diagnostic utility?
Desmoid tumor	Trisomy 8 and/or trisomy 20		25%	?
		APC gene deletion	>75%	?
Hibernoma	Translocation at 11q13		?	?
Lipoblastoma	Rearrangement of 8q		>25%	Yes
Lipoma				
Solitary	Rearrangement of 12q15	*HMGI-C* rearrangement or overexpression	75%	Yes
	Rearrangement of 6p		10%	?
	Deletion of 13q		10%	?
Multiple	None			
Neurofibroma		*NF1* gene deletion	?	?
Uterine leiomyoma	t(12;14)(q15;q24)	*HMGI-C* rearrangement or overexpression	20%	Yes
	Deletion of 7q		15%	No
	Trisomy 12		10%	No

diagnostic methods is beyond the scope of this chapter. However, the principal approaches are summarized here.

Cytogenetic analyses have been instrumental in defining specific chromosome aberrations associated with many soft tissue sarcomas [1–4]. Cytogenetic analyses are performed by first establishing tissue cultures from surgical sarcoma specimens and then harvesting metaphase cells from those cultures. The metaphase cells are stained, typically with Giemsa, to produce banding patterns in the chromosomes. Deviations from normal chromosome banding patterns indicate rearrangements that have occurred during the process of tumor initiation or progression. The cytogenetic approach is extremely broad in scope, being based on morphologic evaluation of the total chromosome complement in individual cells. One often finds novel chromosome aberrations that would be overlooked using more focused detection strategies. Cytogenetic analyses have certain limitations, however. They are quite labor intensive and expensive, they do not detect point mutations, and they require that tissue culture of tumor cells. The last point is key. Conventional cytogenetic analyses cannot be performed using archival (frozen or paraffin-embedded) specimens. In addition, the neoplastic populations in tissue culture are often overgrown by reactive stromal cells, for example, fibroblasts. Virtually all malignant soft tissue tumor cells contain clonal chromosome aberrations [1], and failure to detect such aberrations invariably reflects overgrowth by reactive cells in the tissue cultures.

Molecular cytogenetic analyses generally involve evaluation of particular chromosome regions using DNA probes to those regions. A common approach involves detection of DNA probes using fluorescence markers. This approach is known as fluorescence in situ hybridization (FISH). FISH analyses can be performed in both fresh and archival specimens, and these analyses require relatively little tumor material. For example, FISH evaluations of chromosome copy number and rearrangements can be performed efficiently using touch preparations and cytologic preparations [5].

The diagnostic chromosome rearrangements in various soft tissue sarcomas can also be demonstrated with molecular approaches. Southern blotting is seldom used for diagnostic translocation detection because this approach is less sensitive and often more labor intensive than reverse transcriptase PCR (RT-PCR). In RT-PCR, a cDNA pool is initially transcribed from tumor mRNA, and the cDNA population is then amplified using PCR primers on either side of the chromosome translocation. PCR is the only assay capable of detecting small numbers of translocation-bearing cells amidst predominantly non-neoplastic populations. RT-PCR, has been used, for example, to demonstrate circulating tumor cells in peripheral blood specimens from patients with Ewing's sarcoma. One constraint in RT-PCR is the requirement for reasonably intact mRNA. mRNA in some paraffin-embedded tumors is extensively degraded and cannot be amplified.

Ewing's sarcoma and peripheral primitive neuroectodermal tumor

Ewing's sarcoma and peripheral primitive neuroectodermal tumor (PNET) are both small round-cell tumors, but Ewing's sarcomas are undifferentiated, whereas peripheral PNETs have ultrastructural and immunohistochemical features of neuroectodermal differentiation. Although Ewing's sarcomas and peripheral PNET were originally believed to be unrelated neoplasms, they are regarded as a single neoplastic entity with a spectrum of differentiation. For the sake of simplicity, both Ewing's sarcomas and peripheral PNET will be referred to as Ewing tumors in this chapter. More than 90% of Ewing tumors contain a cytogenetic translocation in which material is exchanged between the long arms of chromosomes 11 and 22. This very characteristic translocation results in fusion of the *FLI1* gene from chromosome 11 with the *EWS* gene from chromosome 22 [6–9]. A smaller subset of cases, perhaps 5–10% of the total, have variant translocations in which the *EWS* gene is fused with the *ETV1* gene from chromosome 7 [10] or the *ERG* gene from chromosome 21 [11].

The chromosome translocations in Ewing tumors are a paradigm for translocations in several other soft tissue sarcomas. This is because the genes activated in the Ewing tumor translocations are functionally related to genes activated by chromosome translocations in rhabomyosarcoma, liposarcoma, clear cell sarcoma, myxoid chondrosarcoma, and intraabdominal desmoplastic small round cell tumor. The *EWS* gene normally encodes a protein containing RNA-binding domains [8,9], and the three genes fused to *EWS* in the different Ewing tumor translocations (*FLI1*, *ETV1*, and *ERG*) are all ETS family transcription factor genes [8–11]. The Ewing tumor *EWS* translocations result in fusion or 'hybrid' genes containing DNA-binding components from an ETS gene together with activation factors from *EWS*. The end result is an activated transcription factor (DNA-binding protein), which promotes expression of yet unidentified genes that are directly responsible for the neoplastic phenotype [12–15]. These findings suggest that activation of regulatory genes is the seminal pathogenetic event in Ewing tumors.

The Ewing tumor *EWS* translocations can be demonstrated diagnostically using cytogenetic, molecular cytogenetic, or polymerase chain reaction (PCR) methods. Cytogenetic analyses require tissue culture of tumor cells for at least 1–3 days. Metaphase preparations are harvested from the tissue cultures and are then stained to reveal characteristic chromosome translocations (Fig. 1) [1,7]. Cytogenetic analyses of Ewing tumors are quite reliable, although one potential problem is tissue culture overgrowth of the tumor by reactive stromal cells. Ewing tumor cytogenetic analyses require relatively small amounts of tissue, and these analyses have been performed using percutaneous needle biopsy specimens [1,16]. In the molecular cytogenetic approach, DNA probes to *EWS* and one of the ETS family genes, for example, *FLI1*, are cohybridized against tumor cells [17]. These genes are then detected in nuclei by dual-color FISH in which, for example, the *EWS* probe is demonstrated with a yellow fluorescence dye and the *FLI1* probe with a red fluorescence dye. The FISH probes have a distinctive physical distribution in Ewing tumor cells because the chromosome translocation brings one copy of *FLI1* and *EWS* together. PCR detection of the *FLI1-EWS* is accomplished, in contrast, using oligonucleotide primers complemetary to the *FLI1* and *EWS* ends of the fusion gene [9,18]. Successful amplification of a contiguous sequence between these two primers confirms *FLI1-EWS* fusion. Both FISH and PCR detection methods are often more rapid than cytogenetic analyses and can be performed

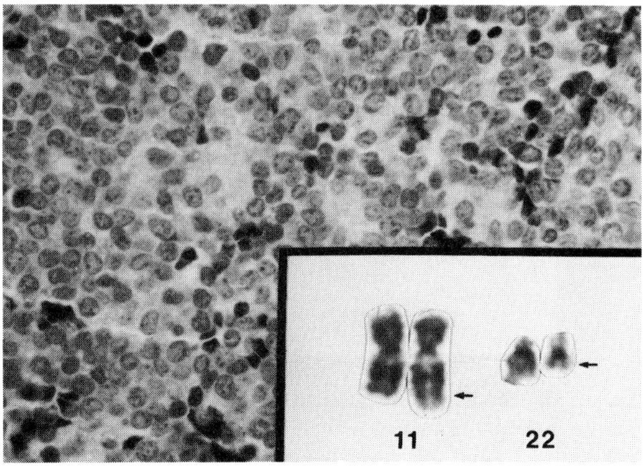

Figure 1. Translocation of chromosomes 11 and 22 supporting a diagnosis of Ewing's sarcoma or peripheral primitive neuroectodermal tumor in an undifferentiated small round-cell pharyngeal tumor from a 7-month-old boy. Arrows indicate translocation breakpoints on the rearranged chromosomes.

readily using tumor materials frozen at −70°C. The exquisite sensitivity of PCR enables detection of circulating tumor cells in patients with newly diagnosed Ewing tumors, and it is likely that PCR detection will have a growing role in evaluation of residual and/or recurrent disease after therapy.

Several additional nonrandom chromosome aberrations have been reported in Ewing tumors. These include trisomy 8, trisomy 12, and a translocation involving chromosomes 1 and 16 [1,19]. Each of these aberrations occurs in fewer than 40% of cases, and the prognostic relevance of these aberrations is unknown.

Clear cell sarcoma (malignant melanoma of soft parts)

Clear cell sarcomas of soft tissues, also referred to as melanoma of soft parts, have many histologic and immunophenotypic features in common with cutaneous melanomas. Hence, it can be difficult to distinguish between clear cell sarcoma and cutaneous melanoma diagnostically. Accurate diagnosis is important, however, because soft tissue clear cell sarcomas typically present as deep-seated masses, and such masses would indicate metastatic disease if the diagnosis was melanoma. It is notable, therefore, that more than 75% of clear cell sarcomas contain a chromosome translocation that has never been reported in cutaneous melanoma [20–27]. This translocation fuses the *ATF1* gene on chromosome 12 with the *EWS* gene on chromosome 22 [28,29]. The *ATF1* gene encodes a transcription factor, and the biologic implications of the translocation are probably similar to those discussed previously in the Ewing tumors. *ATF1-EWS* fusion can be demonstrated readily using cytogenetic (Fig. 2) or PCR methods.

Intraabdominal desmoplastic small round cell tumor

Intraabdominal desmoplastic small round cell tumors typically contain islands of undifferentiated highly malignant small round cells amidst an intense desmoplastic reaction [30]. Most cases have a translocation involving chromo-

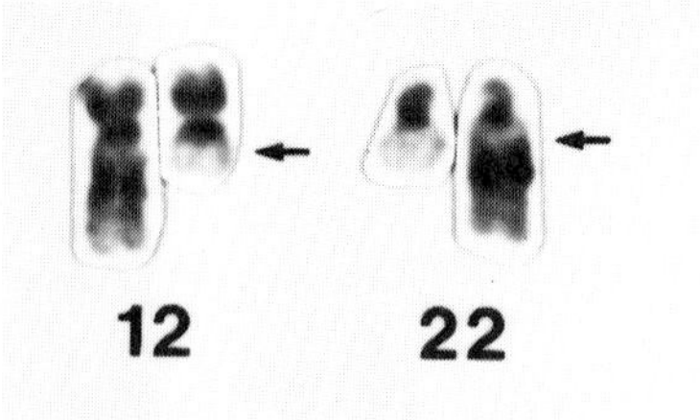

Figure 2. Translocation of chromosomes 12 and 22 from a clear cell sarcoma. Arrows indicate translocation breakpoints on the rearranged chromosomes.

somes 11 and 22, which targets the same gene, *EWS*, involved in Ewing tumors [31,32]. In intraabdominal desmoplastic small round cell tumor, the *EWS* gene from chromosome 22 is fused with the *WT1* gene from chromosome 11 [33,34]. This gene fusion is particularly interesting because *WT1* functions as a tumor suppressor gene — or growth inhibitor — in Wilms tumors. However, activation of this gene, by fusion with *EWS*, appears to promote growth in intraabdominal desmoplastic small round cell tumors.

Rhabdomyosarcoma

Alveolar rhabdomyosarcomas are high-grade neoplasms that are often widely metastatic at diagnosis. Approximately 80% of alveolar rhabdomyosarcomas contain translocations involving the *FKHR* gene on chromosome 13. In most cases the *FKHR* gene is fused with the *PAX3* gene on chromosome 3 [35–37], but a minority of rhadbomyosarcomas contain fusions of *FKHR* with the *RAX7* gene on chromosome 1 [38]. *FKHR*, *PAX3*, and *PAX7* are genes that encode transcription factors, and the *FKHR/PAX3* and *FKHR/PAX7* gene fusions create activated versions of the transcription factors [39,40]. These gene fusions, and the associated chromosome translocations, are diagnostic of alveolar rhabdomyosarcoma and can be demonstrated by cytogenetics, FISH, or PCR [1,41–47]. The recent introduction of multiplex PCR approaches enabled simultaneous appraisal of the *EWS* and *FKHR* gene fusions that are diagnostic, respectively, of alveolar rhabdomyosarcoma and Ewing tumors [46,47]. Embryonal rhabdomyosarcomas lack *FKHR* translocations but invariably have deletion of the short arm of chromosome 11 [48]. Alveolar rhabdomyosarcomas, by contrast, lack chromosome 11 deletions. Hence, assessment of the chromosome 11 deletion has been proposed as a diagnostic method for distinguishing between embryonal rhabdomyosarcoma and alveolar rhabdomyosarcoma [49].

Synovial sarcoma

Virtually all synovial sarcomas contain a translocation involving chromosomes X and 18 [1,50,51]. This translocation results in fusion of the *SSXT* gene from chromosome 18 with one of two highly homologous and closely neighboring genes on chromosome X. The chromosome X genes, designated *SSX1* and *SSX2*, encode DNA-binding proteins that appear to regulate gene transcription [52–54]. Translocation of chromosomes X and 18 is equally common in both monophasic and biphasic synovial sarcomas, and has not been reported in potential histologic mimics, such as hemangiopericytoma, leimyosarcoma, mesothelioma, and malignant peripheral nerve sheath tumor. Thus, the distinctive synovial sarcoma chromosome translocation has substantial diagnostic

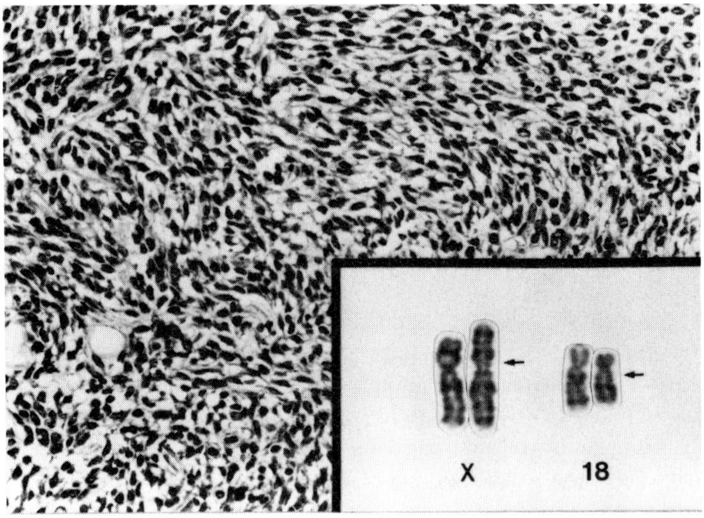

Figure 3. Spindle-cell neoplasm with translocation of chromosomes X and 18 supporting a diagnosis of synovial sarcoma. Arrows indicate translocation breakpoints on the rearranged chromosomes.

relevance. Detection of the translocation can be accomplished by cytogenetic [1,50,51] (Fig. 3), FISH [55,56], or PCR [52,53] methods.

Peripheral nerve sheath tumors

Benign and malignant peripheral nerve sheath tumors are a particular affliction for patients with the hereditary neurofibromatosis syndromes. Malignant peripheral nerve sheath tumors and neurofibromas are especially common in individuals with neurofibromatosis type 1 (NF1), whereas benign schwannomas are particularly common in those with neurofibromatosis type 2 (NF2). Isolation of genes responsible for the neurofibromatosis syndromes has shed light on the genesis of the associated tumors. The *NF1* and *NF2* genes are located on the long arms of chromosomes 17 and 22, respectively, and both of these genes function as tumor suppressors that normally constrain cell proliferation [57–59]. Deletions and inactivations of the *NF1* gene are found in both sporadic malignant peripheral nerve sheath tumors and in cases associated with the NF1 syndrome [57,60,61]. Preliminary studies indicate that novel drugs, particularly farnesyltransferase inhibitors, antagonize the tumorigenic mechanisms of *NF1* gene dysfunction. Neoplastic properties of malignant peripheral nerve sheath tumors can be reversed through farnesyltransferase inhibition or through gene transfer of normal *NF1* [59,62].

The karyotypes in most malignant peripheral nerve sheath tumors (MPNST) are very complex, particularly when contrasted with the relatively

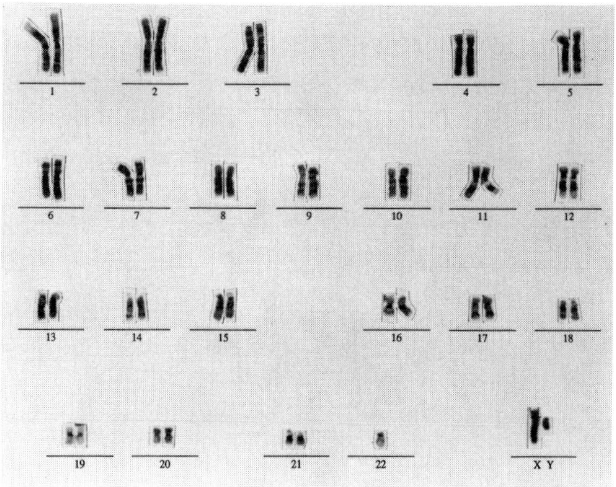

Figure 4. Non–complex karyotype of a benign schwannoma showing loss (monosomy) of chromosome 22 as a solitary chromosome aberration.

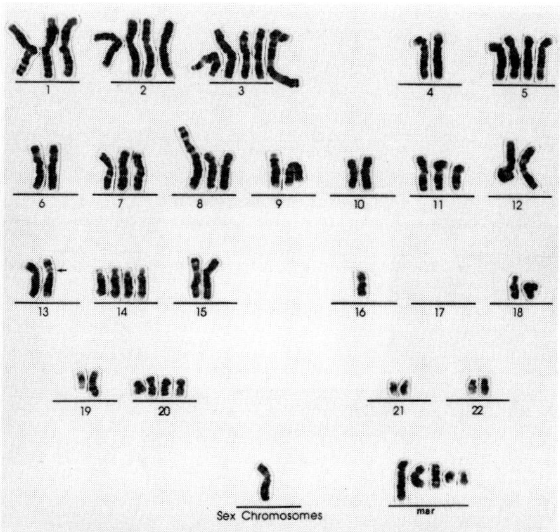

Figure 5. Complex karyotype of a malignant peripheral nerve sheath tumor. The karyotype is aneuploid, with numerous chromosome gains, losses, and rearrangements. Arrow indicates a translocation breakpoint between chromosomes 13 and 17, which resulted in inactivation of the neurofibromatosis type 1 (*NF1*) gene from chromosome 17.

simple karyotypes in benign schwannomas (Figs. 4 and 5) [1,63,64]. One explanation for this complexity is that the numerous chromosome aberrations in malignant peripheral nerve sheath tumors reflect a large number of gene alterations that are responsible collectively for the malignant phenotype. At least one other cancer gene has in fact been implicated in the genesis of malignant peripheral nerve sheath tumors. This is the *p53* tumor suppressor gene, which was mutated in 3 of 4 MPNST from one recent series [65]. As mentioned earlier, benign schwannomas have comparatively simple karyotypes. Loss of chromosome 22 is the sole cytogenetic aberration found in many cases. This chromosome loss, contributing to inactivation of the *NF2* gene, appears to be the central and pivotal cytogenetic aberration in benign schwannomas [66–68]. Chromosome 22 losses and *NF2* inactivations are found in benign schwannomas at all primary sites, whether of vestibular or peripheral nerve sheath origin.

Neurofibromas are NF1-associated lesions that have long been biologic puzzles. Neurofibromas contain a mixture of cell types, including fibroblasts, perineural cells, and Schwann cells, and the overall cell proliferation in individual tumors is polyclonal. It has been unclear, however, whether neurofibromas contain small populations of clonal Schwann cells that initiate and perpetuate the neoplastic growth. A recent study shed light on this question by demonstrating clonal deletion of the *NF1* gene in neurofibromas from patients with the NF1 syndrome [69]. Hence, some neurofibromas contain clonal cell populations, and *NF1* inactivation is probably the key oncogenetic event in those populations. In summary, loss of *NF1* function appears to be a critical event in development of both benign (neurofibroma) and malignant tumors of the peripheral nerve sheath. Loss of *NF2* function, in contrast, is found commonly in benign schwannomas but seldom in malignant peripheral nerve sheath tumors; this observation might explain why benign shwannomas seldom progress to malignancy.

Smooth muscle tumors

It is quite interesting that cancer researchers once regarded the presence of any clonal chromosome aberrations as strong evidence of malignancy. Such views changed during the 1980s when a number of research groups described characteristic cytogenetic aberrations in various benign mesenchymal tumors. The evidence for a clonal origin in entities such as leiomyoma and lipoma is now overwhelming [70–72]. Many leiomyomas contain clonal chromosome aberrations [71], and examples lacking such aberrations probably contain clonal DNA point mutations that are too small to be visualized at the cytogenetic level of resolution [72]. The most distinctive leiomyoma cytogenetic aberration is a translocation of chromosomes 12 and 14 that is found in approximately 20% of cases [70,71]. This translocation activates a high-mobility group gene, *HMGI-C*, which encodes a non–histone DNA-binding protein [73,74]. High-mobility group proteins bind the minor groove of DNA at particular chromosome regions and, is so doing, facilitate the action of DNA transcription factors that bind the same chromosome regions through the DNA major groove. The biologic implications of high-mobility group gene activation are similar to those already discussed for various sarcoma translocations. Many sarcoma chromosome translocations directly activate DNA transcription factors, whereas the leiomyoma translocation activates *HMGI-C*, which in turn activates DNA transcription factors. The end result in either scenario is aberrant regulation of yet unidentified genes. Whereas most leiomyomas have either normal karyotypes or rather simple cytogenetic aberrations, most leiomyosarcomas have extremely complex cytogenetic aberrations [1,75,76]. The translocation (12;14) of leiomyoma has not been reported in leiomyosarcoma, but the complexity of leiomyosarcoma karyotypes has undoubtedly obscured chromosome aberrations occurring non–randomly in these tumors. One cytogenetic aberration found in at least 50% of leiomyosarcomas is deletion of the chromosome 1 short arm [75,76]. This deletion is not useful diagnostically, because it is also found, albeit less frequently, in leiomyomas [77] and in various other soft tissue tumors.

Adipose tumors

Each of the common types of adipose tumor, whether benign or malignant, is associated with distinctive chromosome aberrations. Most solitary lipomas have translocations or other rearrangements involving the mid–portion of the chromosome 12 long arm [78,79]. Those translocations target the high-mobility protein gene, *HMGI-C*, which is the same gene rearranged in many uterine leiomyomas [73]. Lipoblastomas, which are benign pediatric tumors composed of primitive adipocytes, generally contain a rearrangement of the chromosome 8 long arm [80,81]. Well-differentiated liposarcomas, also known as atypical lipomas, contain supernumerary ring chromosomes composed of chromosome 12 material [78,82–86].

Many well-differentiated liposarcomas also contain 'giant marker chromosome,' which are as much as three times the size of the longest normal human chromosomes. The ring chromosomes and giant marker chromosomes in well-differentiated liposarcoma typically contain amplified copies of several genes (*MDM2*, *SAS*, *GLI*, *CDK4*) [87–90], but it is not clear whether any of these genes plays a pivotal role in the genesis of the tumors. More than 75% of myxoid liposarcomas are characterized by a reciprocal translocation between chromosomes 12 and 16: this translocation has not been observed in other varieties of myxoid sarcoma [82,83,91–93]. The myxoid liposarcoma chromosome translocation affects a region on chromosome 12 that is proximal (centromeric) to that rearranged in lipomas, and the biologic implications of the myxoid liposarcoma translocation are similar to those discussed previously for Ewing's sarcoma. Myxoid liposarcoma translocations fuse the *CHOP* gene on chromosome 12 with the *TLS* gene on chromosome 16 [94,95]. The normal *CHOP* gene encodes a DNA transcription factor protein, and the *CHOP-TLS* fusion gene encodes an activated transcription factor that promotes expression of other, yet unidentified genes. Myxoid liposarcoma chromosome translocation can be demonstrated either by cytogenetic analysis [83] or PCR [95].

Fibromatoses, fibrosarcomas, and related lesions

Characteristic cytogenetic aberrations have been reported in both fibromatoses and fibrosarcomas. Many fibrous tumors contain extra copies, often trisomies, of particular chromosomes. These trisomies are not specific for any one histologic type of fibrous tumor. Rather, the trisomies appear to convey proliferative advantage to a wide range of fibrous tumors. For example, trisomies of chromosomes 8, 11, 17, and 20 are found in most infantile fibrosarcomas [96–99], but trisomies of chromosomes 8 and 20 are also found in some desmoid tumors [100–102] (Fig. 6). The molecular significance of chromosome trisomies has not been determined, but it is possible that extra copy number of oncogene(s) on the trisomic chromosomes results in unrestrained cell proliferation.

Most desmoid tumors have deletions of the *APC* (adenomatous polyposis coli) gene on chromosome 5 [103,104]. Deletion and/or inactivation of the *APC* gene is found both in sporadic desmoid tumors and in those associated with Gardner's syndrome. The present cytogenetic and molecular data suggest that loss and/or inactivation of the *APC* gene is the primary and critical event in the genesis of desmoid tumors. As mentioned earlier, approximately 25% of desmoid tumors have trisomies for chromosomes 8 and/or 20; these trisomies are probably acquired after the *APC* mutation and might be associated with an increased risk of local recurrence (see Fig. 6) [100–102].

Most dermatofibrosarcoma protuberans contain ring chromosomes of varying sizes. Ring chromosomes have been the only cytogenetic aberrations found in several dermatofibrosarcoma protuberans (Fig. 7), whereas other examples

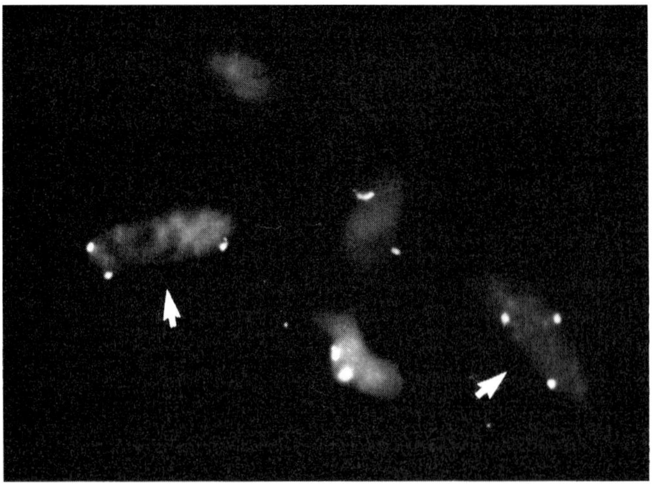

Figure 6. FISH with a chromosome 8 centromere probe in nuclei disaggregated from frozen sections of a desmoid tumor. Two nuclei are trisomic for chromosome 8 (arrows).

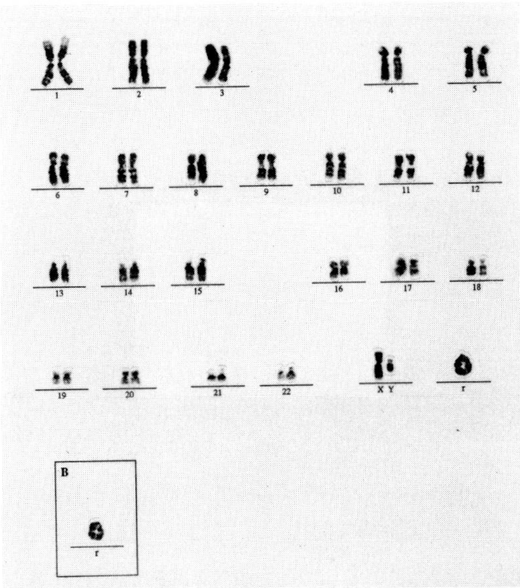

A

B

Figure 7. **A:** Karyotype of a dermatofibrosarcoma protuberans in which the only cytogenetic aberration is a supernumerary ring chromosome (r). **B:** The inset shows a supernumerary ring chromosome from another cell in this tumor.

had somewhat more complex chromosome aberrations, including both ring chromosomes and chromosome trisomies [105,106]. Dermatofibrosarcoma protuberans ring chromosomes are composed of interwoven segments derived from chromosomes 17 and 22 [107,108]. It is likely, therefore, that oncogenes from both these chromosomes participate in dermatofibrosarcoma protuberans tumorigenesis. Rings composed of chromosome 17 and 22 material have not been described in other types of sarcoma, and this cytogenetic finding appears to be useful diagnostically.

Malignant fibrous histiocytoma

Extremely complex karyotypes are the norm in high-grade malignant fibrous histiocytomas. Such complex karyotypes, containing numerous clonal and nonclonal chromosome rearrangements, are challenging for a cytogeneticist to describe accurately. For this reason, it is unclear whether malignant fibrous histiocytoma karyotypes contain diagnostic chromosome rearrangements [1,109,110]. Preliminary studies, however, suggest a prognostic role for certain chromosome rearrangements. Rydholm et al. reported a particularly poor prognosis in high-grade malignant fibrous histiocytomas having rearrangements of chromosome 19 [111]. Most myxoid malignant fibrous histiocytomas are lower grade histologically, and karyotypes in myxoid malignant fibrous histiocytomas are often very simple, contrasting with the cytogenetic complexity in most non–myxoid malignant fibrous histiocytomas. More than 50% of myxoid malignant fibrous histiocytomas contain ring chromosomes, but the constituents of those ring chromosomes have not yet been identified [110,112].

Neuroblastoma

Neuroblastomas are divisible into two principal genetic and clinicopathologic categories. The first category includes neuroblastomas with near-diploid or near-tetraploid DNA content, deletion of the chromosome 1 short arm, and, in some cases, amplification of the N-*myc* oncogene [113,114] (Fig. 8). Patients with such neuroblastoma features are rarely curable, although multimodality treatment with intensive chemotherapy, surgery, and radiation therapy has enabled complete remissions. The second neuroblastoma category includes cases with near-triploid DNA content, absence of chromosome 1 short arm deletion, and absence of N-*myc* amplification [113,114]. Such cases are generally cured with non–intensive therapy and sometimes undergo spontaneous regression. The independent prognostic value of DNA ploidy and N-*myc* amplification are well established, and these parameters are now being used to determine therapy in clinical trials.

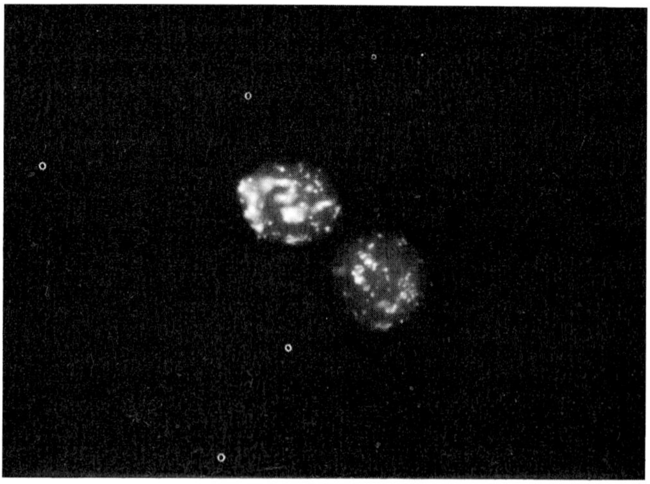

Figure 8. FISH with an N-*myc* probe in nuclei from a neuroblastoma. High-level N-*myc* amplification is seen in both nuclei.

Conclusions

Characteristic cytogenetic aberrations have been identified in many soft tissue sarcomas, and such aberrations, for example, the translocation of chromosomes X and 18 in synovial sarcoma, will likely play an increasing role in sarcoma diagnosis. It is fascinating that soft tissue sarcoma chromosome translocations often result in fusion oncoproteins. These novel oncoproteins probably regulate the expression of various genes relevant to malignant progression of sarcoma progenitor cells. Thus, soft tissue sarcoma chromosome translocations are pivotal genetic events — 'master switches' — contributing to deregulated tumor cell growth.

References

1. Fletcher JA, Kozakewich HP, Hoffer FA, Lage JM, Weidner N, Tepper R, Pinkus GS, Morton CC, Corson JM. Diagnostic relevance of clonal cytogenetic aberrations in malignant soft-tissue tumors. N Engl J Med 324:436–442, 1991.
2. Sandberg AA, Bridge JA. The Cytogenetics of Bone and Soft Tissue Tumors. Austin, TX: R.G. Landes Company, 1995.
3. Sreekantaiah C, Ladanyi M, Rodriguez E, Chaganti RS. Chromosomal aberrations in soft tissue tumors. Relevance to diagnosis, classification, and molecular mechanisms. Am J Pathol 144:1121–1134, 1994.
4. Heim S, Mitelman F. Cancer Cytogenetics. New York: Wiley-Liss, 1995.
5. Xiao S, Renshaw AA, Cibas ES, Hudson TJ, Flecher JA. Novel fluorescence in situ hybridization approaches in solid tumors: Characterization of frozen specimens, touch preparations, and cytologic preparations. Am J Pathol 147:896–904, 1995.
6. Turc-Carel C, Philip I, Berger MP, Philip T, Lenoir GM. Chromosome study of Ewing's sarcoma (ES) cell lines. Consistency of a reciprocal translocation t(11;22)(q24;q12). Cancer Genet Cytogenet 12:1–19, 1984.
7. Turc-Carel C, Aurias A, Mugneret F, Lizard S, Sidaner I, Volk C, Thiery JP, Olschwang S, Philip I, Berger MP, et al. Chromosomes in Ewing's sarcoma. I. An evaluation of 85 cases of remarkable consistency of t(11;22)(q24;q12). Cancer Genet Cytogenet 32:229–238, 1988.
8. Delattre O, Zucman J, Plougastel B, et al. Gene fusion with an ETS DNA-binding domain caused by chromosome translocation in human tumors. Nature 359:162–165, 1992.
9. Delattre O, Zucman J, Melot T, et al. The Ewing family of tumors — a subgroup of small-round-cell tumors defined by specific chimeric transcripts. N Engl J Med 331:294–299, 1994.
10. Jeon IS, Davis JN, Braun BS, Sublett JE, Roussel MF, Denny CT, Shapiro DN. A variant Ewing's sarcoma translocation (7;22) fuses the EWS gene to the ETS gene ETV1. Oncogene 10:1229–1234, 1995.
11. Sorensen PH, Lessnick SL, Lopez-Terrada D, Liu XF, Triche TJ, Denny CT. A second Ewing's sarcoma translocation, t(21;22), fuses the EWS gene to another ETS-family transcription factor, ERG. Nature Genet 6:146–151, 1994.
12. Ohno T, Rao VN, Reddy ES. EWS/Fli-1 chimeric protein is a transcriptional activator. Cancer Res 53:5859–5863, 1993.
13. May WA, Lessnick SL, Braun BS, Klemsz M, Lewis BC, Lunsford LB, Hromas R, Denny CT. The Ewing's sarcoma EWS/FLI-1 fusion gene encodes a more potent transcriptional activator and is a more powerful transforming gene than FLI-1. Mol Cell Biol 13:7393–7398, 1993.

14. Lessnick SL, Braun BS, Denny CT, May WA. Multiple domains mediate transformation by the Ewing's sarcoma EWS/FLI-1 fusion gene. Oncogene 10:423–431, 1995.
15. May WA, Gishizky ML, Lessnick SL, Lunsford LB, Lewis BC, Delattre O, Zucman J, Thomas G, Denny CT. Ewing sarcoma 11;22 translocation produces a chimeric transcription factor that requires the DNA-binding domain encoded by FLI1 for transformation. Proc Natl Acad Sci USA 90:5752–5756, 1993.
16. Hoffer FA, Gianturco LE, Fletcher JA, Grier HE. Percutaneous biospy of peripheral primitive neuroetocdermal tumors and Ewing's sarcomas for cytogenetic analysis. Am J Roentgenol 162:1141–1142, 1994.
17. Desmaze C, Zucman J, Delattre O, Melot T, Thomas G, Aurias A. Interphase molecular cytogenetics of Ewing's sarcoma and peripheral neuroepithelioma t(11;22) with flanking and overlapping cosmid probes. Cancer Genet Cytogenet 74:13–18, 1994.
18. Downing JR, Head DR, Parham DM, Douglass EC, Hulshof MG, Link MP, Motroni TA, Grier HE, Curcio-Brint AM, Shapiro DN. Detection of the (11;22)(q24;q12) translocation of Ewing's sarcoma and peripheral neuroectodermal tumor by reverse transcription polymerase chain reaction. Am J Pathol 143:1294–1300, 1993.
19. Mugneret F, Lizard S, Aurias A, Turc-Carel C. Chromosomes in Ewing's sarcoma. II. Non–random additional changes, trisomy 8 and der(16)t(1;16). Cancer Genet Cytogenet 32:239–245, 1988.
20. Fletcher JA. Translocation (12;22)(q13–14;q12) is a non–random aberration in soft-tissue clear-cell sarcoma. Genes Chromosom Cancer 5:184, 1992.
21. Bridge JA, Borek DA, Neff JR, Huntrakoon M. Chromosomal abnormalities in clear–cell sarcoma. Implications for histogenesis. Am J Clin Pathol 93:26–31, 1990.
22. Mrozek K, Karakousis CP, Perez-Mesa C, Bloomfield CD. Translocation t(12;22)(q13;q12.2–12.3) in a clear–cell sarcoma of tendons and aponeuroses. Genes Chromosom Cancer 6:249–252, 1993.
23. Peulve P, Michot C, Vannier JP, Tron P, Hemet J. Clear–cell sarcoma with t(12;22)(q13–14;q12). Genes Chromosom Cancer 3:400–402, 1991.
24. Reeves BR, Fletcher CD, Gusterson BA. Translocation t(12;22)(q13;q13) is a non–random rearrangement in clear–cell sarcoma. Cancer Genet Cytogenet 64:101–103, 1992.
25. Speleman F, Colpaert C, Goovaerts G, Leroy JG, Van Marck E. Malignant melanoma of soft parts. Further cytogenetic characterization. Cancer Genet Cytogenet 60:176–179, 1992.
26. Stenman G, Kindblom LG, Angervall L. Reciprocal translocation t(12;22)(q13;q13) in clear-cell sarcoma of tendons and aponeuroses. Genes Chromosom Cancer 4:122–127, 1992.
27. Travis JA, Bridge JA. Significance of both numerical and structural chromosomal abnormalities in clear–cell sarcoma. Cancer Genet Cytogenet 64:104–106, 1992.
28. Zucman J, Delattre O, Desmaze C, Epstein AL, Stenman G, Speleman F, Fletchers CD, Aurias A, Thomas G. EWS and ATF-1 gene fusion induced by t(12;22) translocation in malignant melanoma of soft parts. Nature Genet 4:341–345, 1993.
29. Brown AD, Lopez-Terrada D, Denny C, Lee KA. Promoters containing ATF-binding sites are de-regulated in cells that express the EWS/ATF1 oncogene. Oncogene 10:1749–1756, 1995.
30. Gerald WL, Miller HK, Battifora H, Miettinen M, Silva EG, Rosai J. Intra-abdominal desmoplastic small round-cell tumor. Report of 19 cases of a distinctive type of high-grade polyphenotypic malignancy affecting young individuals. Am J Surg Pathol 15:499–513, 1991.
31. Rodriguez E, Sreekantaiah C, Gerald W, Reuter VE, Motzer RJ, Chaganti RS. A recurring translocation, t(11;22)(p13;q11.2), characterizes intra-abdominal desmoplastic small round-cell tumors. Cancer Genet Cytogenet 69:17–21, 1993.
32. Beiegel JA, Conard K, Brooks JJ. Translocation (11;22)(p13;q12): Primary change in intraabdominal desmoplastic small round cell–tumor. Genes Chromosom Cancer 7:119–121, 1993.
33. Ladanyi M, Gerald W. Fusion of the EWS and WT1 genes in the desmoplastic small round–cell tumor. Cancer Res 54:2837–2840, 1994.

34. Gerald WL, Rosai J, Ladanyi M. Characterization of the genomic breakpoint and chimeric transcripts in the EWS-WT1 gene fusion of desmoplastic small round–cell tumor. Proc Natl Acad Sci USA 92:1028–1032, 1995.
35. Galili N, Davis RJ, Fredericks WJ, Mukhopadhyay S, Rauscher FJ, 3d, Emanuel BS, Rovera G, Barr FG, Rauscher FJ. Fusion of a fork–head domain gene to PAX3 in the solid tumour alveolar rhabdomyosarcoma. Nature Genet 5:230–235, 1993.
36. Barr FG, Galili N, Holick J, Biegel JA, Rovera G, Emanuel BS. Rearrangement of the PAX3 paired box gene in the paediatric solid tumor alveolar rhabdomyosarcoma. Nature Genet 3:113–117, 1993.
37. Shapiro DN, Sublett JE, Li B, Downing JR, Naeve CW. Fusion of PAX3 to a member of the fork–head family of transcription factors in human alveolar rhabdomyosarcoma. Cancer Res 53:5108–5112, 1993.
38. Davis RJ, D'Cruz CM, Lovell MA, Biegel JA, Barr FG. Fusion of PAX7 to FKHR by the variant t(1;13)(p36;q14) translocation in alveolar rhabdomyosarcoma. Cancer Res 54:2869–2872, 1994.
39. Fredericks WJ, Galili N, Mukhopadhyay S, Rovera G, Bennicelli J, Barr FG, Rauscher FJ, 3rd. The PAX3-FKHR fusion protein created by the t(2;13) translocation in alveolar rhabdomyosarcomas is a more potent transcriptional activator than PAX3. Mol Cell Biol 15:1522–1535, 1995.
40. Bennicelli JL, Fredericks WJ, Wilson RB, Rauscher FJ, 3rd, Barr FG. Wild type PAX3 protein and the PAX3-FKHR fusion protein of alveolar rhabdomyosarcoma contain potent, structurally distinct transcriptional activation domains. Oncogene 11:119–130, 1995.
41. Turc-Carel C, Lizard-Nacol S, Justrabo E, Favrot M, Philip T, Tabone E. Consistent chromosomal translocation in alveolar rhabdomyosarcoma. Cancer Genet Cytogenet 19:361–362, 1986.
42. Parham DM, Shapiro DN, Downing JR, Webber BL, Douglass EC. Solid alveolar rhabdomyosarcomas with the t(2;13). Report of two cases with diagnostic implications. Am J Surg Pathol 18:474–478, 1994.
43. Wang-Wuu S, Soukup S, Ballard E, Gotwals B, Lampkin B, Sheng WW. Chromosomal analysis of sixteen human rhabdomyosarcomas. Cancer Res 48:983–987, 1988.
44. Whang-Peng J, Knutsen T, Theil K, Horowitz ME, Triche T. Cytogenetic studies in subgroups of rhabdomyosarcoma. Genes Chromosom Cancer 5:299–310, 1992.
45. Biegel JA, Nycum LM, Valentine V, Barr FG, Shapiro DN. Detection of the t(2;13)(q35;q14) and PAX3-FKHR fusion in alveolar rhabdomyosarcoma by fluorescence in situ hybridization. Genes Chromosom Cancer 12:186–192, 1995.
46. Barr FG, Chatten J, D'Cruz CM, Wilson AE, Nauta LE, Nycum LM, Biegel JA, Womer RB. Molecular assays for chromosomal translocations in the diagnosis of pediatric soft tissue sarcomas. JAMA 273:553–557, 1995.
47. Downing JR, Khandekar A, Shurtleff SA, Head DR, Parham DM, Webber BL, Pappo AS, Hulshof MG, Conn WP, Shapiro DN. Multiplex RT-PCR assay for the differential diagnosis of alveolar rhabdomyosarcoma and Ewing's sarcoma. Am J Pathol 146:626–634, 1995.
48. Fletcher JA, Kozakewich HP, Pavelka K, Grier HE, Shamberger RC, Korf B, Morton CC. Consistent cytogenetic aberrations in hepatoblastoma: A common pathway of genetic alterations in embryonal liver and skeletal muscle malignancies? Genes Chromosom Cancer 3:37–43, 1991.
49. Scrable H, Witte D, Shimada H, Seemayer T, Sheng WW, Soukup S, Koufos A, Houghton P, Lampkin B, Cavenee W. Molecular differential pathology of rhabdomyosarcoma. Genes Chromosom Cancer 1:23–35, 1989.
50. Limon J, Mrozek K, Mandahl N, et al. Cytogenetics of synovial sarcoma: Presentation of ten new cases and review of the literature. Genes Chromosom Cancer 3:338–345, 1991.
51. Dal Cin P, Rao U, Jani-Sait S, Karakousis C, Sandberg AA. Chromosomes in the diagnosis of soft tissue tumors. I. Synovial sarcoma. Mod Pathol 5:357–362, 1992.
52. Clark J, Rocques PJ, Crew AJ, Gill S, Shipley J, Chan AM, Gusterson BA, Cooper CS.

Identification of novel genes, SYT and SSX, involved in the t(X;18)(p11.2;q11.2) translocation found in human synovial sarcoma. Nature Genet 7:502–508, 1994.
53. Crew AJ, Clark J, Fisher C, Gill S, Grimer R, Chand A, Shipley J, Gusterson BA, Cooper CS. Fusion of SYT to two genes, SSX1 and SSX2, encoding proteins with homology to the Kruppel-associated box in human synovial sarcoma. EMBO J 14:2333–2340, 1995.
54. Renwick PJ, Reeves BR, Dal Cin P, Fletcher CD, Kempski H, Sciot R, Kazmierczak B, Jani K, Sonobe H, Knight JC. Two categories of synovial sarcoma defined by divergent chromosome translocation breakpoints in Xp11.2, with implications for the histologic subclassification of synovial sarcoma. Cytogenet Cell Genet 70:58–63, 1995.
55. de Leeuw B, Suijkerbuijk RF, Olde Weghuis D, Meloni AM, Stenman G, Kindblom LG, Balemans M, van den Berg E, Molenaar WM, Sandberg AA, Geurts van Kessel A. Distinct Xp11.2 breakpoint regions in synovial sarcoma revealed by metaphase and interphase FISH: Relationship to histologic subtypes. Cancer Genet Cytogenet 73:89–94, 1994.
56. Poteat HT, Corson JM, Fletcher JA. Detection of chromosome 18 rearrangement in synovial sarcoma by fluorescence in situ hybridization: FISH diagnosis of t(X;18) in synovial sarcoma. Cancer Genet Cytogenet 84:76–81, 1995.
57. Legius E, Marchuk DA, Collins FS, Glover TW. Somatic deletion of the neurofibromatosis type 1 gene in a neurofibrosarcoma supports a tumor suppressor gene hypothesis. Nature Genet 3:122–126, 1993.
58. Basu TN, Gutmann DH, Fletcher JA, Glover TW, Collins FS, Downward J. Aberrant regulation of ras proteins in malignant tumour cells from type 1 neurofibromatosis patients. Nature 356:713–715, 1992.
59. DeClue JE, Papageorge AG, Fletcher JA, Diehl SR, Ratner N, Vass WC, Lowy DR. Abnormal regulation of mammalian p21ras contributes to malignant tumor growth in von Recklinghausen (type 1) neurofibromatosis. Cell 69:265–273, 1992.
60. Reynolds JE, Fletcher JA, Lytle CH, Nie L, Morton CC, Diehl SR. Molecular characterization of a 17q11.2 translocation in a malignant schwannoma cell line. Hum Genet 90:450–456, 1992.
61. Glover TW, Stein CK, Legius E, Andersen LB, Brereton A, Johnson S. Molecular and cytogenetic analysis of tumors in von Recklinghausen neurofibromatosis. Genes Chromosom Cancer 3:62–70, 1991.
62. Yan N, Ricca C, Fletcher J, Glover T, Seizinger BR, Manne V. Farnesyltransferase inhibitors block the neurofibromatosis type I (NF1) malignant phenotype. Cancer Res 55:3569–3575, 1995.
63. Jhanwar SC, Chen Q, Li FP, Brennan MF, Woodruff JM. Cytogenetic analysis of soft tissue sarcomas. Recurrent chromosome abnormalities in malignant peripheral nerve sheath tumors (MPNST). Cancer Genet Cytogenet 78:138–144, 1994.
64. Mertens F, Rydholm A, Bauer HF, Limon J, Nedoszytko B, Szadowska A, Willen H, Heim S, Mitelman F, Mandahl N. Cytogenetic findings in malignant peripheral nerve sheath tumors. Int J Cancer 61:793–798, 1995.
65. Legius E, Dierick H, Wu R, Hall BK, Marynen P, Cassiman JJ, Glover TW. TP53 mutations are frequent in malignant NF1 tumors. Genes Chromosom Cancer 10:250–255, 1994.
66. Lekanne Deprez RH, Bianchi AB, et al. Frequent NF2 gene transcript mutations in sporadic meningiomas and vestibular schwannomas. Am J Hum Genet 54:1022–1029, 1994.
67. Merel P, Hoang-Xuan K, Sanson M, Moreau-Aubry A, Bijlsma EK, Lazaro C, Moisan JP, Resche F, Nishisho I, Estivill X, Delattre JY, Poisson M, Theillet C, Hulsebos T, Delattre O, Thomas G. Predominant occurrence of somatic mutations of the *NF2* gene in meningiomas and schwannomas. Genes Chromosom Cancer 13:211–216, 1995.
68. Bijlsma EK, Merel P, Bosch DA, Westerveld A, Delattre O, Thomas G, Hulsebos TJ. Analysis of mutations in the SCH gene in schwannomas. Genes Chromosom Cancer 11:7–14, 1994.
69. Colman SD, Williams CA, Wallace MR. Benign neurofibromas in type 1 neurofibromatosis (NF1) show somatic deletions of the *NF1* gene. Nature Genet 11:90–92, 1995.

70. Rein MS, Friedman AJ, Barbieri RL, Pavelka K, Fletcher JA, Morton CC. Cytogenetic abnormalities in uterine leiomyomata. Obstet Gynecol 77:923–926, 1991.
71. Pandis N, Heim S, Bardi G, Floderus UM, Willen H, Mandahl N, Mitelman F. Chromosome analysis of 96 uterine leiomyomas. Cancer Genet Cytogenet 55:11–18, 1991.
72. Mashal RD, Fejzo ML, Friedman AJ, Mitchner N, Nowak RA, Rein MS, Morton CC, Sklar J. Analysis of androgen receptor DNA reveals the independent clonal origins of uterine leiomyomata and the secondary nature of cytogenetic aberrations in the development of leiomyomata. Genes Chromosom Cancer 11:1–6, 1994.
73. Ashar HR, Fejzo MS, Tkachenko A, Zhou X, Fletcher JA, Weremowicz S, Morton CC, Chada K. Disruption of the architectural factor HMGI-C: DNA-binding A-T hook motifs fused in lipomas to distinct transcriptional regulatory domains. Cell 82:57–65, 1995.
74. Schoenmakers EFPM, Wanschura S, Mols R, Bullerdiek J, Van Den Berghe H, Van de Ven WJM. Recurrent rearrangements in the high mobility group protein gene, *HMGI-C*, in benign mesenchymal tumors. Nature Genet 10:436–443, 1995.
75. Fletcher JA, Morton CC, Pavelka K, Lage JM. Chromosome aberrations in uterine smooth muscle tumors: Potential diagnostic relevance of cytogenetic instability. Cancer Res 50:4092–4097, 1990.
76. Sreekantaiah C, Davis JR, Sandberg AA. Chromosomal abnormalities in leiomyosarcomas. Am J Pathol 142:293–305, 1993.
77. Nilbert M, Heim S, Mandahl N, Floderus UM, Willen H, Akerman M, Mitelman F. Ring formation and structural rearrangements of chromosome 1 as secondary changes in uterine leiomyomas with t(12;14)(q14–15;q23–24). Cancer Genet Cytogenet 36:183–190, 1988.
78. Mandahl N, Hoglund M, Mertens F, Rydholm A, Willen H, Brosjo O, Mitelman F. Cytogenetic aberrations in 188 benign and borderline adipose tissue tumors. Genes Chromosom Cancer 9:207–215, 1994.
79. Sreekantaiah C, Leong SP, Karakousis CP, et al. Cytogenetic profile of 109 lipomas. Cancer Res 51:422–433, 1991.
80. Fletcher JA, Kozakewich HP, Schoenberg ML, Morton CC. Cytogenetic findings in pediatric adipose tumors: Consistent rearrangement of chromosome 8 in lipoblastoma. Genes Chromosom Cancer 6:24–29, 1993.
81. Dal Cin P, Sciot R, De Wever I, Van Damme B, Van Den Berghe H. New discriminative chromosomal marker in adipose tissue tumors. The chromosome 8q11–q13 region in lipoblastoma. Cancer Genet Cytogenet 78:232–235, 1994.
82. Karakousis CP, Dal Cin P, Turc-Carel C, Limon J, Sandberg AA. Chromosomal changes in soft-tissue sarcomas. A new diagnostic parameter. Arch Surg 122:1257–1260, 1987.
83. Sreekantaiah C, Karakousis CP, Leong SP, Sandberg AA. Cytogenetic findings in liposarcoma correlate with histopathologic subtypes. Cancer 69:2484–2495, 1992.
84. Heim S, Mandahl N, Kristoffersson U, Mitelman F, Rooser B, Rydholm A, Willen H. Marker ring chromosome — a new cytogenetic abnormality characterizing lipogenic tumors? Cancer Genet Cytogenet 24:319–326, 1987.
85. Pedeutour F, Suijkerbuijk RF, Van Gaal J, Van de Klundert W, Coindre JM, Van Haelst A, Collin F, Huffermann K, Turc-Carel C. Chromosome 12 origin in rings and giant markers in well-differentiated liposarcoma. Cancer Genet Cytogenet 66:133–134, 1993.
86. Suijkerbuijk RF, Olde Weghuis DE, Van den Berg M, Pedeutour F, Forus A, Myklebost O, Glier C, Turc-Carel C, Geurts van Kessel A. Comparative genomic hybridization as a tool to define two distinct chromosome 12-derived amplification units in well-differentiated liposarcomas. Genes Chromosom Cancer 9:292–295, 1994.
87. Nilbert M, Rydholm A, Willen H, Mitelman F, Mandahl N. MDM2 gene amplification correlates with ring chromosome in soft tissue tumors. Genes Chromosom Cancer 9:261–265, 1994.
88. Smith SH, Weiss SW, Jankowski SA, Coccia MA, Meltzer PS. SAS amplification in soft tissue sarcomas. Cancer Res 52:3746–3749, 1992.
89. Forus A, Florenes VA, Maelandsmo GM, Meltzer PS, Fodstad O, Myklebost O. Mapping of

amplification units in the q13–14 region of chromosome 12 in human sarcomas: Some amplica do not include MDM2. Cell Growth Differ 4:1065–1070, 1993.
90. Pedeutour F, Suijkerbuijk RF, Forus A, et al. Complex composition and co-amplification of SAS and MDM2 in ring and giant rod marker chromosomes in well-differentiated liposarcoma. Genes Chromosom Cancer 10:85–94, 1994.
91. Turc-Carel C, Limon J, Dal Cin P, Rao U, Karakousis C, Sandberg AA. Cytogenetic studies of adipose tissue tumors. II. Recurrent reciprocal translocation t(12;16)(q13;p11) in myxoid liposarcomas. Cancer Genet Cytogenet 23:291–299, 1986.
92. Altungoz O, Meloni AM, Peier A, Zalupski M, Spanier S, Brooks JS, Sandberg AA. Deletion 6q in three cases of mixed-type liposarcoma in addition to t(12;16)(q13;p11). Cancer Genet Cytogenet 79:104–110, 1195.
93. Gibas Z, Miettinen M, Limon J, Nedoszytko B, Mrozek K, Roszkiewicz A, Rys J, Niezabitowski A, Debiec-Rychter M. Cytogenetic and immunohistochemical profile of myxoid liposarcoma. Am J Clin Pathol 103:20–26, 1995.
94. Aman P, Ron D, Mandahl N, Fioretos T, Heim S, Arheden K, Willen H, Rydholm A, Mitelman F. Rearrangement of the transcription factor gene CHOP in myxoid liposarcomas with t(12;16)(q13;p11). Genes Chromosom Cancer 5:278–285, 1992.
95. Panagopoulos I, Mandahl N, Ron D, Hoglund M, Nilbert M, Mertens F, Mitelman F, Aman P. Characterization of the CHOP breakpoints and fusion transcripts in myxoid liposarcomas with the 12;16 translocation. Cancer Res 54:6500–6503, 1994.
96. Schofield DE, Fletcher JA, Grier HE, Yunis EJ. Fibrosarcoma in infants and children. Application of new techniques. Am J Surg Pathol 18:14–24, 1994.
97. Mandahl N, Heim S, Rydholm A, Willen H, Mitelman F. Non–random numerical chromosome aberrations (+8, +11, +17, +20) in infantile fibrosarcoma. Cancer Genet Cytogenet 40:137–139, 1989.
98. Speleman F, Dal Cin P, De Potter K, Laureys G, Roels HJ, Leroy J, Van Den Berghe H. Cytogenetic investigation of a case of congenital fibrosarcoma. Cancer Genet Cytogenet 39:21–24, 1989.
99. Sankary S, Dickman PS, Wiener E, Robichaux W, Swaney WP, Malone PS, Gollin SM. Consistent numerical chromosome aberrations in congenital fibrosarcoma. Cancer Genet Cytogenet 65:152–156, 1993.
100. Fletcher JA, Naeem R, Xiao S, Corson JM. Chromosome aberrations in desmoid tumors. Trisomy 8 may be a predictor of recurrence. Cancer Genet Cytogenet 79:139–143, 1995.
101. Dal Cin P, Sciot R, Aly MS, Delabie J, Stas M, De Wever I, Van Damme B, Van Den Berghe H. Some desmoid tumors are characterized by trisomy 8. Genes Chromosom Cancer 10:131–135, 1994.
102. Dal Cin P, Sciot R, Van Damme B, De Wever I, Van Den Berghe H. Trisomy 20 characterizes a second group of desmoid tumors. Cancer Genet Cytogenet 79:189, 1995.
103. Miyaki M, Konishi M, Kikuchi-Yanoshita R, Enomoto M, Tanaka K, Takahashi H, Muraoka M, Mori T, Konishi F, Iwama T. Coexistence of somatic and germ-line mutations of APC gene in desmoid tumors from patients with familial adenomatous polyposis. Cancer Res 53:5079–5082, 1993.
104. Sen-Gupta S, Van der Luijt RB, Bowles LV, Meera Khan P, Delhanty JD. Somatic mutation of APC gene in desmoid tumor in familial adenomatous polyposis. Lancet 342:552–553, 1993.
105. Stephenson CF, Berger CS, Leong SP, Davis JR, Sandberg AA. Ring chromosome in a dermatofibrosarcoma protuberans. Cancer Genet Cytogenet 58:52–54, 1992.
106. Mandahl N, Heim S, Willen H, Rydholm A, Mitelman F. Supernumerary ring chromosome as the sole cytogenetic abnormality in a dermatofibrosarcoma protuberans. Cancer Genet Cytogenet 49:273–275, 1990.
107. Pedeutour F, Coindre JM, Nicolo G, Bouchot C, Ayraud N, Carel CT. Ring chromosomes in dermatofibrosarcoma protuberans contain chromosome 17 sequences: Fluorescence in situ hybridization. Cancer Genet Cytogenet 67:149, 1993.

108. Pedeutour F, Simon M, Minoletti F, Sozzi G, Peirotti MA, Hecht F, Turc-Carel C. Ring 22 chromosomes in dermatofibrosarcoma protuberans are low-level amplifiers of chromosome 17 and 22 sequences. Cancer Res 55:2400–2403, 1995.
109. Orndal C, Mandahl N, Carlen B, Willen H, Wennerberg J, Heim S, Mitelman F. Near-haploid clones in a malignant fibrous histiocytoma. Cancer Genet Cytogenet 60:147–151, 1992.
110. Mandahl N, Heim S, Willen H, Rydholm A, Eneroth M, Nilbert M, Kreicbergs A, Mitelman F. Characteristic karyotypic anomalies identify subtypes of malignant fibrous histiocytoma. Genes Chromosom Cancer 1:9–14, 1989.
111. Rydholm A, Mandahl N, Heim S, Kreicbergs A, Willen H, Mitelman F. Malignant fibrous histiocytomas with a 19p+ marker chromosome have increased relapse rate. Genes Chromosom Cancer 2:296–299, 1990.
112. Orndal C, Mandahl N, Rydholm A, Willen H, Brosjo O, Heim S, Mitelman F. Supernumerary ring chromosomes in five bone and soft tissue tumors of low or borderline malignancy. Cancer Genet Cytogenet 60:170–175, 1992.
113. Brodeur GM, Azar C, Brother M, et al. Neuroblastoma. Effect of genetic factors on prognosis and treatment. Cancer 70:1685–1694, 1992.
114. Kaneko Y, Kanda N, Maseki N, Sakurai M, Tsuchida Y, Takeda T, Okabe I. Different karyotypic patterns in early and advanced stage neuroblastomas. Cancer Res 47:311–318, 1987.

3. Molecular genetics of soft tissue sarcomas

Colin S. Cooper and Paul Cornes

During the past decade considerable progress has been made in elucidating the mechanisms underlying the development of human soft tissue sarcomas. It has been established that certain genetic disorders can predispose to the development of soft tissue sarcomas, and in many cases the individual genes containing the inherited mutation have been cloned and characterized. Cytogenetic studies have identified specific chromosomal translocations in certain types of soft tissue sarcoma, and most of the genes that become altered by these rearrangements have now been isolated. Progress has also been made in identifying genes that control the differentiation of some mesenchymal lineage (e.g., striated muscle). These recent developments are reviewed in this chapter, with particular emphasis being placed on (1) recent advances that have been made in understanding precisely how the genetic alteration found in soft tissue sarcomas may lead to tumor formation and (2) the potential use of genetic markers in tumor diagnosis and prognosis.

Role of oncogenes and suppressor genes

Tumor development involves the accumulation of genetic alterations in two classes of genes called *protooncogenes* and *suppressor genes*. Protooncogenes become converted by mutation into oncogenes that act in a dominant fashion to transform cells. This process of oncogene formation in human tumors may occur by a variety of mechanisms, including point mutation (e.g., K-*RAS*, N-*RAS*), amplification (e.g., N-*MYC*, C-*MYC*), and translocation (e.g., *ABL*, *TLS*, *PAX3*). It is the altered or overexpressed proteins resulting from these changes that are responsible for initiation or maintenance of the malignant phenotype. By comparison, for tumor suppressor genes loss or inactivation of both copies of the gene is usually required for tumor development. This alteration results in complete removal of the normal protein encoded by the gene. In some cases (e.g., for *p53* and *RB1*) the suppressor function has been clearly demonstrated by showing that reintroduction of the gene into tumor cells results in suppression of the malignant phenotype.

J. Verweij, H.M. Pinedo, and H.D. Suit (eds). SOFT TISSUE SARCOMAS: PRESENT ACHIEVEMENTS AND FUTURE PROSPECTS.

RB1 pathway

During the past 5 years remarkable progress has been made in understanding the events regulating cell division, and these advances have provided important insights into precisely how alterations in protooncogenes and suppressor genes act to cause transformation. Transition through the cell cycle is regulated by a family of protein kinases called *cyclin dependent kinases* (CDKs) that are bound to cyclins in their active state. In particular, progress through the G1 phase of the cell cycle prior to entry into the S or DNA replication phase is controlled by D-type cyclins in association with the cyclin-dependent kinases CDK4 or CDK6. These proteins act by phosphorylating the RB1 protein. The presence of hypophosphorylated RB1 arrests cells in G1, while phosphorylation of RB1 relieves this inhibition, allowing the cell cycle to proceed. A further level in control is provided by a protein such as p16 and p15 that can bind to and inhibit the activities of CDK4 and CDK6 kinases [1]. The mechanism of control of the phosphorylation status of the RB1 protein is shown in Figure 1.

Alterations in genes that regulate several steps in this control pathway have been found in human sarcomas, and in each case it is predicted that the alteration would result in removal or reduction of the dephosphorylated form of the RB1 protein, allowing the cells to proceed unchecked through to the next stage of the cell cycle. Abnormalities in expression and homozygous loss (loss of both copies) of the *RB1* gene itself is observed in some tumors [2–4]. In addition, loss of a single copy of chromosome 13 in the general region of the *RB1* gene was found in around 35% of sarcomas [2]. These abnormalities have been found in many types of sarcomas but were found most commonly in malignant fibrous histiocytoma (MFH), leiomyosarcomas, and rhabdomyosarcomas. Recently homozygous deletion (loss of both gene cop-

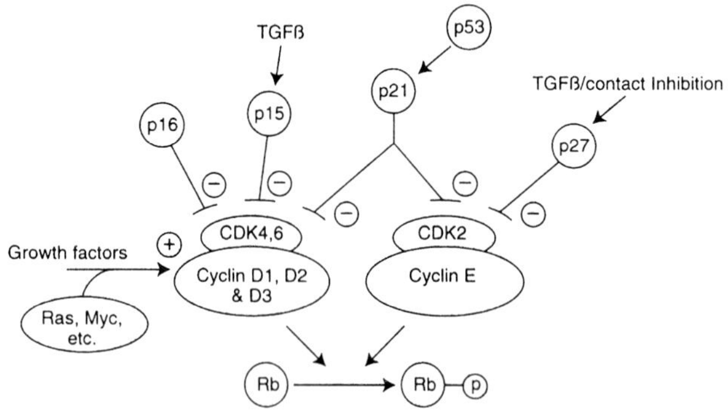

Figure 1. Control of Rb protein phosphorylation during the G1 phase of the cell cycle. The phosphorylation status of RB1 is controlled as shown schematically here by cyclin–CDK complexes. The components implicated in the development of soft tissue sarcomas through mutation, overexpression, or deletion include CDK4, p53, cyclinD1, p16, and RB1 itself.

ies) of the *CDKN2* gene, which encodes p16, been reported in malignant peripheral nerve sheath tumors, rhabdomyosarcomas, and leiomyosarcomas [5]. In the same study, amplification and overexpression of the *CDK4* and *cyclin D1* genes were observed in some sarcomas. The latter observation agreed with an immunological study showing that the cyclin D1 protein level is elevated in up to 40% of soft tissue sarcomas [6] and with an early report of *CDK4* gene amplification in a rhabdomyosarcoma [7]. Direct evidence that *cyclin D1* can have a role in cell transformation is provided by experiments showing that overexpression of this gene can (1) confer transformed properties on established fibroblast lines and (2) cooperate with other protooncogenes, including activated *RAS* and *MYC* genes, to transform primary cells. The detection of *CDK4* amplification and overexpression is of interest because for some cell types it has been proposed that overexpression of CDK4 protein may act by rendering cells insensitive to the CDK inhibitor protein p15 that is induced following exposure to transforming growth factor beta (TGF-β). If removal of the TGF-β control pathway acting through p15 is indeed important in sarcoma induction, then it should also be possible to find alteration of the *p15* gene, and the results of such studies are awaited with interest.

p53 suppressor pathway

The p53 protein acts, at least in part, as a transcriptional regular that can activated genes by binding specific DNA sequences. At least two key functions contribute to the ability of p53 to act as a tumor suppressor. First, it has been shown that following DNA damage, the level of p53 protein is elevated, leading to cell cycle arrest at the border between G1 and S [8]. The effect appears to be mediated as a consequence of the ability of p53 to induce expression of the gene *WAF1* that encodes the p21 inhibitor of G1 cyclin-dependent kinases (see Fig. 1). Secondly, in several systems it has been demonstrated that p53 overexpression can induce apoptosis [9]. Thus it is believed that in response to DNA damage p53 produces the arrest of cells prior to the S phase of the cell cycle to allow for DNA repair to take place, and may also play a role in inducing apoptosis in cells that are too severely damaged to be repaired correctly. Removal of p53 would therefore promote genetic instability, both by allowing cells to accumulate mutations in the genome and by helping these cells to survive as the level of genomic alteration gradually accumulates.

Inactivation of the *p53* gene, resulting in the removal of the normal p53 protein, has been detected in many types of human cancers. The *p53* gene is located on a region of chromosome 17 that is frequently lost during tumor development, and the *p53* allele that remains in these tumors usually contains point mutations. Loss of chromosome 17 and inactivating point mutations have frequently been observed in soft tissue sarcomas, particularly in MFHs, rhabdomyosarcomas, and leiomyosarcomas [10–12]. However, in contrast to the results obtained with most other cancer types but in common with osteosarcoma and blast crisis chronic myeolgenous leukemia, homozygous deletion of the *p53* gene was also frequently observed [13,14].

Mis-sense mutation usually induces conformational changes in the p53 protein that dramatically prolong its half-life, resulting in the accumulation of p53 protein in the tumor cells to levels that can be detected by immunohistochemical methods. In analyses of 211 soft tissue sarcomas using this approach, an overall frequency of 20% p53 overexpression was observed [15]. By comparison, in a smaller study on a series of 29 leiomyosarcoma revealed p53 overexpression in 17% of tumors, and in this study all tumors overexpressing p53 protein were also shown to contain point mutations in the p53 gene [16].

Cooperation between *p53* and *RB1*

Abnormalities of the *p53* gene have been found, together with alterations of the *RB1* gene in soft tissue sarcomas, indicating that coincident loss of these two suppressor genes may be required for tumor development [10]. This pattern of alteration of *p53* and *RB1* is similar to that observed following infection of cells with transforming viruses such as SV40, papilloma virus, and adenovirus. For example, papilloma virus encodes two proteins, called E6 and E7, that bind to and abrogate the function of the p53 and RB1 proteins, respectively. Similarly, the large T antigen of SV40 binds to both p53 and RB1 proteins. Thus the pattern of genetic alteration observed in human soft tissue sarcomas appear to reproduce that which occurs at the level of protein–protein interaction during viral infection.

Recent studies on transgenic mice where *p53* and/or *RB1* expression has been eliminated in specific tissue have shed some light on the way in which the *RB1* and *p53* deletions may interact during tumorigenesis [17]. In mice that lack *RB1* expression, the lens cells that would normally withdraw from the cell cycle and differentiate instead continue to divide and then die by apoptosis. By comparison, in mice lacking both functional RB1 and p53, apoptosis in the lens cells is dramatically reduced and lens tumors develop. These results are interpreted as indicating that the cell proliferation that results from *RB1* deletion can only be sustained in the absence of the *p53* safeguard mechanism, which would normally result in the death of cells engaged in untimely DNA synthesis. Both the *p53* and *RB1* functions must therefore be removed for tumors to develop.

MDM2 gene

The *MDM2* protooncogene is found amplified and overexpressed in a variety of sarcoma types [18], and it has been demonstrated that overproduction of *MDM2* is both tumorigenic and capable of immortalizing primary rat embryo fibroblasts [19,20]. The oncogenic capacity of overexpressed MDM2 protein is ascribed to its ability to bind to and inhibit the growth-regulating functions of both p53 and RB1 [21]. The *MDM2* gene was originally reported to be amplified in over a third of a group of 47 sarcomas that included both bone and soft tissue tumors [18]. Amplification was seen in 7 of 13 liposarcomas and 7 of 22 MFHs, and overexpression of the MDM2 protein was observed in tumors containing the amplification. In a study by Cordon-Cardo et al. [15] on a larger series of adult soft tissue sarcomas, 5 to 35-fold amplification was detected in 11 of 73 (15%) tumors. In immunostaining studies, only 6 of the 11 *MDM2*-amplified cases showed *MDM2* overexpression. In addition, 17 of the 62 (27%) cases with no detectable amplified *MDM2* gene also showed elevated levels of *MDM2* protein. These observations suggest that amplification of *MDM2* is not necessarily accompanied by overexpression, and that overexpression can occur by a mechanism that does not require amplification. In a recent study by Florenes et al. [22], *MDM2* amplification and/or overexpression was found in 1 of 20 MFHs, 0 of 14 leiomyosarcomas, 2 of 2 fibrosarcomas, 3 of 6 malignant peripheral nerve sheath tumors, 3 of 19 liposarcomas, and 1 hemangiopericytoma examined.

It is important to remember that amplification in human tumors often involves large stretches of the genome encompassing up to 1000–2000 kb. It is therefore possible that other genes in the *MDM2* amplification could be responsible for the transforming effect of the amplification event. The transforming effects introducing cloned *MDM2* into certain cell types mentioned earlier argues for the importance of *MDM2*. However, observation that amplification of *MDM2* is apparently not always accompanied by overexpression could support the hypothesis that other genes are important. Genes closely linked to *MDM2* include the *GLI* protooncogene and *CDK4*. In some tumors *GLI* and *CDK4* were amplified together with *MDM2*, but in particular in one rhabdomyosarcoma amplification included *CDK4* and *GLI* but not *MDM2* [7]. These observations suggest that *CDK4* and/or *GLI* may also have a role in sarcoma formation. Amplification of another gene called *SAS* that maps to the same region on chromosome 12 has also been reported [23].

Activation of *RAS*

Activation of members of the *RAS* gene family (H-*RAS*, K-*RAS*, and N-*RAS*) have been detected in several types of human cancer. RAS proteins lie on a key pathway that transduces signals from cell surface receptors. Binding of ligands such as epidermal growth factor receptors results in conversion of the inactive GDP-bound form of RAS to the active GTP-bound form. Activation of RAS that occurs by point mutation at codons 12, 13, and 61 fixes RAS in the active conformation, resulting in constitutive activation of the RAF protein serine kinase. This leads, in turn, to activation of MAP kinase, which is believed to modulate the G0/G1 phase of the cell cycle.

Activated *RAS* genes were originally detected in human tumors using a biological assay in which the ability of tumor DNA to transform NIH3T3 mouse fibroblasts was examined. Of 46 soft tissue sarcomas and tumor cell lines examined using this method, four were found to contain activated *RAS* genes. Activated N-*RAS* was detected in rhabdomyosarcoma and fibosarcoma cell lines [24], while K-*RAS* was activated in a primary embryonal rhabdomyosarcoma [25] and a leiomyosarcoma [26]. Activated genes unrelated to *RAS* were detected in a liposarcoma and a leiomyosarcoma [26,27]. Using oligonucleotide probes to screen for alterations in codons 12, 13, and 61, Stratton et al. [28] detected point mutations of N-*RAS* and K-*RAS* in 35% (5 of 14) embryonal rhabdomyosarcomas. When considered together, these observations indicated that *RAS* activation is common in one class of childhood sarcoma but is relatively rare in adult soft tissue sarcomas.

***MYC* gene family**

Members of the *MYC* family of cellular protooncogenes (C-*MYC*, N-*MYC*, and L-*MYC*) have been implicated in the control of cellular growth, differentiation, and programmed cell death. The nuclear proteins encoded by these genes are believed to function as sequence-specific transciptional factors. Although their precise mechanism of action is unknown, it is apparent that MYC may influence the expression of many growth-promoting genes in a positive fashion. The importance of MYC in regulating cellular proliferation is illustrated by the observation that removal of functional C-*MYC* RNA can block proliferation and by the fact that introduction of deregulated *MYC* genes into culture cells and transgenic mice can facilitate malignant transformation.

Deregulation of *MYC* expression, either as a consequence of specific chromosomal translocations or gene amplification, has frequently been demonstrated in human sarcomas. Double minute chromosomes (DMs) and homogeneously staining regions (HSRs), the cytogenetic hallmarkers of gene amplification, have frequently been observed in rhabdomyosarcomas as well as in malignant fibrous histiocytomas and liposarcomas [29–33]. In agreement with these observations, amplification of N-*MYC* and/or C-*MYC* genes was observed in embryonal and alveolar rhabdomyosarcomas, and in one study N-*MYC* amplification was found in a tumor recurrence but not in the original tumor, suggesting that N-*MYC* amplification may have been involved in tumor regrowth [34–37].

Chromosomal translocations

One of the most interesting genetic features of soft tissue sarcomas is the occurrence of specific chromosomal translocations in several sarcoma types. The detection of specific chromosome translocations in leukemias is used

Table 1. Tumor-specific chromosomal translocations in soft tissue sarcomas

Tumor type	Translocation	Genes	References
Synovial sarcoma	t(X;18)(p11.2;q11.2)	*SSX1, SSX2, SYT*	38,39
Alveolar rhabdomyosarcoma	t(2;13)(q37;q14)	*PAX3, FKHR*	40
	t(1;13)(p36;q14)	*PAX7, FKHR*	41
Myxoid liposarcoma	t(12;16)(q13;p11)	*CHOP, TLS*	42, 43
Soft tissue clear cell sarcoma	t(12;22)(q13;q12)	*ATF1, EWS*	44
Myxoid chondrosarcoma (extraskeletal)	t(9;22)(q22–31;q11–12)	*CHN, EWS*	45
Desmoplastic small round cell tumor	t(11;22)(p13;q12)	*WT1, EWS*	46

widely in diagnosis and in distinguishing subclasses of the disease that have different prognoses. Similarly, the identification of specific chromosomal abnormalities in sarcomas offers the prospect of their use in diagnosis and prognosis. In many cases the genes involved in these translocations have now been identified. These are listed in Table 1. What has emerged is that the genes that becomes fused as a consequence of these translocations often encode transcription factors. For example, in the t(2;13) translocation found in alveolar rhabdomyosarcoma, the *FKHR* gene, a member of the forkhead family of developmentally regulated transcription factor genes, becomes joined to the *PAX3* gene, a member of the PAX family of transcription factors, which contain a paired box DNA-binding domain. Similarly, *CHOP*, the gene involved in the t(12;16) liposarcoma translocation, encodes a negative regulator of transcription that is inducible by DNA damage and that has been implicated in fat cell development. Other genes that appear to encode transcription factor are *SSX1* and *SSX2*, which are involved in the t(X;18) synovial sarcoma translocation, and the *WT1* (Wilms tumor) gene, involved in the t(11;22) translocation found in desmoplastic small round cell tumours.

MET protooncogene

The *MET* protooncogene encodes a tyrosine kinase receptor that, together with its ligand, hepatocyte growth factor/scatter factor (HGF), constitute a paracrine signaling pathway, in which cells of mesenchymal origin produce HGF that binds to a receptor that is predominantly expressed in cells of epithelial origin. Studies in human sarcomas demonstrate that they abnormally produce the MET receptor as well as expressing HGF, indicating that an autocrine loop may have been set up in which the sarcomas produce a ligand that stimulates their own growth [47]. In support of this model for cell transformation, it has been reported that mesenchymal cells in culture (NIH3T3 mouse fibroblasts) can be transformed by overexpression of normal MET protein.

Genetic predisposition

It is generally accepted that the development of cancer is a multistep process requiring the accumulation of genetic alteration or mutation of several loci before a neoplastic clone can develop. A genetic predisposition to cancer may occur if one of the mutations is inherited in the germline, thus reducing the number of mutations that need to be acquired by somatic mutation. Alternatively, the inherited abnormality may predispose to the accumulation of such a mutation, for example, by encoding a defective DNA repair protein. There is evidence of a genetic predisposition to both malignant and benign soft tissue tumors but the latter are less well characterized and will not be considered here.

Inherited mutations in the p53 and RB1 genes

Since abnormalities in both the *p53* and *RB1* genes have been implicated in the development of soft tissue sarcomas, it is perhaps not surprising to find that inherited alterations in both of these genes can predispose to sarcoma development. The Li-Fraumeni syndrome was first identified as an autosomal dominant familial cancer syndrome that in its classic form is defined by the existence of both a proband with a sarcoma and two other first-degree relatives with cancer by age 45 years [48,49]. In these families affected members may develop a variety of early-onset cancers, including breast carcinoma, sarcomas, brain tumors, leukemias, and adrenocortical carcinoma. Germline mutations of the *p53* gene have been identified in a high proportion of Li-Fraumeni families [50,51]. Furthermore, a high incidence of diverse tumor types in transgenic mice deficient for *p53* has confirmed that germline mutation of the *p53* gene can result in a genetic predisposition to cancer [52]. Germline *p53* mutations have also been reported in patients who develop multiple primary cancers, including sarcomas [53].

Retinoblastoma, which is usually found in children under 5 years of age, occurs in both sporadic and hereditary forms. Notably, the hereditary form is almost always bilateral and multifocal. Ten to 20% of patients with the hereditary disease develop secondary tumors, usually osteosarcomas and soft tissue tumors, later in life [54,55]. Based on analysis of the epidemiological characteristics of retinoblastoma, Knudson proposed that the development of this tumor requires two hits or mutation [56]. He proposed that individuals with the inherited form of the disease carry one hit as a germline mutation and require only one further mutation in a retinal cell for a tumor to develop. By comparison, in sporadic retinoblastoma both hits must be acquired by somatic mutation. Based on analysis of constitutional chromosomal deletions in a small proportion of patients and from genetic linkage analysis, the gene mutated in the germline in hereditary retinoblastoma was localized to 13q14. Chromosome analysis in retinoblastoma further suggested that the second hit was in the same region of chromosome 13. The gene located at 13q14 that is responsible for the inherited predisposition to the development of retinoblastoma in children and osteosarcoma and soft tissue sarcomas is the *RB1* gene described in detail earlier.

NF1 gene

Von Recklinghausen's neurofibromatosis (type I neurofibromatosis NF1) is an autosomal dominant disorder affecting around 1 in 3500 newborns, 30–50% of which are thought to arise from spontaneous mutations. Characteristics of this disorder are the presence of cafe-au-lait spots, skin neurofibromas, Lisch nodules, and orthopedic abnormalities. In addition, 5% of individuals with *NF1* develop Schwannomas of the peripheral nerves and 2% of cases develop malignant peripheral nerve sheath tumors [57]. The gene for NF1 was identified on chromosome 17 by using the chromosome translocation breakpoints in two unique NF1 patients to pinpoint the gene [58–60]. Support for the idea that the *NF1* gene may act as a tumor suppressor gene was provided by the detection of germline point mutations within this gene in NF1 patients, and in particular by the documentation of activation of both copies of the *NF1* gene in a neurofibrosarcoma from an NF1 patient [6]. Somatic mutation of the *NF1* gene has also been detected in colon carcinoma and osteocytomas specimens. The *NF1* gene encodes a protein, neurofibroma, which exhibits homology to the mammalian RAS-GTPase-activating protein (GAP) and has been established as an important regulator of the RAS signal transduction pathway [62]. Point mutation or removal of the *NF1* gene would be predicted to produce activation of this pathway by reducing RAS GTPase activation, thus preventing the conversion of the active GTP-bound form of RAS to its inactive GDP-bound form.

APC gene

Fibromatoses are rare fibromatous lesions that are intermediate in character between benign fibrous lesions and fibrosarcomas [63]. The deep fibromatoses (desmoids) are found as a complication in around 10% of patients with adenomatous polyposis (FAP), an autosomal dominant disease in which affected patients develop multiple adenomatous polyps in the colon and rectum. The association between FAP with desmoids and other conditions, including ostemata, cutaneous cysts, and other soft tissue tumors, including lipomas and leiomyomas, is known in *Gardener's syndrome*. Both FAP and Gardner's syndrome are now known to result from inherited mutations in a gene called *APC* at the chromosomal location 5q21–22 [64–66].

However, a detailed analysis of mutation of the *APC* gene FAP and Gardner's patient failed to reveal any correlation between the type of mutation in the APC gene and desmoid formation. Indeed, Nishisho et al. [65] found that individuals with a G→T transition of codon 302 in the *APC* gene can either have the range of symptoms associated with GS or have FAP with no evidence of extracolonic manifestation. These observations suggest that other genetic factors may control the conditions specifically associated with GS. Support for the idea that the *APC* gene acts as a suppressor gene that must be removed during the development of fibromatosis has been provided by genetic analysis of eight desmoid tumours taken from seven FAP patients [67]. In addition to the presence of germline mutations in the *APC* gene, evidence was presented that all eight tumors contained a somatically acquired mutation in the second copy of the *APC* allele.

Beckwith-Wiedemann syndrome

The Beckwith-Wiedemann syndrome (BWS) is characterized by anterior abdominal wall defects, macroglossia, and gigantism, and is associated with a range of less commonly encountered clinical features, including a greatly increased risk of developing Wilms' tumor, hepatoblastoma, and rhabdomyosarcoma. The majority of cases are sporadic, but several families with an autosomal dominant mode of inheritance have been described and used in linkage studies to locate the predisposing gene to 11p15 [68]. Constitutional abnormalities of this chromosomal region have also been observed in this condition [69], and loss of the short arm of chromosome 11 has been detected in tumors arising in BWS patients [70]. Further support for the idea that this region is important for the development of embryonal tumors is provided by the observation of the consistent loss of the short arm of chromosome 11 in embryonal rhabdomyosarcomas accompanied by duplication of the remaining allele [71].

Analysis of the Beckwith-Wiedemann syndrome demonstrated that constitutional uniparental paternal disomy (both alleles derived from the father) occurred at the 11p15 region [72]. This observation, together with the finding that the degree of penetrance in familial cases depends on whether the defect is inherited from the father or mother, suggests that the BWS gene(s) may be imprinted. In this regard, particular attention has focused on the gene for insulin-like growth factor II (IGFII), which is exclusively silent at the maternal allele in normal human tissue. Recent studies have demonstrated biallelic expression (expression of both maternal and paternal copies) of this gene in some BWS patients as well as in sporadic rhabdomyosarcoma and Wilms' tumor specimens that have retained both 11p15 alleles [73–75]. These findings implicate the overexpression of IGFII in the BWS condition and in the development of embryonal tumors.

In principle, the detection of inherited mutations that predispose to cancer development could be extremely useful in the management of sarcomas through identification of individuals at high risk of tumor development. For example, it is now possible to screen Li-Fraumeni families for mutations in the *p53* gene. This procedure identifies both carriers who have a high risk of cancer development and normal individuals within Li-Fraumeni families who do not harbour *p53* gene mutations. If screening is to be undertaken, then it is important to develop strategies for counseling care and treatment of carriers of *p53* mutations.

Mismatch repair genes

Several studies have implicated defects in DNA mismatch repair in the pathogenesis of hereditary non-polyposis colorectal cancer (HNPCC). Evidence showing changes in microsatellite sequences consisting of dinucleotide and trinucleotide repeats in colorectal cancer provided the first indication that HNPCC may result from abnormalities in the DNA repair system [76]. Subsequently inherited mutations have been detected in mismatch repair genes such as *PMS1*, *PMS2*, *hMSH2*, and *hMLH1* in HNPCC kindreds [77]. In addition to the observed abnormalities in colorectal cancer, a high frequency of genetic instability in microsatellites (the mutator phenotype) has also been observed in other classes of human cancer, including endometrial, pancreatic, gastric, esophageal, and small-cell lung cancers. In contrast, analysis of soft tissue sarcomas revealed only a low frequency of microsatellite instability (2 abnormalities in 216 typings), indicating that mutation in microsatellite repair genes is not of major importance in sarcoma development [78].

Molecular diagnosis of soft tissue sarcomas

Soft tissue sarcomas present frequent diagnostic problems. For example, the existence of one of the major categories of classification, malignant fibrous histiocytoma, is still debated, and difficulty is often encountered in distinguishing rhabdomyosarcomas from other classes of small round cell tumours. The recent cloning of genes involved in the chromosome-specific translocations found in some sarcoma groups and the identification of genes that take control of the development of specific lineages has suggested new strategies that may assist in sarcoma diagnosis.

Chromosomal translocations

Cytogenetic studies have identified specific chromosomal translocations in several classes of soft tissue sarcoma (see Table 1). These abnormalities can be found as the only cytogenetic alteration, indicating that their formation may be a key event in tumor development, and they usually occur in a high proportion of tumors, thus offering the prospect of their use in tumor diagnosis. A consistent feature of these translocations is the result of the fusion of genes present in two different chromosomes. The new chimeric genes created by these fusions are expressed in chimeric transcripts, which in turn encode novel fusion proteins in which functional domains usually found in distinct proteins are combined. These discoveries have led to the development of RT-PCR procedures that can be used to detect the hybrid transcripts found by each individual translocation. RNA from the tumor is initially incubated with reverse transferase to produce a DNA copy. This DNA copy is then subject to the polymerase chain reaction using primers corresponding to the separate genes involved in the translocation so that only fused gene sequences are amplified. Because of difficulties in growing soft tissue sarcomas in culture, it is often difficult or impossible to obtain a karyotype, and where karyotypes are obtained it can in some cases take 2–3 weeks to complete the analysis. The RT-PCR approach for detecting translocations overcomes these problems of reliability and speed of analysis, allowing rapid and sensitive analysis of samples in 1–2 days.

The t(X;18)(p11.2;q11.2) translocation detected in both monophasic and biphasic variants of synovial sarcoma was found to result in the fusion of the *SYT* gene on chromosome 18 to two closely related genes, *SSX1* and *SSX2*, located at Xp11.2. Notably, *SYT-SSX1* and *SYT-SSX2* transcripts were detected by RT-PCR in 29 of 31 synovial sarcomas examined, emphasizing the potential usefulness of this approach in tumor diagnosis [39]. In particular, the RT-PCR technology may be useful in distinguishing the monophasic tumour subtype from other types of spindle cell tumors that fall within its differential diagnosis, such as fibrosarcomas, leiomyosarcomas, malignant peripheral nerve sheath tumors, MFHs, and hemangiopericytomas. The translocations t(2;13)(q37;q14) and t(1;13)(p36;q14) have been detected during cytogenetic studies on alveolar rhabdomyosarcomas. These translocations result in the fusion of either the *PAX3* and *PAX7* gene, present, respectively, on chromosomes 2 and 1, to the *FKHR* gene on chromosome 13 [41,42]. Using RT-PCR strategies to detect *PAX3-FKHR* and *PAX7-FKHR* hybrid transcripts, these gene fusions were found in 18 of 21 alveolar tumors but in only 2 of 30 embryonal rhabdomyosarcomas, suggesting that this approach may be very useful in identifying alveolar rhabdomyosarcomas [79]. In addition, Scrable et al. [80] found that all embryonal tumors had lost one copy of this chromosomal region, while alveolar tumors retained both copies.

The consistent translocation t(12;16)(q13;p11) identified in liposarcomas involves the fusion of the *FUS/TLS* gene on chromosome 16 to the *CHOP* gene on chromosome 12 [42,43]. Although this translocation was originally identified in cytogenetic and molecular studies on myxoid liposarcomas, recent evidence shows that it also occurs in the rarer round cell liposarcomas and in mixed tumors containing both round cell and myxoid regions [81]. This was particularly interesting because these tumor subgroups have different clinical characteristics. Myxoid liposarcomas are rarely metastatic and are associated with a favorable survival, while round cell liposarcomas are highly metastatic high-grade tumors. Because no evidence of progression from myxoid to round cell morphology was obtained, it was suggested that progenitor cells containing the t(12;16) translocation may evolve into either phenotype depending on the presence of other (unidentified) factors. This translocation may therefore have particular diagnostic use in distinguishing myxoid and round cell liposarcomas from other tumors that fall within their differential diagnosis (e.g., myxoid chondrosarcomas).

Use of lineage-specific markers in the diagnosis of rhabdomyosarcoma

The development of striated muscle is controlled by a family of genes called the *myf* (*MyoD1*) genes. The proteins encoded by these genes are closely related helix-loop-helix transcription factors that control the expression of muscle-specific genes. Because rhabdomyosarcomas are tumors that show differentiation towards striated muscle, they would be expected to express members of this gene family. In agreement with this prediction, it has been demonstrated that *myf* genes are expressed in >90% of alveolar and embryonal rhabdomyosarcomas. Cavenee and colleagues [80,82] found expression of all four *myf* genes (*myf3*, *myf4*, *myf5*, and *myf6*) in these tumors, while Clark et al. [83] found that *myf3* and *myf4* were expressed in a high proportion of tumors, while *myf5* and *myf6* were expressed in a lower proportion of tumours (55% and 33%, respectively). Both groups failed to observe the expression of *myf* genes in other types of pediatric round cell tumors, indicating that expression of members of this family may provide extremely useful diagnostic markers. In these studies, expression of *myf* genes was determined by Northern analysis of tumor RNA. However, the production of antibodies that recognize myf proteins in formalin-preserved specimens will be necessary if this approach is to be adopted for routine use in histopathology laboratories.

Use as prognostic markers

There has been considerable interest in using the presence of genetic abnormalities to predict tumor response to the treatment and survival of individual patients. For example, in breast cancer amplification and overexpression of the *c-erbB-2* gene is correlated with poor survival and shorter times to relapse [84], while amplification and overexpression of *N-myc* is restricted to stage III and IV neuroblastoma and is not commonly found in stage I and stage II tumors [85].

Abnormalities of RB1

Attempts have been made to correlate the presence of abnormalities in the *RB1* gene and its expression with clinical parameters in soft tissue sarcomas. In a combined study of soft tissue and bone sarcomas, Wunder et al. [86] found that the *RB1* gene was altered in 10 of 25 high-grade tumors but in only 1 of 11 low-grade tumours. Wang et al. [87] used an antibody against the DNA binding region of the RB1 protein to assess levels of this protein in a series of 68 soft tissue sarcomas. Complete or partial loss of RB1 protein was found in 11

(17%) of sarcomas, with 6 of 7 sarcomas showing complete loss. Loss or partial loss of RB1 immunostaining correlated with increased tumor grade.

p53 and MDM2 genes

There has been considerable interest in examining the potential use of abnormalities in the *p53* and *MDM2* gene as prognostic markers. Kawai et al. [88] used an anti-*p53* antibody to screen for nuclear accumulation of *p53*, an indirect indicator of the presence of point mutations in the *p53* gene in soft tissue sarcomas from 96 patients. The percentage of tumors with a positive immunoreaction was high in patients with MPNSTs (100%), rhabdomyosarcoma (71%), and synovial sarcoma (50%) but low in patients with liposarcoma (14%) and fibrosarcoma (0%). Notably, there was a close association between immunostaining and histological grade of malignancy (grade 1, 12%; grade 2, 31%; grade 3, 44%) and patient age (<40 years, 47%; >40 years, 25%). In addition, both overall and metastatic free survival were lower for patients with a nuclear p53 immunoreactivity. In agreement with these observations, Toffoli et al. [89] in a study of tumors from 61 patients found evidence that *p53* overexpression is found mainly in the most aggressive forms of soft tissue sarcomas. In a study of 73 soft tissue sarcomas, Latres et al. [90] found allelic loss of 17p, the location of the *p53* gene, in 53% and 29% of informative cases and p53 nuclear overexpression in 34% of tumors. 17p deletions and p53 overexpression were both more frequent in metastatic than primary tumors, while *p53* overexpression was also associated with tumor grade and size.

A cohort of over 200 adult soft tissue sarcomas has been examined for molecular alteration and altered patterns of expression of *MDM2* and *p53* genes [15]. Using monoclonal antibodies that detect the proteins encoded by these genes, 76 of 207 tumors had high levels of MDM2 proteins and 56 of 211 tumors overexpressed the p53 protein. Twenty-two cases have abnormally high levels of both MDM2 and *p53* proteins. There was a notable correlation between overexpression of the two proteins on the same tumor and poor survival. In a separate study on a group of 29 leiomyosarcomas, genetic alteration of either the *MDM2* gene or *p53* genes were observed in 10 tumors, and there was a significant correlation between the presence of these alterations and a more advanced clinicopathological stage [16].

Other markers

Limited evidence suggests that cytogenetic abnormalities may also be of use as prognostic markers. Thus in studies on malignant fibrous histiocytomas, correlations have been found between tumor behavior and the presence of in 19p+ marker chromosome or the presence of ring chromosomes [32,91]. Thus metastases and/or local recurrence occurred in 8 of 9 patients with the 19p+ marker but in only 4 of 13 without it. In addition, relapse occurred in 2 of 8 patients with ring chromosomes compared with 10 of 14 patients without them. There have been unconfirmed reports of a dramatic correlation between the expression of the *mdr-1*–encoded protein, P-glycoprotein, and resistance to treatment with chemotherapeutic agents in childhood sarcoma [92]. Remarkably, all nine patients who had tumors expressing P-glycoprotein relapsed after the initial response, and only 1 of 20 tumors were consistently P-glycoprotein negative. P-glycoprotein is an energy-dependent pump that removes drugs from cells and can confer resistance to classes of structurally and functionally unrelated drugs. Based on these results, clinical trials have been initiated to determine whether drugs that inhibit the activity of P-glycoprotein can improve the response of childhood sarcomas to chemotherapy.

Future developments

Studies on human colon cancer have demonstrated that the sequential alteration of at least one oncogene (*RAS*) and inactivation of three suppressor genes (*APC*, *DCC*, and *p53*) may be required for malignant transformation. Although impressive advances have been made in pinpointing the genes involved in sarcoma developments, in many cases only a single or at most two genes (e.g., alterations in *p53* together with *RB1*) have been identified. In future studies it will therefore be important to continue the search for genes involved in sarcoma development and analyses of the way in which these genes interact to cause transformation. In this regard, the new technique of comparative genomic hybridization, which can be used to identify and refine regions of amplification and deletion within the genome of individual tumors, offers the prospect of providing completely fresh insights into types of genetic alterations involved in sarcoma development [93].

The identification of genes involved in chromosome-specific translocation that are found in several types of soft tissue sarcoma have provided important insights into the mechanisms of tumor induction. In addition, this work is leading to the development of PCR-based procedures for detecting translocations in synovial sarcomas, rhabdomyosarcomas, and liposarcomas. A thorough assessment of the value of these techniques in tumor diagnosis and prognosis is an important subject that must now be addressed. The use of *myf* gene lineage-specific markers in the diagnosis of rhabdomyosarcoma illustrates a general approach that could, in principle, be used in the diagnosis of other sarcoma types. Identification of genes that determine differentiation towards, for example, fat, smooth muscle, and cartilage, may therefore be a key step in further improving diagnostic methods.

Acknowledgments

We would like to thank Christine Bell for typing this manuscript. We are grateful to the Cancer Research Campaign and the John Glees Research Fund for supporting our research.

References

1. Hunter T, Pines J. Cyclins and cancer II: Cyclin D and CDK inhibitors come of age. Cell 79:573–582, 1994.
2. Stratton MR, Williams S, Fisher C, Ball A, Westbury G, Gusterson BA, Fletcher CDM, Knight JC, Fung Y-K, Reeves BR, Cooper CS. Structural alterations of the RB1 gene in human soft tissue tumours. Br J Cancer 60:202–205, 1989.
3. Friend SH, Horowitz JM, Gerber MR, Wand XF, Bogenmann E, Li FP, Weinberg RA. Deletions of a DNA sequence in retinoblastomas and mesenchymal tumours: Organisation of the sequence and its encoded protein. Proc Natl Acad Sci USA 84:9059–9063, 1987.
4. Mendoza AE, Shew JY, Lee EY, Brookstein R, Lee WH. A case of synovial sarcoma with abnormal expression of the human retinoblastoma susceptibility gene. Hum Pathol 19:487–489, 1988.
5. Maelandsmo GM, Berner J-M, Florenos JA, Forus A, Hovig E, Fodstad O, Myklebust O. Homozygous deletion frequency and expression levels of the CDKN2 gene in human sarcomas—relationship to amplification and MRNA levels of CDK4 and CCND1. Br J Cancer 72:393–398, 1995.
6. Bartkova J, Lukas J, Strauss M, Bartek J. Cyclin D1 oncoprotein aberrantly accumulates in malignancies of diverse histogenesis. Oncogene 10:775–778, 1995.
7. Khatib ZA, Matsushime H, Valentine M, Shapiro DN, Sherr CJ, Look AT. Coamplification of the CDK4 gene with MDM2 and GL1 in human sarcomas. Cancer Res 53:5535–5541, 1993.
8. Mercer WE, Shields MT, Amin M, Sauve GJ, Appella E, Romano JW, Ullrich SJ. Negative growth regulation in a glioblastoma in tumour cell line that conditionally expresses human wild-type p53. Proc Natl Acad Sci USA 87:6166–6170, 1990.
9. Shaw P, Bovey R, Tardy S, Sahli R, Sordat B, Costa J. Induction of apoptosis by wild-type p53 in a human colon tumor-derived cell line. Proc Natl Acad Sci USA 89:4495–4499, 1992.
10. Stratton MR, Moss S, Warren W, Patterson H, Clark J, Fisher C, Fletcher CDM, Ball A, Thomas M, Gusterson BA, Cooper CS. Mutation of the p53 gene in human soft tissue sarcomas: Association with abnormalities of the RB1 gene. Oncogene 5:1297–1301, 1990.
11. Mulligan LM, Matlashewski GJ, Scrable HJ, Cavenee WK. Mechanisms of p53 loss in human sarcomas. Proc Natl Acad Sci USA 87:5863–5867, 1990.
12. Leach FS, Tokino T, Meltzer P, Burrell M, Oliner JD, Smith S, Hill DE, Sidransky D, Kinzler KW, Vogelstein B. p53 mutation and MDM2 amplification in human soft tissue sarcomas. Cancer Res 52:2231–2234, 1993.
13. Ahuja H, Bar-Eli M, Advani SH, Benchimol S, Cline M. Alterations in the p53 gene and the clonal evolution of the blast crisis of chronic myelocytic leukemia. Proc Natl Acad Sci USA 86:6783–6787, 1989.
14. Masuda H, Miller C, Koeffler HP, Battifora H, Cline MJ. Rearrangement of the p53 gene in human osteogenic sarcomas. Proc Natl Acad Sci USA 84:7716–7719, 1987.
15. Cordon-Cardo C, Latres E, Drobnjak M, Oliva MR, Pollack D, Woodroff JM, Marechal V, Chen J, Brennan MF, Levine AJ. Molecular abnormalities of mdm2 and p53 genes in adult soft tissue sarcomas. Cancer Res 54:794–799, 1994.
16. Patterson H, Gill S, Fisher C, Law MG, Jayatilake H, Fletcher CD, Thomas M, Grimer R, Gusterson BA, Cooper CS. Abnormalities of the p53, MDM2 and DCC genes in human leiomyosarcomas. Oncogene 69:1052–1058, 1994.
17. White E. p53, guardian of Rb. Nature 371:21–22, 1994.
18. Oliner JD, Kinzler KW, Meltzer PS, George DL, Vogelstein B. Amplification of a gene encoding a p53-associated protein in human sarcomas. Nature 358:80–83, 1992.
19. Fakharzadeh SS, Trusko SP, George DL. Tumourigenic potential associated with enhanced expression of a gene that is amplified in a mouse tumor cell line. EMBO J 10:1565–1569, 1991.
20. Finlay CA. The mdm-2 oncogene can overcome wild-type p53 suppression of transformed cell growth. Mol Cell Biol 13:301–306, 1993.

21. Xlao Z-X, Chen J, Levine AJ, Modjtahedi N, Xing J, Sellers WR, Livingston DM. Interaction between the retinoblastoma protein and the oncoprotein MDM2. Nature 375:694–697, 1995.
22. Florenes VA, Moelandsmo GM, Fours A, Andreassen A, Myklebost O, Fodstad O. MDM2 gene amplification and transcript levels in human sarcomas: Relationship to TP53 gene status. J Natl Cancer Inst 87:1297–1302, 1994.
23. Smith SH, Weiss SW, Jankowski SA, Coccia MA, Meltzer PS. SAS amplification in soft tissue sarcomas. Cancer Res 52:3746–3749, 1992.
24. Marshall CJ, Hall A, Weiss RA. A transforming gene present in human sarcoma lines. Nature 299:171–173, 1982.
25. Pulciani S, Santos E, Lauver AV, Long LK, Aaronson SA, Barbacid M. Oncogenes in solid tumours. Nature 300:539–542, 1982.
26. Gill S, Stratton MR, Patterson H, Spurr NK, Fisher C, Gusterson B, Cooper CS. Detection of transforming genes by transfection of DNA from primary soft tissue tumours. Oncogene 6:1651–1656, 1991.
27. Fukui MT, Yamamoto T, Kawai S, Maruo K, Toyoshima K. Detection of a raf-related and two other transforming DNA sequences in human tumors maintained in nude mice. Proc Natl Acad Sci USA 82:5954–5958, 1985.
28. Stratton MR, Fisher C, Gusterson BA, Cooper CS. Detection of point mutations in N-ras and K-ras genes of human embryonal rhabdomyosarcomas using oligonucleotide probes and the polymerase chain reaction. Cancer Res 49:6324–6327, 1989.
29. Mertens F, Johansson B, Mandahl N, Heim S, Bennet K, Pydholom A, Willen H, Mitelman F. Clonal Chromosome abnormalities in two liposarcomas. Cancer Genet Cytogenet 28:137–144, 1987.
30. Douglass EC, Valentine M, Etcubanas E, Parham D, Webber BL, Houghton PJ, Green AA. A specific chromosoaml abnormality in rhabdomyosarcoma. Cytogenet Cell Genet 45:148–155, 1987.
31. Sheng WW, Soukup S, Ballard E, Gotwals B, Lampkin B. Chromosomal analysis of sixteen human rhabdomyosarcomas. Cancer Res 48:983–987, 1998.
32. Mandahl N, Heim S, Willen H, Rydholm A, Eneroth M, Nilbert M, Kreicbergs A, Mitelman F. Characteristic karyotypic anomalies identify subtypes of malignant fibrous histiocytoma. Genes Chromosom Cancer 1:9–14, 1989.
33. Coccia M, Meltzer P, Dal Cin P, Turc-Carel C, Sait S, Sandberg AA, Trent J. DNA sequence amplification in malignant fibrous histiocytoma (meeting abstract). Proc Annu Meet Am Assoc Cancer Res 30:A1682, 1989.
34. Garson JA, Clayton J, McIntyre P, Kemshead JT. N-myc oncogene amplification in rhabdomyosarcoma at release. Lancet 1:1496–1497, 1986.
35. Mitani K, Kurosawa H, Suzuki A, Hayashi Y, Hanada R, Yanamoto K, Komatsu A, Kobayashi N, Nakagome Y, Yanada M. Amplification of N-myc in a rhabdomyosarcoma. Jpn J Cancer Res 77:1062–1065, 1986.
36. Tsuda H, Shimosato Y, Upton MP, Yokota J, Terada M, Ohira M, Sugimura T, Hirohashi S. Retrospective study on amplification of N-myc and c-myc genes in paediatric solid tumours and its association with prognosis and tumour differentiation. Lab Invest 59:321–327, 1988.
37. Dias P, Kumar P, Marsden HB, Gattamaneni HR, Heighway J, Kumar S. N-myc gene is amplified in alveolar rhabdomyosarcoma (RMS) but not in embryonal RMS. Int J Cancer 45:593–596, 1990.
38. Clark J, Rocques PJ, Crew AJ, Gill S, Shipley J, Chan AM, Gusterson BA, Cooper CS. Identification of novel genes, SYT and SSX, involved in the t(X;18)(p11.2;q11.2) translocation found in human synovial sarcoma. Nature Genet 7:502–508, 1994.
39. Crew AJ, Clark J, Fisher C, Gill S, Grimer R, Chand A, Shipley J, Gusterson BA, Cooper CS. Fusion of SYT to two genes, SSX1 and SSX2, encoding proteins with homology to the Kruppel-associated box in human synovial sarcomas. EMBO J 14:2333–2340, 1995.
40. Galili N, Davies RJ, Fredericks WJ, Mukhopadhyay S, Rauscher FJ, Emanuel BS, Rovera G,

Barr FG. Fusion of a forkhead domain gene to PAX3 in the solid tumour alveolar rhabdomyosarcoma. Nature Genet 5:230–235, 1993.
41. Davis RJ, D'Cruz CM, Lovell MA, Biegel JA, Barr FG. Fusion of PAX7 to FKHR by the variant t(1;13)(p36;q14) translocation in alveolar rhabdomyosarcoma. Cancer Res 54:2869–2872, 1994.
42. Aman P, Ron D, Mandahl N, Fioretos T, Heim S, Arheden K, Willen H, Rydholm A, Mitelman F. Rearrangement of the transcription factor gene CHOP in myxoid liposarcomas with t(12;16)(q13;p11). Genes Chromosom Cancer 5:278–285, 1992.
43. Crozat A, Aman P, Mandahl N, Ron D. Fusion of CHOP to a novel RNA-binding protein in human myxoid lipsosarcoma. Nature 363:640–644, 1993.
44. Zucman J, Delattre O, Desmaze C, Epstein AL, Stenman G, Speleman F, Fletchers CDM, Aurias A, Thomas G. EWS and ATF-1 gene fusion induction by t(12;22) translocation in malignant melanoma of soft parts. Nature Genet 4:341–344, 1993.
45. Gill S, McManus AP, Crew AJ, Benjamin H, Shear D, Gusterson BA, Pinkerton CR, Patel K, Cooper CS, Shipley JM. Fusion of the EWS gene to a DNA segment from 9q22–31 in a human myxoid chondrosarcoma. Genes Chromosomes Cancer 12:307–310, 1995.
46. Ladanyi M, Gerald W. Fusion of the EWS and WT1 genes in desmoplastic small round cell tumor. Cancer Res 54:2837–2840, 1994.
47. Rong S, Jeffers M, Resau JH, Tsarfaty I, Oskarsson M, Vande-Woude GF. Met expression and sarcoma tumorgenicity. Cancer Res 53:5355–5360, 1993.
48. Li FP, Fraumeni JF. Soft tissue sarcomas, breast cancer and other neoplasms. A familial syndrome? Ann Intern Med 71:747–752, 1969.
49. Li FP, Fraumeni JF. Rhabdomyosarcoma in children: Epidemiologic study and identification of a familial cancer syndrome. J Natl Cancer Inst 43:1365–1373, 1969.
50. Malkin D, Li FP, Strong LC, Fraumeni JF, Nelson CE, Kim DH, Kassel J, Gryka MA, Bischoff FZ, Tainsky MA, Friend SH. Germ line p53 mutations in a familial syndrome of breast cancer, sarcomas and other neoplasms. Science 250:1233–1238, 1990.
51. Frebourg T, Barbier N, Yan Y-X, Garber JE, Dreyfus M, Fraumeni J, Jr., Li FP, Frined SH. Germ-line p53 mutations in 15 families with Li-Fraumeni syndrome. Am J Hum Genet 56:608–615, 1995.
52. Donehower LA, Harvey M, Slagle BL, McArthur MJ, Montgomery CA, Jr., Butel JS, Bradley A. Mice deficient for p53 are developmentally normal but susceptible to spontaneous tumours. Nature 356:215–221, 1992.
53. Eeles RA, Warren W, Knee G, Bartek J, Averill D, Stratton MR, Blake PR, Tait DM, Lane DP, Easton DF, Yarnold JR, Cooper CS, Sloane JP. Constitutional mutation of exon 8 of the p53 gene in a patient with multiple primary tumours. Molecular and immunohistochemical findings. Oncogene 8:1269–1276, 1993.
54. Draper GJ, Sanders BM, Kingston JE. Secondary primary neoplasms in patients with retinoblastoma. Br J Cancer 53:661–671, 1986.
55. DerKinderen DJ, Koten JW, Nagelkerke NJ, Tan KE, Beemer FA, Den-Otter W. Non-ocular cancer in patients with hereditary retinoblastoma and their relatives. Int J Cancer 41:499–504, 1988.
56. Knudson AG. Mutation and cancer: Statistical study of retinoblastoma. Proc Natl Acad Sci USA 68:820–832, 1971.
57. Ponder B. Neurofibromatosis gene cloned. Nature 34:703–704, 1990.
58. Cawthon RM, Weiss R, Xu G, Viskochil D, Culver M, Stevens J, Robertson M, Dunn D, Gesteland R, O'Connell P, White R. A major segment of the neurofibromatosis type I gene: cDNA sequence, genomic structure and point mutations. Cell 62:193–201, 1990.
59. Viskochil D, Buchberg AM, Xu G, Cawthon RM, Stevens J, Wolff RK, Culver M, Carey JC, Copeland NG, Jenkins NA, White R, O'Connell P. Deletions and a translocation interrupt a cloned gene at the neurofibromatosis type 1 locus. Cell 62:187–192, 1990.
60. Wallace MR, Marchuk DA, Andersen LB, Letcher R, Odeh HM, Saulino AM, Fountain JW, Brereton A, Nicholson J, Mitchell AL, Brownstein BH, Collins FS. Type 1 neurofibromatosis

gene: Identification of a large transcript disrupted in three NF1 patients. Science 249:181–186, 1990.
61. Legius E, Marchuk DA, Collins FS, Glover TW. Somatic deletion of the neurofibromatosis type 1 gene in a neurofibrosarcoma supports a tumour suppressor gene hypothesis. Nature Genet 3:122–126, 1993.
62. McCormick F. Ras signalling and NF1. Curr Opin Genet Dev 5:51–55, 1995.
63. Enzinger FM, Weiss SW. Soft Tissue Tumours, 2nd ed. St Louis, MO: Mosby, 1988.
64. Kinzler KW, Nilbert MC, Su LK, Vogelstein B, Bryan TM, Levy DB, Smith KJ, Preisinger AC, Hedge P, McKechnie D, Finniear R, Markham A, Groffen J, Boguski MS, Altschul SF, Horu A, Ando H, Miyoshi Y, Miki Y, Nishisho I, Nakamura Y. Identification of FAP locus genes from chromosome 5q21. Science 253:661–665, 1961.
65. Nishisho I, Nakamura Y, Miyoshi Y, Miki Y, Ando H, Horii A, Koyama K, Utsunomiya J, Baba S, Hedge P, Markham A, Krush AJ, Petersen G, Hamilton SR, Nilbert MC, Levy DB, Bryan TM, Pressinger AC, Smith KJ, Su Li-K, Kinzler KW, Vogelstein B. Mutations of chromosome 5q21 genes in FAP and colorectal cancer patients. Science 253:665–669, 1991.
66. Groden J, Thliveris A, Samowitz W, Carlson M, Gelbert L, Albertsen H, Joslyn G, Stevens J, Spirio L, Robertson M, Sargeant L, Krapcho K, Wolff E, Burt R, Hughes JP, Warrington J, McPherson J, Wasmuth J, La Pasher D, Abderrahim H, Cohen D, Leppert J, White R. Identification and characterization of the familial adenomatus polyposis coli gene. Cell 66:589–600, 1991.
67. Miyaki M, Konishi M, Kikuchi-Yanoshita R, Enomoto M, Tanaka K, Takahashi H, Muraoka M, Mori T, Konishi F, Iwana T. Coexistence of somatic and germ-line mutations of APC gene in desmoid tumours from patients with familial adenomatous polyposis. Cancer Res 53:5079–5082, 1993.
68. Ping AJ, Reeve AE, Law DJ, Young MR, Boehnke M, Feinberg AP. Genetic linkage of Beckwith-Wiedemann syndrome to 11p15. Am J Hum Genet 44:720–723, 1989.
69. Pettenati MJ, Haines JL, Higgins RR, Wappner RS, Palmer CG, Weaver DD. Wiedemann-Beckwith syndrome: Presentation of clinical and cytogenetic data on 22 new cases and review of the literature. Hum Genet 74:143–154, 1986.
70. Grundy P, Kaufos A, Morgan K, Li FP, Meadows AT, Cavenee WK. Familial predisposition to Wilms tumour does not map to the short arm of chromosome 11. Nature 336:374–376, 1988.
71. Scrable HJ, Witte DP, Lampkin BC, Cavenee WK. Chromosomal localization of the human rhabdomyosarcoma locus by mitotic recombination mapping. Nature 329:645–647, 1987.
72. Henry I, Bonaiti-Pellie C, Chehensee V, Beldjord C, Schwatz C, Utermann G, Junien C. Uniparental paternal disomy in a genetic cancer — predisposing syndrome. Nature 351:665–667, 1991.
73. Zhan S, Shapiro DN, Helman LJ. Activation of an imprinted allele of the insulin-like growth factor II gene implicated in rhabdomyosarcoma. J Clin Invest 94:445–448, 1994.
74. Rainier S, Johnson LA, Dobry CJ, Ping AJ, Grundy PE, Feinberg AP. Relaxation of imprinted genes in human cancer. Nature 362:747–749, 1993.
75. Slatter RE, Elliott M, Welham K, Carrera M, Schofield PN, Barton DE, Maher ER. Mosaic uniparental disomy in Beckwith-Wiedemann syndrome. J Med Genet 31:749–753, 1994.
76. Ionov Y, Peinado MA, Malkhosayn S, Shibata D, Perucho M. Ubiquitous somatic mutations in simple repeat sequences reveal a new mechanism for colonic carcinogenesis. Nature 363:558–561, 1993.
77. Papadopoulos N, Nicolaides NC, Wei Y-F, Ruben SN, Carter KC, Rosen CA, Haseltine WA, Fleischmann RD, Fraser CM, Adams MD, Venter JC, Hamilton SR, Petersen GM, Watson P, Lynch HT, Peltomaki P, Mecklin JP, De la Chapelle, Kinzler KW, Vogelstein B. Mutation of a mutL homolog in hereditary colon cancer. Science 263:1625–1629, 1993.
78. Wooster R, Cleton-Jansen AM, Collins N, Mangion J, Cornelis RS, Cooper CS, Gusterson BA, Ponder BAJ, Von Deimling A, Wiestler OD, Cornelisse CJ, Devilee P, Stratton MR. Instability of short tandem repeats (microsatellites) in human cancer. Nature Genet 6:152–156, 1994.

79. Barr FG, Chatten J, D'Cruz CM, Wilson AE, Nauta LE, Nycum LM, Biegel JA, Womer RB. Molecular assays for chromosomal translocations in the diagnosis of paediatric soft tissue sarcomas. JAMA 273:553–557, 1995.
80. Scrable H, Witte D, Shimada H, Seemayer T, Wang-Wuu S, Soukup S, Koufos A, Houghton P, Lampkin B, Cavenee W. Molecular differential pathology of rhabdomyosarcoma. Genes Chromosom Cancer 1:23–35, 1989.
81. Knight JC, Renwick PJ, Cin PD, Van den Berghe H, Fletcher CD. Translocation t(12;16)(q13;p11) in myxoid liposarcoma and round cell liposarcoma: Molecular and cytogenetic analysis. Cancer Res 55:24–27, 1995.
82. Tonin PN, Scrable H, Shimada H, Cavenee WK. Muscle-specific gene expression in rhabdomyosarcomas and stages of human skeletal muscle development. Cancer Res 51:5100–5106, 1991.
83. Clark J, Rocques PJ, Braun T, Bober E, Arnold HH, Fisher C, Fletcher C, Brown K, Gusterson BA, Carter RL, Cooper CS. Expression of members of the *myf* gene family in human rhabdomyosarcomas. Br J Cancer 64:1039–1042, 1991.
84. Slamon DJ, Clark GM, Wong SG, Levin WJ, Ullrich A, McGuire WL. Human breast cancer: Correlation of relapse and survival with amplification of the HER-2/neu oncogene. Science 235:177–182, 1987.
85. Seeger R, Brodeur G, Salter M, Dutton A, Siegel S, Wang K, Hammond O. Association of multiple copies of *N-myc* with the rapid progression of neuroblastomas. N Engl J Med 313:1111–1116, 1985.
86. Wunder JS, Czitrom AA, Kandel R, Andrulis IL. Analysis of alterations in the retinoblastoma gene and tumour grade in bone and soft tissue sarcomas. J Natl Cancer Inst 83:194–200, 1991.
87. Wang J, Gown AM, Wen SF, Coltrera MD. Loss of p110 RB expression in tissue sections of human soft tissue sarcomas correlates with tumor grade and cell proliferation index. Proc Ann J Meet Am Assoc Cancer Res 35:A1424, 1994.
88. Kawai A, Noguchi M, Beppu Y, Yokoyama R, Mukai K, Hirohashi S, Inoue H, Fukuma H. Nuclear immunoreaction of p53 protein in soft tissue sarcomas: A possible prognostic factor. Cancer 73:2499–2505, 1994.
89. Toffoli G, Doglioni C, Cernigoi C, Frustaci S, Perin T, Canal B, Boiocchi M. p53 overexpression in human soft tissue sarcomas: Relation to biological aggressiveness. Ann Oncol 5:167–172, 1994.
90. Latres E, Drobnjak M, Pollack D, Oliva MR, Ramos M, Karpeh M, Woodruff JM, Cordon-Cardo C. Chromosome 17 abnormalities and TP53 mutations in adult soft tissue sarcomas. An J Pathol 145:345–355, 1994.
91. Rydholm A, Mandahl N, Heim S, Kreicbergs A, Willen H, Mitelman F. Malignant fibrous histiocytomas with a 19p+ marker chromosome have increased relapse rate. Genes Chromosom Cancer 2:296–299, 1990.
92. Chan HS, Thorner PS, Haddad G, Ling V. Immunohistochemical detection of P-glycoprotein: Prognostic correlation in soft tissue sarcoma of childhood. J Clin Oncol 8:689–704, 1990.
93. Kallioniemi A, Kallioniemi OP, Sudar D, Rutovitz D, Grey JW, Waldman F, Pinkel D. Comparative genomic hybridisation for molecular cytogenetic analysis fo solid tumors. Science 258:818–821, 1992.

4. PET imaging in soft tissue sarcomas

Floro Miraldi, Lee P. Adler, and Peter Faulhaber

Introduction

Positron emission tomography (PET) was conceived in the early years of nuclear medicine; however, until about 1980 the technology was insufficiently developed to allow its routine application. Furthermore, the high cost of construction and operation of a PET facility delayed its use in the clinical arena and also limited the number of sites available for its development. Today, only 15 years later, PET instrumentation is very sophisticated, costs are decreasing relative to other clinical studies, and clinical PET procedures are proliferating rapidly. In the last few years the application of PET to oncology has proven to be very successful, and there is now a significant literature on PET imaging of many different cancers [1–18].

In this chapter we describe the PET technique as well as how it has been applied to oncological problems and, in particular, in the evaluation of sarcomas. A summary of the literature of PET sarcoma studies follows, and finally we venture into predictions of its future applications.

PET technique

The PET concept is based on the administration of a positron emitting radionuclide in the form of a biological tracer followed by the reconstruction of an image from externally detected radiations. One of the important features of PET is that most of the radionuclides used are isotopes of the common biological elements: carbon, oxygen, and nitrogen. Because of common use of fluorinated biologicals, F-18 is also a frequently used radionuclide. Table 1 lists some of the radionuclides that have been used in the study of tumors and their chemical forms.

The advantage of using such radionuclides in nuclear imaging cannot be overemphasized. The development of nuclear imaging has relied on chemistry to provide tagged compounds that could mimic various physiological functions. These compounds are frequently quite exotic and are not common biological compounds. This process has been very successful, as is well known;

J. Verweij, H.M. Pinedo, and H.D. Suit (eds). SOFT TISSUE SARCOMAS: PRESENT ACHIEVEMENTS AND FUTURE PROSPECTS.

however, the potential to explore in vivo biochemistry and physiology with more ordinary compounds tagged with nuclides of common biological elements is extraordinary. A simple example will suffice to illustrate: Consider the problem of tracing water. There exists no possibility of 'tagging' water that would not completely alter its behavior. However, synthesizing water with a radionuclide of oxygen (O^{15}) would produce H_2O^{15}, water that chemically and biologically behaves exactly as ordinary water. Similarly, many ordinary biologically interesting compounds can be synthesized with the substitution of an element by its radioactive isotope. This has been the great strength of PET and the reason for the interest it has generated.

The use of positron emitters is really not a choice; isotopes of carbon, oxygen, nitrogen, and fluorine do not exist that are suitable to use for ordinary gamma imaging. Either the gamma emissions do not exist, the emissions are of energies not easily imaged, or the half-life of the isotope is too short. All of these elements do have isotopes that are positron emitters, however, and this makes gamma imaging possible. When positron emitters decay, the positrons (positive electrons) travel on the order of a millimeter or less before interacting with a negative electron. The interaction results in the annihilation of both particles and the creation of two 511-KEV photons that are emitted at approximately 180 degrees to each other (Fig. 1).

The use of these radioisotopes does present a difficulty because of their relatively short half-life (Table 2). Some longer lived positron emitters, such as

Table 1. Positron radionuclides with their chemical form and uses in oncology

Radionuclide	Chemical form	Use
Carbon-11	Carbon monoxide	Blood volume
	Methionine	Amino acid uptake
	BCNU	Tumor drug level
	Thymidine	DNA turnover
Oxygen-15	Oxygen	Oxygen utilization
	Water	Blood flow
	Butanol	Blood flow
Nitrogen-13	Amino acids	Amino acid uptake
Fluorine-18	Deoxyglucose	Glucose utilization
Iodine-124	Monoclonal antibody	Tumor detection

Table 2. Common PET radionuclides

Isotope	Half-life (min)
O-15	2
N-13	10
C-11	20
F-18	110

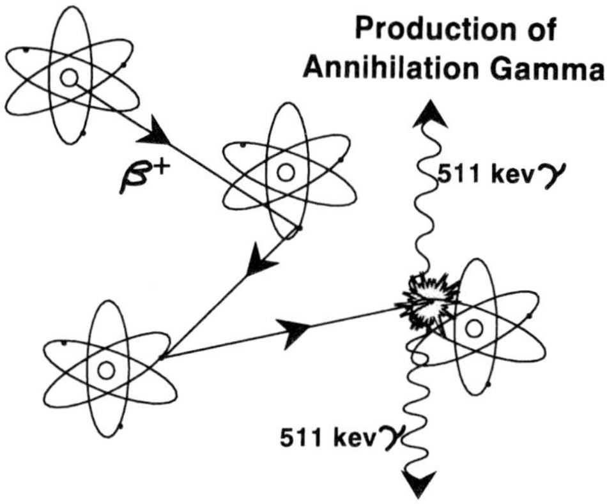

Figure 1. A positron is created and ejected from the nucleus and, after numerous collisions with orbital electrons, loses its kinetic energy and annihilates with an electron to yield two back-to-back 511-KEV gamma rays.

iodine-124 [19] and copper-64 [20], have been studied but have not attracted extensive interest. Because of their short half-life, these isotopes must be generated and incorporated into the desired compound quickly. This, in turn, requires that the production of the radiopharmaceutical take place close to the site of use. Most facilities have therefore constructed on-site cyclotrons for isotope production and chemical laboratories for radiopharmaceutical synthesis. Facility costs are accordingly very high. Recently, as more interest has been generated and more sites are being developed, the concept of regional shared production facilities has emerged and in the future will probably be the construction of choice.

Short half-lives not only present disadvantage, but also have the advantage of short study times, which allow repetition of studies or sequential studies. For example, in our institution a blood perfusion tumor study may be performed with O^{15}-labeled water followed by a receptor or amino acid study labeled with C^{11}, which in turn may be followed by a sugar metabolism study with F-18–labeled fluorodeoxyglucose. Because of the short half-lives of the O^{15} and the relatively short half-life of the C^{11}, all three studies can be performed in one patient visit.

Coincidence detection of the paired photons created during the annihilation process forms the basis of positron emission tomography (Fig. 2). The imaging device, the PET scanner, consists of a large number of paired detectors in a ring encompassing the body that allows simultaneous acquisition of data from all angles. Because the simultaneous (coincidence) detection of two gammas by the paired detectors signals that the annihilation process has occurred along the line joining the two detectors, image reconstruction of the spatial distribution of radioactivity in the transaxial plane can be accomplished using a standard line reconstruction technique such as filtered backprojection [21,22]. Modern instruments acquire multiple slices simultaneously, and these slices can be reformatted to yield coronal or sagittal slices.

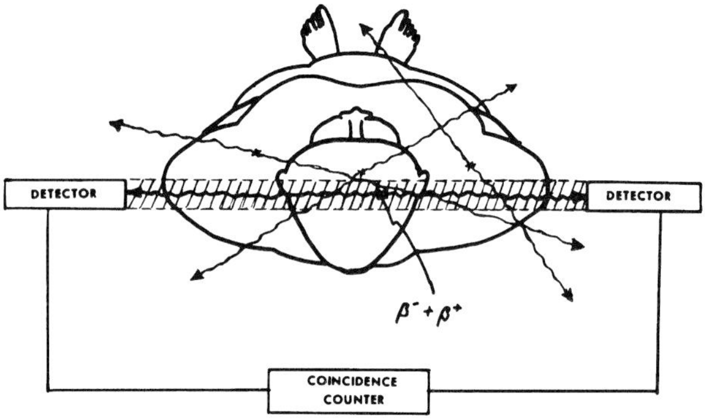

Figure 2. Paired gamma detectors connected in coincidence determine the line along which an annihilation event has occurred. The summation of multiple lines from paired detectors surrounding the body, using a reconstruction technique such as filtered backprojection, yields the transverse slice PET image.

Two important aspects of this imaging system that separate it from other radionuclide scanning procedures are the ability to correct for loss of signal by tissue attenuation and the relatively uniform resolution throughout the scanning field. This permits the regional concentration of the tracer to be measured in absolute units, a feat that is extremely difficult in either planar or SPECT nuclear imaging. If one combines these measured activities with the pharmacokinetics of the tracer compound, a kinetic model can be formulated that allows the derivation of equations that convert the radionuclide distribution into a regional tissue function map. The PET image is thus converted into an image that represents a physiological function. A PET scan is then a true functional image in which a functional image is defined as a picture in which each pixel has an anatomical correspondence to the body and also represents the numerical value of a measured biochemical or physiological parameter.

A large number of models have been developed, but only a few have been established and proven. These include the determination of regional tissue blood flow [23–25], blood volume [26], oxygen use [23], and glucose use [27–29]. Many other factors have been studied in a more qualitative manner and still others are based on models that have not been firmly established or accepted. Because metabolism provides a basis for understanding the function and physiology in living systems, any method, such as PET oxygen or glucose utilization, that can provide localized metabolic information noninvasively is of extreme importance in medicine. Many models, including those listed earlier, have been applied to oncological problems, but most of the studies to date have been primarily feasibility studies meant to demonstrate the potential. Thus, they are not of clinical importance yet, and their general use must wait until they have been proven useful in the clinical setting. The exception is glucose utilization using [fluorine-18]-2-deoxy-2-fluoro-D-glucose (FDG).

Fluorine-labeled FDG

Neoplastic tissue usually takes up more glucose and has a highter rate of glycolysis then normal tissue [30,31]. This difference is exploited in tumor detection by using labeled glucose or glucose analogues. Som et al. [32] first proposed FDG as a tumor imaging agent in 1980, and since then a variety of different neoplasms have been imaged with PET using this radiopharmaceutical. Because the active transport mechanism cannot distinguish between glucose and FDG, the amount of labeled tracer transported intracellularly is greater in cells with a high metabolic rate. Both glucose and FDG can be phosphorylated by hexokinase to glucose-6-phosphate and FDG-6-phosphate, respectively, but only glucose-6-phosphate can be stored as glycogen or can undergo aerobic or anaerobic glycolysis (Fig. 3). The only way that the labeled FDG-6-phosphate can leave the cell is for it to be dephosphorylated by glucose-6-phosphatase. FDG localization within tissue is therefore a function of the rate of glucose utilization and the ratio of the enzymes hexokinase and glucose-6-phosphatase [33].

The operational equation for using FDG is based on the work of Sokoloff et al. [34], which uses a compartmental model that assumes that the uptake of the glucose analogue is the same as glucose, with little loss from the cell because of back hydrolysis, which has been shown to be true for deoxyglucose. Although this model has only been established successfully for the study of brain, it has generally been assumed to be true in most neoplastic tissue. Else-Maj Suolinna et al. [35] demonstrated that the conditions for the Sokoloff model are maintained in Rous sarcoma tumors implanted in rats; however, it has not been established that the model applies in most neoplastic tissue. Thus,

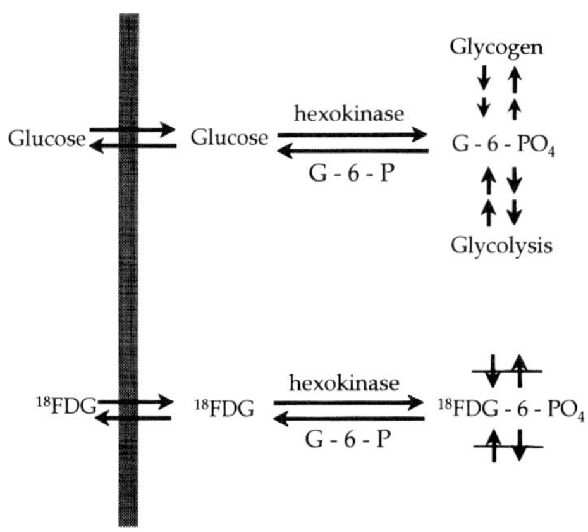

Figure 3. The vertical line denotes the cell boundary. Transport and phosphorylation is the same for glucose and FDG. The enzymes necessary to carry FDG-6-PO_4 along a glycolytic pathway or into a storage mode do not exist, and, therefore, FDG accumulates in the cell. PET imaging with FDG works in tissues in which dephosphorylation is slow compared with phosphorylation.

although this model has been applied in selected situations, absolute metabolic values have generally not been calculated in clinical tumor studies with FDG.

The techniques, in general, are much too difficult to apply in routine clinical situations, and the common practice has been divided along two paths. In one camp are those who examine images in the traditional qualitative manner, while in the other camp are those who insist that some form of quantification is necessary to interpret a study adequately. Most published clinical reports present quantitative data, even though these data are usually questionable because of the many sources of error that exist.

In clinical PET oncology, the common practice today is to present a measure of the glucose trapped in the neoplasm in terms of an uptake ratio. These uptake ratios go by many names, such as the dose uptake ratio (DUR) or the standard uptake value (SUV). They are defined as the PET measured radioactivity in the tissue normalized by body weight and the amount of tracer administered. The biggest problem with these ratios is that they have not been standardized. Because they are dependent on many parameters, including blood glucose levels, body habitus, lesion size, and timing, to mention a few, interlaboratory comparisons are very difficult and usually meaningless. They are useful for any given facility provided that the same conditions are used when comparing tissues within a patient or when comparing the same patient at different times. Interpatient comparison is difficult, even in the same laboratory, because of the variations of the dependent parameters. In general, the quantitative values are best used when comparing changes in a patient when the patient is used as his or her own control.

PET imaging of sarcomas

PET sarcoma studies reported to date have generally been performed to prove a point of feasibility. Clinical trials of many patients have not been accomplished, and therefore accurate indices such as sensitivity, specificity, etc. are not available. The PET literature on sarcomas is quite sparse, even though the first report, by Brownell et al. [36], came out many years ago. These researchers measured blood flow and oxygen utilization in human sarcomas implanted in small animals and demonstrated the feasibility of studying the physiology of these tumors noninvasively with PET. The first reported study of human PET FDG imaging of musculoskeletal tumors was by Kern et al. [4], who described five such tumors, two of which were malignant fibrous histiocytomas and one of which was a myxoid liposarcoma. These authors calculated the glucose utilization rate using the Sokoloff method. Although by the authors' admission their results are only approximate, they suggest that FDG uptake and PET evaluation have the potential of providing a noninvasive malignancy grading.

Adler et al. [6] also showed that FDG uptake in soft tissue sarcomas correlated well with histopathological grades. Measuring the uptake using both tumor-to-background ratios as well as DURs, this group demonstrated that there was a factor of two difference in the uptake ratios between malignant liposarcomas and benign tumors. In a later study [37] in which a large group of different tumors, including angiosarcomas, liposarcomas, osteosarcomas, neurosarcomas, Ewing's sarcoma, chondrosarcomas, and malignant fibrous histiocytomas, were included, a strong correlation was found between tumor grade and the DUR, despite the inclusion of neoplasms originating from many different types of tissue. Their report indicated that normalized uptake of FDG by musculoskeletal tumors could be used to separate lesions into three groups: low-uptake tumors that are likely to be benign, high-uptake tumors that are likely to be malignant, and lesions that fall in between these two groups and may be either malignant or benign. In an article on neoplasms in the pediatric population, Shulkin et al. [38] reported high uptake of FDG in several sarcomas, including Ewing's sarcoma and a hepatic sarcoma. However, they did not show any abnormal uptake of FDG in a cardiac angiosarcoma or in rhabdomyosarcomas.

Two studies of interest on the use of PET imaging of soft tissue sarcomas showed the potential use of this technique in the evaluation of therapy. Nieweg et al. [39] demonstrated high FDG uptake with PET before treatment of an advanced liposarcoma of the left thigh. Treatment consisted of isolated regional limb perfusion with tumor necrosis factor-α, interferon-γ, and melphalan. Following therapy the glucose metabolism of the tumor, as measured by PET, was absent. Subsequent excision demonstrated complete necrosis of the tumor, confirming the PET evaluation of the treatment results. Daemen et al. [40] demonstrated the radiotherapeutic effects of tumors using C-11 tyrosine and F-18 FDG. These researchers used rhabdomyosarcoma tumors growing in the flank of rats and compared the PET results with measured values of growth of tumors following radiotherapy. They demonstrated that the C-11 tyrosine and FDG uptake into the tumor tissue correlated well with the radiation effects on tumor volume and concluded that PET was suitable for investigations of tumor growth kinetics during and after radiotherapeutic treatment. Also, they showed in this work that both C-11 tyrosine and FDG uptake were equivalent in their potential for assessing radiotherapy effects.

Some examples of PET sarcoma images are presented in Figures 4 through 9. Figure 4 illustrates a benign lesion, a lipoma, that shows no abnormal accumulation of FDG. The opposite situation is illustrated in Figure 5, which is an image of a malignant fibrous histiocytoma of the thigh. The strong tumor uptake correlates well with the MRI study. Note that the marked increased uptake of FDG is primarily in the rim of the tumor, and the central portion has very little metabolic activity. The non-avid central portion represents necrosis and nonmalignant cell types. This scan demonstrates a useful feature of PET imaging in such cases; namely, it serves as a guide for the surgeon in obtaining a biopsy. The DUR was calculated for this case because the patient was to undergo chemotherapy. The DUR went from 14 pertherapy to 7.4 post-therapy, indicating a rather good response to therapy.

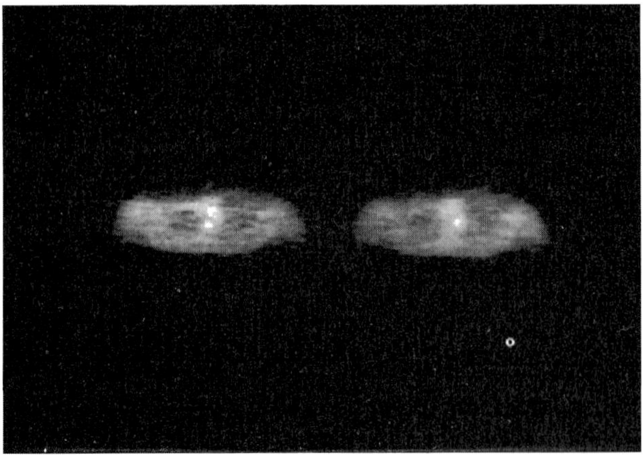

Figure 4. Patient with a 5 cm lipoma of the posterior right shoulder. FDG-PET images through the mass in the transaxial plane demonstrate no significant tracer accumulation.

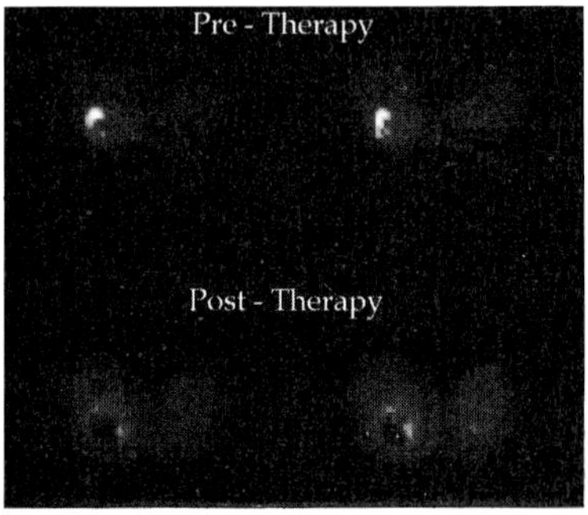

A

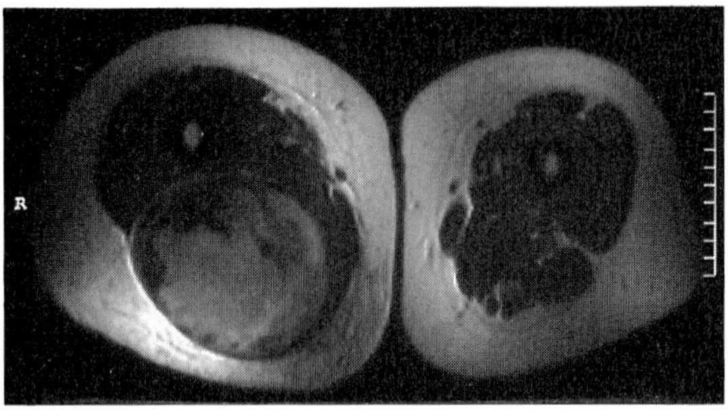

B

Figure 5. **A:** Thirty-two–year-old male with malignant fibrous histiocytoma of the right thigh. FDG-PET studies were acquired prior to and following three cycles of chemotherapy. The pretherapy images show FDG avidity in the medial and posterior compartments of the right thigh with a central photopenic area. The post-therapy images show a similar pattern with less intense avidity. The peak DUR pretherapy was 14 and post-therapy it was 7.4. The decreased avidity indicates a response to treatment. **B:** Corresponding transaxial proton density MRI through the right thigh mass. The central portion of the mass has the high signal of fluid and corresponds to the photopenic area seen on FDG-PET images.

The ability to monitor the response to therapy may prove to be the best use of PET imaging in sarcoma lesions and is again illustrated in Figures 6 and 7. Figure 6 shows strong uptake preradiation therapy with a DUR of 14.7 and a post-therapy DUR of 5.9, again, an excellent response. A second example of chemotherapy response is shown in Figure 7, which illustrates a Ewing's sarcoma tumor in the distal left fibula. DUR values are not presented here, but it is clear that the images reflect a rather dramatic decrease in overall tumor avidity.

The third possible useful function of PET imaging in soft tissue sarcomas is the detection of distant metastases. Figures 8 and 9 are examples of total body images in patients with thigh lesions. Figure 8 illustrates metastatic lesions in the anterior abdomen and retroperitoneum. No demonstrable metastasis is shown in Figure 9. It must be noted that these images are only part of the entire series of images for these patients. In both cases, successive 6mm

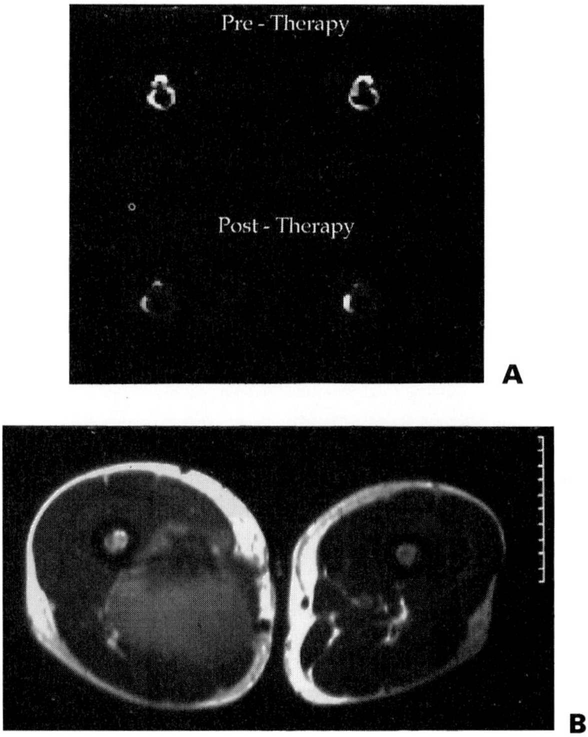

Figure 6. **A:** Sixty-two–year-old female with a liposarcoma of the right thigh: FDG-PET studies were acquired prior to and following radiation therapy. Transaxial images show a mass with a rim of intense FDG avidity and a photopenic center prior to therapy with a similar, less intense pattern post-therapy. The pretherapy peak DUR was 14.7 and post-therapy it was 5.9. This change indicates a therapeutic response. **B:** Corresponding transaxial MRI image, showing the proton density through the right thigh mass. There is increased signal in the central area of the fluid, corresponding to the photopenic area on FDG-PET images.

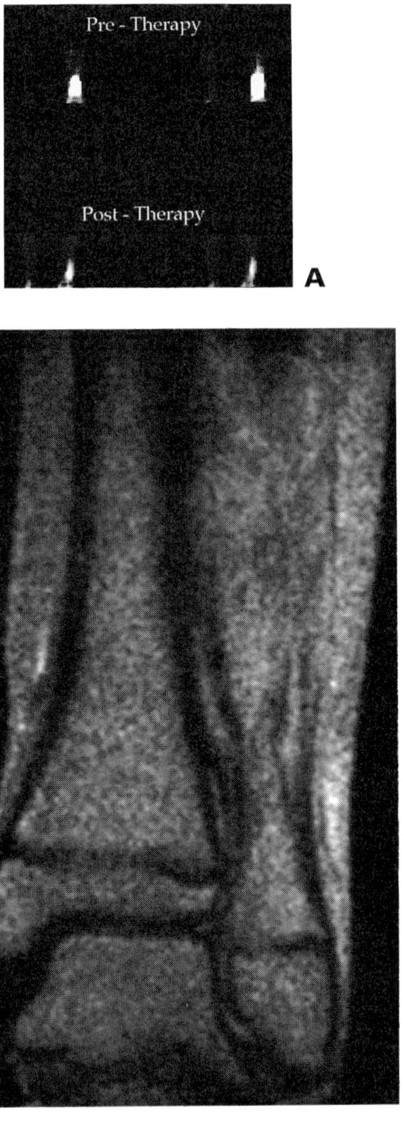

A

B

Figure 7. **A:** Ten-year-old child with Ewing's sarcoma of the distal left fibula. FDG-PET images were acquired prior to and following chemotherapy. The pretherapy coronal images demonstrate intense FDG avidity of the distal fibula. The post-treatment scan shows a marked decrease in avidity, indicating a therapeutic response. **B:** Corresponding T1-weighted MRI images in the coronal plane show a low signal mass involving the distal fibula.

coronal, sagittal, and transverse slices of the entire body were examined. Only representative slices are presented in Figures 8 and 9. Note the strong concentration of activity in the brain, heart, kidneys, and bladder. As is well known, the brain derives its energy from sugar, as can the myocardium. FDG is

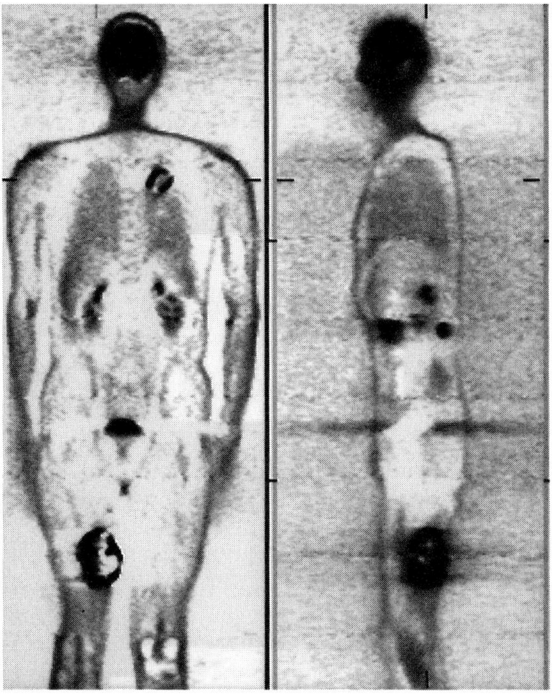

Figure 8. Whole-body FDG-PET scan on a 57-year-old male with right thigh MFH. The coronal slice is taken through the right thigh mass and includes a focus of FDG avidity in the left apex. The sagittal slice again demonstrates the primary tumor and two additional foci of FDG avidity: one in the anterior abdomen and the other in the retroperitoneum.

excreted via the urine, which accounts for the kidney and bladder concentrations.

Role of PET imaging in soft tissue sarcoma management

In general, the use of PET imaging for the identification of these tumors is not necessary. Identification is usually quite obvious and is usually detectable by clinical or other simpler imaging modalities. Obtaining biopsy specimens is also relatively routine today, and the use of PET imaging for tumor grading is also of question. PET imaging does have a biopsy role, however. Because many of these tumors have large areas of necrosis, the PET image may guide the surgeon to the correct biopsy site.

The use of total body imaging for the detection of metastases would seem to be valid, and this may prove to be one of the more useful applications of PET in sarcoma management. As illustrated in Figure 8, the detection of

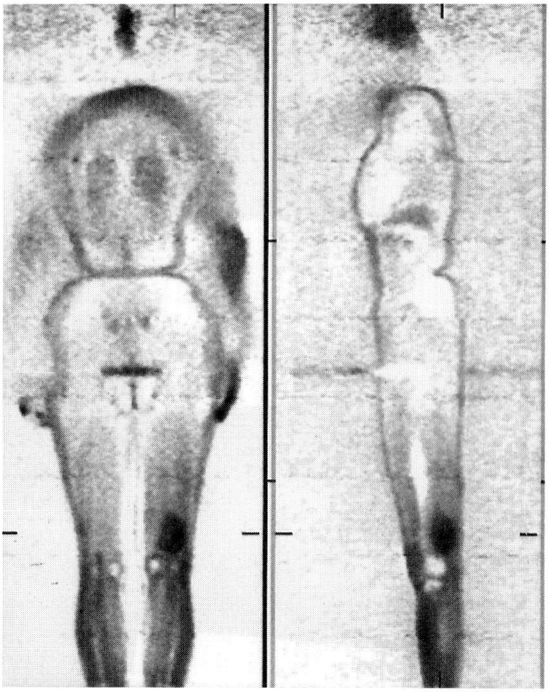

Figure 9. Whole-body FDG-PET scan on a 32-year-old female with a left thigh leiomyosarcoma. Coronal and sagittal slices taken through a focus of intense FDG avidity in the distal left thigh, posterior compartment. No additional abnormal foci of FDG avidity are present.

distant metastases is quite good. Even though sensitivity and specificity measures for detection of sarcoma metastases by PET are not available, in our experience the uptake in sarcomas is very high and the ability to detect metastatic lesions should be excellent. Finally, the potential use of PET imaging to follow the effects of therapy appears to have potential. The cases shown in Figures 5–7 demonstrate the sensitive nature of FDG uptake in therapy of these tumors, and it is our prediction that this will develop into PET's greatest application in the management of such tumors.

References

1. Di Chiro G, De LaPaz RL, Brooks RA, Sokoloff L, Kornblith PL, Smith BH, Patronas NJ, Kufta CV, Kessler RM, Johnston GS, Manning RG, Wolf AP. Glucose utilization of cerebral gliomas measured by [^{18}F]fluorodeoxyglucose and positron emission tomography. Neurology 32:1323–1329, 1982.
2. Yonekura Y, Benua RS, Brill AB, Som P, Yeh SDJ, Kemeny NE, Fowler JS, MacGregor RR, Stamm R, Christman DR, Wolf AP. Increased accumulation of 2-deoxy-2-[^{18}F]Fluoro-D-glucose in liver metastases from colon carcinoma. J Nucl Med 23:1133–1137, 1982.

3. Kiyosawa M, Ohmura M, Mizuno K, Fukuda H, Hatazawa J, Ito M, Abe Y, Matsuzawa T, Ido T. ^{18}F-FDG positron emission tomography in orbital lymphoid tumor. Nippon Ganka Gakkai Zasshi 89:1329–1333, 1985.
4. Kern KA, Brunetti A, Norton JA, Chang AE, Malawer M, Lock E, Finn RD, Rosenburg SA, Larson SM. Metabolic imaging of human extremity musculoskeletal tumors by PET. J Nucl Med 29:181–186, 1988.
5. Strauss LG, Clorius JH, Schalg P, Lehner B, Kimmig B, Engenhart R, Morin-Grey M, Helus F, Oberdorfer F, Schmidlin P, Von Kaich G. Recurrence of colorectal tumors: PET evaluation. Radiology 170:329–332, 1989.
6. Adler LP, Blair H, Williams RP, Pathria MN, Makley JT, Joyce MJ, Al-Kaisi N, Miraldi F. Noninvasive grading of liposarcomas using PET with FDG. J Comput Assist Tomogr 14:960–962, 1990.
7. Adler LP, Blair HF, Makley JR, Pathria MN, Miraldi F. Comparison of PET with MR and conventional scintigraphy in a benign and in a malignant soft-tissue tumor. Orthopaedics 14:892–895, 1991.
8. Costa J, Wesley RA, Gladstein E, Rosenberg SA. The grading of soft-tissue sarcomas. Cancer 54:530–541, 1984.
9. Kubota K, Matsuzawa T, Ito M, Ito K, Fujiwara T, Abe Y, Yoshieka S, Fukuda H, Hatazawa J, Iwata R, Watanuki S, Ido T. Lung tumor imaging by positron emission tomography using C-11-L-methionine. J Nucl Med 26:37–42, 1985.
10. Gupta NC, Bowman BM, Frank AL, Thorson AB, Shiue CY, Frick MP. PET-FDG imaging for follow-up evaluation of treated colorectal cancer (abstr). Radiology 199:181P, 1991.
11. Gupta N, Frank A, Mailliard J, Rysavy J, Chandramouli B, Boman B. Accurate detection of liver metastases in patients (PTS) with primary malignancies using PET-FDG imaging (abstr). J Nucl Med 34:6P, 1993.
12. Gupta NC, Frank AR, Dewan NA, Redepenning LS, Rothberg ML, Maillaird JA, Phalen JJ, Sunderland JJ, Frick MP. Solitary pulmonary nodules: Detection of malignancy with PET with 2-[F-18]-fluoro-2-deoxy-D-glucose. Radiology 184:441–444, 1992.
13. Gupta NC, Dewan NA, Frank A. Diagnostic evaluation of suspected solitary nodules (SPN) using PET FDG imaging. Chest 104:119S, 1993.
14. Kubota K, Matsuzawa T, Fujiwara T, Ito M, Hatazawa J, Ishiwata K, Iwata R, Ido T. Differential diagnosis of lung tumor with positron emission tomography: A prospective study. J Nucl Med 31:1927–1933, 1990.
15. Wahl RL, Quint LE, Greenough RL, Meyer CR, White RL, Orringer MB. Staging of mediastinal non-small cell lung cancer with FDG PET, CT, and fusion images preliminary prospective evaluation. Radiology 191:371–377, 1994.
16. Tse N, Hoh CK, Hawkins RA, Zinner MJ, Dahlbom M, Choi Y, Maddahi J, Brunicardi C, Phelps ME, Glaspy JA. The application of positron emission tomographic imaging with fluorodeoxyglucose to the evaluation of breast disease. Ann Surg 216:27–34, 1992.
17. Hoh CK, Hawkins RA, Glaspy J, Dahlbom M, Nielson YT, Hoffman EJ, Schiepers C, Choi Y, Rege S, Nitzsche E. Cancer detection with whole-body PET using 2-[F-18]-fluoro-2-deoxy-D-glucose. J Comput Assist Tomogr 1777:582–589, 1993.
18. Nieweg OE, Kim EE, Wong WH, Broussard WF, Singletary SE, Hortobagyi GN, Tilbury RS. Positron emission tomography with fluorine-18-deoxyglucuose in the detection and staging of breast cancer. Cancer 71:3920–3925, 1993.
19. Miraldi F. Monoclonal antibodies and neuroblastoma. Semin Nucl Med 19:282–294, 1989.
20. Philpott GW, Schwarz SW, Anderson CJ, Griffeth LK, Connett JM, Zinn KR, Meares CF, Siegel BA, Welch MJ. Initial clinical study of Cu-64-labeled anticolon-carcinoma monoclonal antibody (MAB 1A3) in colorectal cancer. J Nucl Med 34:81P(322), 1993.
21. Ter-Pergossian MM, Phelps ME, Brownell GL, Cox JR, Davis DO, Evans RG, eds. Reconstruction Tomography in Diagnostic Radiology and Nuclear Medicine. Baltimore, MD: University Park Press, 1977.
22. Brooks RA, Di Chiro G. Theory of image reconstruction in computed tomography. Radiology 117:561–572, 1975.

23. Frackowiak RSJ, Lenzi GL, Jones T, Heather JD. Quantitative measurements of regional cerebral blood flow and oxygen metabolism in man using O-15 and positron emission tomography: Theory, procedure and normal values. J Comput Assist Tomogr 4:727–736, 1980.
24. Raichle ME. Quantitative in vivo autoradiography with positron emission tomography. Brain Res Rev 1:47–68, 1979.
25. Muzic RF, Nelson AD, Miraldi F. Mathematical simplification of a PET blood flow model. IEEE Trans Med Imag 9:172–176, 1990.
26. Phelps ME, Huang SC, Hoffman EJ, Kuhl DE. Validation of tomographic measurement of cerebral blood volume with C-11 labeled carboxyhemoglobin. J Nucl Med 20:328–334, 1979.
27. Brooks RA. Alternative formula for glucose utilization using labelled deoxyglucose. J Nucl Med 23:538–539, 1982.
28. Phelps ME, Huang SC, Hoffman EJ, Selin C, Sokoloff L, Kuhl DE. Tomographic measurement of local cerebral glucose metabolic rate in humans with (F-18) 2-fluoro-2-deoxy-D-glucose: Validation of method. Ann Neurol 6:371–388, 1979.
29. Reivich M, Kuhl DE, Wolf A, Greenberg J, Phelps M, Ido T, Casella V, Fowler J, Hoffman E, Alavi A, Som P, Sokoloff L. The F-18 fluorodeoxyglucose method for the measurement of local cerebral glucose utilization in man. Circ Res 44:127–137, 1979.
30. Warburg O. On the origin of cancer cells. Science 123:309–314, 1956.
31. Weber G. Enzymology of cancer cells (part 1). N Engl J Med 296:486–541, 1977.
32. Som P, Atkins HL, Bandoypadhyay D, Fowler JS, MacGregor RR, Matsui K, Oster ZH, Sacker DF, Shive CY, Turner H, Won C-N, Wolf HP, Zabinski SV. A fluorinated glucose analog, 2-fluro-2-fluocse(F-18): Nontoxic tracer for rapid tumor detection. J Nucl Med 21:670–675, 1980.
33. Gallagher BM, Fowler JS, Gutterson NI, MacGregor RR, Won C-N, Wolf AP. Metabolic trapping as a principle of radiopharmaceutical design: Some factors responsible for the biodistribution of [^{18}F]2-deoxy-2-fluoro-D-glucose. J Nucl Med 19:1154–1161, 1978.
34. Sokoloff L, Reivich M, Kennedy C, Des Rosiers MH, Patlak CS, Pettigrew KD, Sakurada O, Shinohara M. The [^{14}C] deoxyglucose method for the measurement of local cerebral glucose utilization: Theory, procedure, and normal values in the conscious and anesthetized albino rat. J Neurochem 28:897, 1977.
35. Suolinna EM, Haaparanta M, Paul R, Harkonen P, Solin O, Sipila H. Metabolism of 2-[^{18}F]fluoro-2-deoxyglucose in tumor-bearing rats: Chromatographic and enzymatic studies. Nucl Med Biol 13:577–581, 1986.
36. Brownell G, Kairento AL, Swartz M, Elmaleh DR. Positron emission tomography in oncology — the Massachusetts General Hospital experience. Semin Nucl Med 25:201–209, 1985.
37. Adler LP, Blair HF, Makley JT, Williams RP, Joyce MJ, Leisure G, Al-Kaisi N, Miraldi F. Noninvasive grading of musculoskeletal tumors using PET. J Nucl Med 32:1508–1512, 1991.
38. Shulkin BL, Mitchell DS, Ungar DR, Prahash D, Dole MG, Castle VP, Hernandez RJ, Koeppe RA, Hutchinson RJ. Neoplasms in a pediatric population: 2-[F-18]-fluoro-2-deoxy-D-glucose PET studies. Radiology 194:495–500, 1995.
39. Nieweg OE, Pruim J, Hoekstra HJ, Paans AMJ, Vaalburg W, Oldhoff J, Koops HS. Positron emission tomography with fluorine-18-fluorodeoxyglucose for the evaluation of therapeutic isolated regional limb perfusion in a patient with soft-tissue sarcoma. J Nucl Med 35:90–92, 1994.
40. Daemen BJG, Elsinga PH, Paans AMJ, Wieringa AR, Konings AWT, Vaalburg W. Radiation-induced inhibition of tumor growth as monitored by PET using L-[1-^{11}C]tyrosine and fluorine-18-fluorodeoxyglucose. J Nucl Med 33:373–379, 1992.

5. Metastasectomy for soft tissue sarcomas

Ugo Pastorino

Introduction

Complete surgical resection of isolated lung metastases is now considered an essential component of the multimodality treatment of soft tissue sarcomas. However, the recognition of the curative potential of metastasectomy occurred relatively slowly, and only in the last decade has lung metastasectomy been accepted as a standard therapeutic procedure. Many years after the first resection of a single lung metastasis, discovered intraoperatively during the excision of a chest wall sarcoma [1], elective surgery has been occasionally offered to selected cases [2] with single pulmonary metastases and or a long disease-free interval [3].

It was only in the late seventies that metastasectomy was applied systematically to multiple or bilateral lesions with favorable results [4]. Various elements justify a more aggressive therapeutic management for soft tissue sarcomas. In a significant proportion of patients with distant metastases, either at presentation or following curative treatment of the primary tumor, the lungs represent the only site of spread of the disease. In the absence of complete resection, lung metastases are associated with a median survival of 6–8 months, rarely exceeding 2 years. New chemotherapy regimens, potentially more effective on micrometastatic foci but unable to eradicate the component of the disease that is clinically detectable, may expand the role of adjuvant or salvage surgery in order to excise the residual tumor after induction chemotherapy and/or confirm a complete pathological remission.

Biology of metastases

The natural history of sarcomas provides a solid rational basis for lung metastasectomy. The clinical evidence of organ-restricted spread is reinforced by autopsy data showing that the lungs are often the only site of progression of the disease. Notwithstanding the overall improvement of survival achieved with multimodality treatments, lung metastases represent the main reason for ultimate treatment failure.

J. Verweij, H.M. Pinedo, and H.D. Suit (eds). SOFT TISSUE SARCOMAS: PRESENT ACHIEVEMENTS AND FUTURE PROSPECTS.

Long-term survival in soft tissue sarcomas ranges in the literature from 40% to 60% [5]. The crude incidence of lung metastases in soft tissue is lower than in osteosarcoma but similar to that observed in other bone sarcomas. In the experience of the National Cancer Institute (NCI), of 307 localized soft tissue sarcomas (grade III) that underwent radical resection, only 56 (18%) developed isolated lung metastases, representing 52% of all the observed recurrences and 67% of all distant relapses [6].

The prognosis of those patients who develop pulmonary metastases not suitable for complete resection, or receiving medical treatment only, is extremely poor. Even though adjuvant chemotherapy may result in a longer disease-free interval, a more limited extent of pulmonary relapse and a prolongation of median survival on the order of a few months, the vast majority of patients die within 2 years, with no survivors after the third year [7,8]. In the NCI study [9], the median survival of patients with unresected lung metastases was 7.4 months, a figure entirely consistent with previous reports on metastatic soft tissue sarcomas [10].

Clinical staging

A more extensive application of metastasectomy has increased the requirements of preoperative intrathoracic staging in order to reduce the risk of exploratory thoracotomy or incomplete resection and to choose the optimal surgical approach for every patient. In cases of proven or suspicious lung metastases, clinical staging should provide the most accurate information on each of the following aspects: (a) probability of a false positive, (b) single versus multiple lesions, (c) unilateral versus bilateral disease, (d) involvement of hilar or mediastinal lymph nodes, and (e) the total volume of lung resection required.

Computed tomography (CT) and nuclear magnetic resonance (NMR) of the chest have significantly improved the radiological diagnosis, particularly in the assessment of lesion number. Chest CT can identify up to 80% of all pulmonary nodules greater than 3 mm detected at surgical exploration (25% more than linear tomography), but a few such lesions may ultimately prove benign, whilst other radiologically occult nodules may be discovered in critical areas such as the costophrenic angles. It has been estimated that the final diagnostic accuracy of radiological staging is on the order of 40% for plain chest x-rays and 60–80% for CT [11–13]. As for most thoracic malignancies, CT has completely replaced linear tomography in the assessment of lung metastases [14,15]. The probability of false-positive lesions is higher in patients who underwent previous lung resections due to lung distortion and fibrosis [16].

New developments in CT technology, such as continuous spiral scanning, have further improved the diagnostic yield of radiological staging, both in terms of the minimum size parenchymal nodules (less than 3 mm) and significant hilar or mediastinal adenopathies. NMR offers no advantages over CT in the staging of lung metastases, but its longer scanning time expands the risk respiratory artifacts and false-negative results [17].

In the experience of the Istituto Nazionale Tumori of Milano, the accuracy of radiological diagnosis of single versus multiple metastases in soft tissue sarcomas was 76%. However, assessment of the real number of lesions was accurate only in 57% of cases, with 33% false-negative and 10% false-positive results. As far as the site of disease was concerned, the frequency of occult contralateral metastases was 55% in patients undergoing median sternotomy for unilateral disease and 47% for patients with single lesions, thus confirming the advantage of the bilateral surgical approach. The role of other diagnostic examinations such as PET scanning or the use of targeted monoclonal antibodies is still under evaluation.

Preoperative histological confirmation of metastatic disease is not necessary in patients with prior soft tissue sarcoma because surgical excision provides reliable diagnosis and potentially curative treatment. Clearly, for those patents who are being offered preoperative chemotherapy and achieve a complete remission with treatment, the lack of pathological confirmation may create some doubt in the assessment of the total result of treatment. Because soft tissue sarcomas mainly metastasize to the lungs, only limited further screening (e.g., site of the primary; liver for GI sarcomas) is mandatory.

Local recurrence at the site of the primary tumor should always be excluded, or deemed resectable, before undertaking lung metastasectomy. Particularly for soft tissue sarcomas, with which the probability of local relapse is very high, preoperative staging should include CT or NMR of the primary tumor site.

Selection criteria

In general terms, eligibility criteria for curative resection of lung metastases include the following: (a) primary tumor previously cured or curable, (b) no evidence of extrapulmonary metastases, (c) complete resectability of all pulmonary metastases, (d) planned resection volume tolerable by the patient, and (e) no valid therapeutic alternatives available.

Patients presenting with synchronous metastases at the time of initial diagnosis, as well as patients with concurrent local relapse and lung metastases after primary treatment, may still be eligible for metastasectomy provided that the primary tumor or local relapse are amenable to curative management. The most appropriate timing for surgery of the primary and metastases (simultaneous or sequential), as well as the need for primary chemotherapy, have to be decided for each individual case. Clinical features, such as the histological type and grading, disease-free interval, doubling time, or number of lesions, represent potential prognostic factors but cannot be used to select patients for surgery. Incomplete resection of extensive lung disease with macroscopic intrathoracic residual disease (debulking) does not appear to improve patient prognosis, nor is it justifiable as palliative management.

Surgical technique

In soft tissue sarcomas the optimal surgical approach is represented by sequential exploration of both lungs, both inflated and deflated, for screening of radiologically occult lesions, even in the case of single or unilateral metastases. Some authors prefer a bilateral thoracotomy (simultaneous or staged), and others favor a median sternotomy [18]. It has been demonstrated that in 30–40% of cases presenting with unilateral lesions, median sternotomy revealed bilateral lung metastases [12,19,20]. In addition to one-stage resection of all palpable lesions, a median sternotomy offers other advantages, such as less functional damage and postoperative pain, early mobilization of the patient, and limited morbidity and mortality [21–23]. In redo surgery for recurrent lung metastases, the choice of the best approach has to be based on the specific clinical features that characterize the individual patient (age, lung function, number and location of lesions, prior resections, pleural adhesions) and may necessitate a monolateral or bilateral incision.

The appropriate resection volume depends on the number, site, and dimensions of secondary lung lesions. A sublobar resection (segmentectomy, atypical tangential or wedge resection) is generally adequate in sarcomas. In these tumors it is important to preserve as much lung as possible in view of future resections: in the experience of the Memorial Sloan-Kettering Cancer Center, 60% patients underwent more than one thoracotomy and nearly 30% underwent more than two thoracotomies [24]. If multiple lesions are present, the margin of healthy tissue must be sufficient to minimize the risk of local relapse, while in solitary lesions the lobectomy may be preferred when the possibility of a primary lung tumor cannot be excluded. A wedge resection and frozen section may help to choose the proper resection volume. The presence of nodal metastases may necessitate a lobectomy, or even a larger volume of resection, but such an event is rare in soft tissue sarcomas.

Mechanical staplers have contributed to the development of this type of surgery by providing a quick, safe, and standardized technique for sublobar lung resection. However, the so-called precision resection may be more volume effective in the case of multiple bilateral metastases. This technique consists of cutting out a uniform layer (5–10 mm) of normal lung tissue around the nodule, using a YAG laser, argon beam, or simply a diathermy needle. Experience acquired with the use of the various available surgical options has reduced the morbidity and mortality of metastasectomy considerably. The overall mortality reported in the literature ranges from 0 to 4% [25–27]. In our experience, total perioperative mortality (within 30 days) is less than 1%.

For all the above-mentioned reasons, we do not recommend the use of video-assisted thoracoscopy for metastasectomy. In fact, the thoracoscopic technique precludes thorough palpation of the lungs and proper intra-operative staging. Moreover, in the frequent cases of multiple metastases, the use of endoscopic staplers without palpatory control may result in inappropriate resection margins, with either insufficient or excessive resection volumes.

Long-term results

The overall 5-year survival after metastasectomy reported in the literature, regardless of the type, free interval, and number of lesions, ranges from 25% to 45% [24]. The experience of the Istituto Nazionale Tumori of Milan includes 136 patients with metastatic soft tissue sarcomas who underwent surgical exploration during the period 1975–1994. Of these 110 (81%) were amenable to macroscopic complete resection of all pulmonary metastases. Table 1 summarizes the main clinical features of the 110 patients who received radical metastasectomy. Long-term survival is illustrated in Figure 1. The actuarial survival after complete resection was 48% at 3 years, 36% at 5 years, and 30% at 10 years, with a median survival of 35 months. The probability of survival was significantly lower for incomplete resections, with a median survival of only 16 months.

Our results have been recently confirmed by the data from the EORTC Soft Tissue Sarcoma Group [28]. They performed a restrospective analysis on 255 patients with soft tissue sarcomas (excluding chondrosarcoma and small round cell sarcomas) who underwent complete resection of lung metastases. The overall post-metastasectomy survival in this study was 54% at 3 years, 38% at 5 years, and 27% at 10 years. The corresponding values for disease-free survival were 42% at 3 years, 35% at 5 years, and 28% at 10 years. Using a Cox regression model, favorable prognostic factors for survival (Table 2) were a

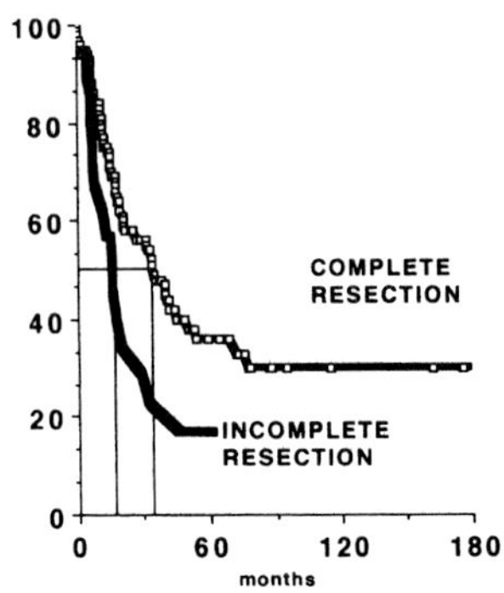

Figure 1. Actuarial survival after metastasectomy for soft tissue sarcomas at the Istituto Nazionale Tumori of Milan. Complete resection (110 patients) versus incomplete resection (26 patients) are shown.

Table 1. Lung metastasectomies for soft tissue sarcomas: Istituto Nazionale Tumori of Milan, 1975–1994

		Single	Multiple	Total
Age	Mean (range)	41 (8–80)	39 (6–75)	39 (6–80)
Sex	Male	25	36	61
	Female	14	35	49
Rx	Single	30	17	47
	Multiple	9	54	63
Interval (DFI)	0–11 mos	7	21	28
	12–35 mos	16	32	48
	36+ mos	16	18	34
Number	2–3	—	33	33
	4+	—	38	38
Lymph nodes	Positive	2	0	2
Approach	Thoracotomy	19	10	29
	Sternotomy	20	61	81
Resection	Sublobar	28	41	69
	Lobar	10	30	40
	Pneumo	1	—	1
Chemotherapy	Adjuvant	12	42	54
Total		39	71	110

DFI = disease-fill interval.

Table 2. Lung metastasectomies for soft tissue sarcomas: EORTC Soft Tissue Sarcoma Group (255 cases) — Results of multivariate analysis

		p	S.E.	t
Free interval	≤2.5 yr	0.003	19	−2.9
Grade II	Yes/no	0.031	46	2.1
Grade III	Yes/no	0.003	43	2.9
Radical resection	Yes/no	0.025	24	−2.2
Age	≥40 yr	0.005	18	2.8

disease-free interval greater than 2.5 years before the development of lung metastases, age less than 40 years, and grade I–II tumors.

An even greater effort to provide reliable data on the ultimate outcome of patients undergoing lung metastasectomy is represented by the International Registry of Lung Metastases. This cooperative project, established in 1991, has collected clinical data on 5207 patients from 18 major departments of thoracic surgery in Europe, the United States, and Canada. The preliminary results were discussed during a two-day workshop held in London in October 1995. The subset of 938 patients who underwent complete metastasectomy for soft tissue sarcomas within the International Registry showed an overall 5-year survival of 30%, a 10-year survival of 22%, and a median survival of 27 months. All these independent analyses have unequivocally demonstrated the curative potential of metastasectomy in soft tissue sarcomas.

Prognostic factors

Achievement of a macroscopically complete resection is probably the most important independent prognostic factor for lung metastasectomy. The disease-free interval, defined as the time elapsed between treatment of the primary tumour and diagnosis of lung metastases, represents a more prominent prognostic factor in soft tissue sarcomas then in other tumor types. In the majority of reports from the literature, a longer disease-free interval is associated with better survival, but the cutoff ranges between 12 and 36 months [5,29]. In our experience in Milan, a significant improvement in prognosis is observed when the disease-free interval exceeds 2 years. This observation does not imply that patients with resectable metastases should be excluded from surgery on the grounds of a short free interval.

The number of pathologically proven lung metastases is another determinant of prognosis. An early report from the NCI, based on 106 cases of sarcoma, showed a dismal prognosis for patients with more than four lesions, with a median survival of 6 months after metastasectomy [5]. However, this observation was not confirmed by other authors [26,30]. In some experiences a favorable outcome can be identified only for single lesions of less than 3 cm in diameter (50% vs. 25% 5-year survival) [24]. Other authors report a better survival for pulmonary metastases with a maximum diameter of less than 3 cm [31] or less than 1.5 cm [30] indepent of the total number of resected lesions.

As for primary tumors of the lung, secondary involvement of the hilar or mediastinal lymph nodes is a poor prognostic factor after metastasectomy. However, this is an extremely rare condition in soft tissue sarcomas. The volume of resection does not represent an independent prognostic factor, but the need for pneumonectomy for metastatic sarcomas generally indicates very extensive disease and a dismal prognosis, even after radical resection.

In the European cooperative study, multivariate analysis identified disease-free interval, grading, radical resection, and age as significant prognostic factors, but not the number of metastases nor the site or type of primary sarcoma [28]. The data from this multivariate analysis are summarized in Table 2. Analysis of the data from the International Registry is still ongoing, but preliminary results are very similar to those of the European Organization for Research and Treatment of Cancer (EORTC) study. It appears that patients with a disease-free interval of 36 months or longer had a significantly better survival (40% at 5 years, 24% at 10 years, median 40 months) than those with a disease-free interval of less than 12 months (19% at 5 years, 13% at 10 years, median 21 months) (Fig. 2). Patients with single metastases had a better survival (38% at 5 years, 30% at 10 years, median 37 months) than those with four or more metastases (18% at 5 years, 12% at 10 years, median 23 months)

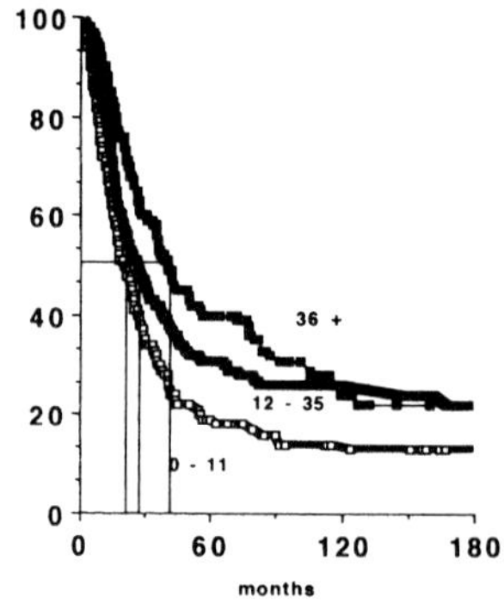

Figure 2. Actuarial survival after metastasectomy for soft tissue sarcomas in the International Registry of Lung Metastases. Disease-free interval 0–11 months (287 patients), 12–35 months (388 patients), and 36 months (255 patients) are shown.

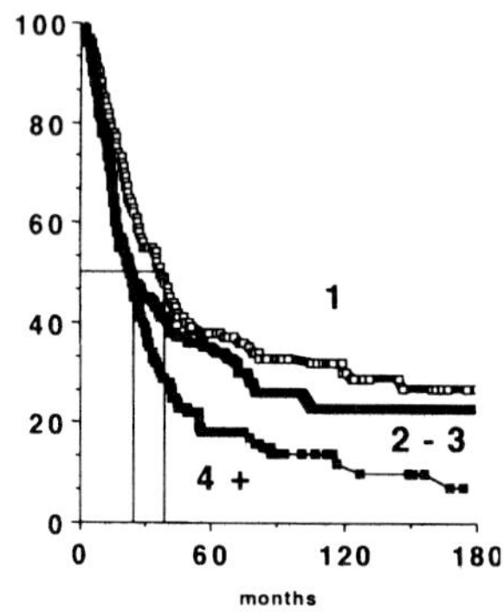

Figure 3. Actuarial survival after metastasectomy for soft tissue sarcomas in the International Registry of Lung Metastases. Single lung metastasis (350 patients), two to three lung metastases (243 patients), and four lung metastases (337 patients) were reported.

(Fig. 3). The improved prognosis for patients with a single lesion compared with those with multiple lesions remained statistically significant on multivariate analysis with the Cox model.

Relapse after metastasectomy and follow-up

The modality of relapse after the first metastasectomy is clearly influenced by the histological type and extent of the primary tumor. In the experience of the Milan group, the majority of relapses (37 of 71) were confined to the lung and were potentially suitable for salvage surgery. In this respect, the limiting factors were extent of pulmonary relapse and residual respiratory function of

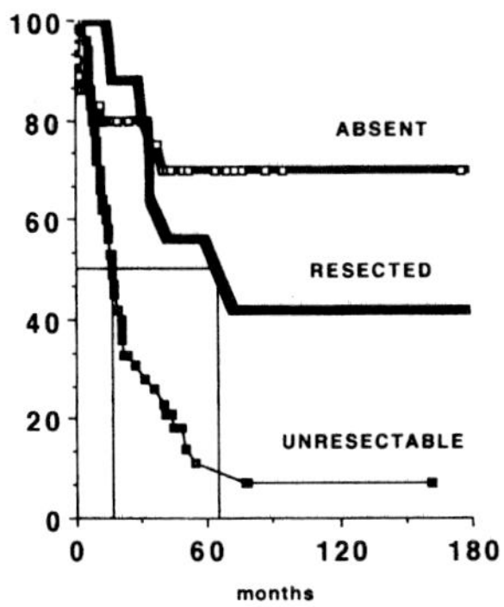

Figure 4. Actuarial survival after metastasectomy for soft tissue sarcomas at the Istituto Nazionale Tumori of Milan. No evidence of recurrence (39 patients), resected lung relapse (20 patients), and unresectable relapse (51 patients) were reported.

the patient. In the NCI experience, based on 23 cases, the average number of operations per patient was 1.9, with a 40% survival at 5 years [6]. In our series, of 37 patients with intrapulmonary relapses, 20 (54% of local or 28% of all relapses) were treated with further resections. The actuarial survival of patients with resected pulmonary relapse is illustrated in Figure 4: a 56% survival at 5 years represents a very encouraging result.

It is therefore essential, in order to apply salvage surgery to a higher proportion of patients, to maintain a strict follow-up after the first metastasectomy. Taking into account the distribution of the second disease-free interval, it appears that the majority of relapses occur during the first 6 months. In practical terms, the follow-up should include a plain chest x-ray every 2 months and a CT scan of the chest every 6 months for a minimum of 12 months. Such intensive screening of lung metastases should be implemented using a similar follow-up protocal for the primary tumor site, with physical examination and CT or NMR, to detect and adequately treat any locoregional recurrences [32].

References

1. Weinlecher. Wiener Med Wrsch 20 & 21, 1882.
2. Barney JD, Churchill EJ. Adenocarcinoma of the kidney with metastasis to the lung. J Urol 42:269, 1939.
3. Alexander J, Haight C. Pulmonary resection for solitary metastatic sarcomas and carcinomas. Surg Gynecol Obstet 85:129, 1947.
4. Martini N, McCormak PM, Bains MS. Indications for surgery for intrathoracic metastases in testicular carcinoma. Semin Oncol 6:99–103, 1979.
5. Roth JA, Putnam JB, Wesley MN, Rosemberg SA. Differing determinants of prognosis following resection of pulmonary metastases from osteogenic and soft-tissue sarcoma patients. Cancer 55:1361–1366, 1985.

6. Potter DA, Kinsella T, Glatstein E, Wesley R, White DE, Seipp CA, Chang AE, Lack EE, Costa J, Rosemberg SA. High grade soft tissue sarcomas of the extremities. Proc ASCO 4:144, 1985.
7. Eilber F, Giuliano A, Eckardt J, Patterson K, Moseley S, Goodnight J. Adjuvant chemotherapy for osteosarcoma: A randomized prospective trial. J Clin Oncol 5:21–26, 1987.
8. Jaffe N, Smith E, Abelson HT, Frei E. Osteogenic sarcoma: Alteration in the pattern of pulmonary metastases with adjuvant chemotherapy. J Clin Oncol 1:251–254, 1983.
9. Potter DA, Glenn J, Kinsella T, Glatstein E, Lack EE, Restrepo C, White DE, Seipp CA, Wesley R, Rosemberg SA. Patterns of recurrence in patients with high-grade soft-tissue sarcomas. J Clin Oncol 3:353–366, 1985.
10. McKenna RJ, McKenna RJ, Jr. Patterns of pulmonary metasteses — An orthopedic hospital experience. In L Weiss, HA Gilbert, eds. Pulmonary Metastasis. Boston: GK Hall & Co, 1978.
11. Chang AE, Schaner EC, Conkle DM, et al. Surgical resection of the solitary pulmonary metastasis. In L Weiss, HA Gilbert, eds. Pulmonary Metastasis. Boston: GK Hall & Co, 1978.
12. Roth JA, Pass HI, Wesley MN, White D, Putnam JB, Seipp C. Comparison of median sternotomy and toracotomy for resection of pulmonary metastases in patients with adult soft-tissue sarcomas. Ann Thorac Surg 42:134–138, 1986.
13. Paul KP, Toomes H, Vogt-Moykopf I. Lung volumes following resection of pulmonary metastases in paediatric patients — a retrospective study. Eur J Pediatr 149:862–865, 1990.
14. Chang AE, Schaner EG, Conkle DM, Flyle MW, Doppmann YJL, Rosemberg SA. Evaluation of computed tomography in the detection of pulmonary metastases. Cancer 43:913, 1979.
15. Mintzer RA, Malave SR, Neiman HL, Michaelis LL, Vanecko RM, Sanders JM. Computed vs. conventional tomography in evaluation of primary and secondary pulmonary neoplasms. Radiology 132:653, 1979.
16. Gurtler KF, Riebel TH, Beron G, Heller M, Euler A. Vergleich von Rontgennubersichtsaufnahmen, Rontgenschichtaufnahmen und Computertomogrammen bei pulmonalen Rundherden im Kindes- und Jugendalter. Fortschr Rontgenstr 140:416, 1984.
17. Muller NL, Gamsu G, Webb WR. Pulmonary nodules: Detection using magnetic resonance and computed tomography. Radiology 155:687, 1985.
18. Takita H, Edgerton F, Karakousis C, et al. Surgical management of metastases to the lung. Surg Gynecol Obstet 152:191–194, 1981.
19. Johnston MR, et al. Median sternotomy for resection of pulmonary metastases in patients with soft-tissue sarcomas. Arch Surg 121:1248–1252, 1986.
20. Pastorino U, Valente M, Gasparini M, Azzarelli A, Santoro A, Tavecchio L, Casali P, Ravasi G. Median sternotomy and multiple lung resections for metastatic sarcomas. Eur J Cardiothorac Surg 4:477–481, 1990.
21. Mark JB. Surgical management of metastatic neoplasms to the lungs. In DC Sabiston, FC Spencer, eds. Surgery of the Chest. Philadelphia: WB Saunders, 1983.
22. Regal AM, Reese P, Antkowiak J, Hart T, Takita H. Median sternotomy for metastatic lung lesions in 131 patients. Cancer 55:1334–1339, 1985.
23. Takita H, Merrin C, Didolkar MS, et al. The surgical management of multiple lung metastases. Ann Thorac Surg 24:359–363, 1977.
24. McCormack P. Surgical treatment of pulmonary metastases: Memorial Hospital experience. In L Weiss, HA Gilbert, eds. Pulmonary Metastasis. Boston: GK Hall & Co, 1978.
25. Mountain CF, McMurtrey MJ, Hermes KE. Surgery for pulmonary metastasis: A 20-year experience. Ann Thorac Surg 38:323–330, 1984.
26. Thomford NR, Woolner LB, Claget OT. The surgical treatment of metastatic tumors in the lungs. J Thorac Cardiovasc Surg 49:357–363, 1965.
27. Venn GE, Sarin S, Goldstraw P. Survival following pulmonary metastasectomy. Eur J Cardiothorac Surg 3:105–110, 1989.

28. Van Geel AN, Pastorino U, Jauch KW, et al. Surgical treatment of lung metastases: The EORTC-Soft Tissue and Bone Sarcoma Group study of 255 patients. Cancer 77:675–682, 1996.
29. Putnam JB, Jr., Roth JA. Prognostic indicators in patients with pulmonary metastases. Semin Surg Oncol 6:291–296, 1990.
30. Marincola FM, Mark JB. Selection factors resulting in improved survival after surgical resection of tumors metastatic of the lungs. Arch Surg 125:1387–1393, 1990.
31. Goya T, Miyazawa N, Kondo H, Tsuchiya R, Naruke T, Suemasu K. Surgical resection of pulmonary metastases from colorectal cancer: 10-year follow-up. Cancer 64:1418–1421, 1989.
32. Potter DA, Kinsella T, Glatstein E, Wesley R, White DE, Seipp CA, Chang AE, Lack EE, Costa J, Rosemberg SA. High grade soft tissue sarcomas of the extremities. Cancer 58:190, 1986.

6. Post-treatment limb function in soft tissue sarcomas

Martin H. Robinson

Introduction

It has become clear that a quality of life assessment of anticancer treatment is crucial in measuring its impact. Quality of life assessment in cancers tends to assess side effects of treatment, usually chemotherapy, and therefore contains measures that are inappropriate for the majority of extremity sarcoma patients. Although it is important to measure emotional and social factors, physical factors are also crucial. The European Organization for Research and Treatment of Cancer (EORTC) QLQC30 is a commonly used measure that evaluates pain, fatigue, emotional functions, systemic symptoms, and physical functions [1]. About 40% of its questions assess physical function, but the total score is affected by measures that are not particularly relevant to extremity sarcoma patients. It is therefore not the most appropriate instrument in this group of patients.

Although there have been a large number of reports on the efficacy of limb conservation treatment in soft tissue sarcoma [2–7], most have not included an assessment of the main outcome measure, that is, limb function. The methods of treatment previously reported have also varied considerably. The extent of the surgery carried out often is not clearly reported, and the timing, dose, and fractionation of radiation treatments vary considerably. Most authors have used postoperative radiotherapy [2,4,7], with some centers favoring preoperative radiotherapy [6]. The fractionation schedules vary between weekly doses of 6.6 Gy to twice-daily schedules using 1.2 Gy fractions [8,9]. In American reports many, but not all, of the patients have received chemotherapy either intravenously or intra-arterially [3,10]. All of these parameters impact on the final functional result.

Issue of amputation versus limb conservation

In 1982 Sugarbaker and colleagues threw into doubt the established doctrine that limb conservation inevitably resulted in a better quality of life for patients than amputation [11]. They reported an important study of patients with

J. Verweij, H.M. Pinedo, and H.D. Suit (eds). SOFT TISSUE SARCOMAS: PRESENT ACHIEVEMENTS AND FUTURE PROSPECTS.

extremity sarcoma entered into a randomized trial comparing amputation and adjuvant chemotherapy with limb-sparing surgery, radiotherapy, and chemotherapy [11]. The results were surprising. They concluded that there was no evidence of an improved quality of life in those patients in whom the limb had been spared. Patient numbers were small, there was no pretreatment assessment, and the assessment was done on a single variable time following the treatment. However, they found surprising differences in body care and movement, but because of the small number of patients and the 2:1 randomization, it was not possible to prove that these differences did not occur due to chance alone. Although other workers carrying out a retrospective study using questionnaires have not confirmed these findings [12], this research set the scene for the studies that followed.

Postma et al. [13] compared the quality of life data of 33 long-term survivors of lower extremity bone cancer, 14 of whom were treated with limb salvage and 19 with amputation. Self-report questionnaires, semistructured interviews, and visual analog scales were used to measure psychoneurotic and somatic distress, activities of daily living, self-esteem, and adjustment to illness. The median time after surgery was 10 years. The differences between the two groups were not statistically significant, with physical complaints reported more often by limb salvage patients, whereas amputees showed a trend towards lower self-esteem and isolation in social life due to their disability. Both groups felt equal diminution of quality of life and disability. The authors felt that these findings, which seem inconclusive, could support the cosmetic advantage of limb salvage versus amputation.

A further assessment of the impact of limb-salvage surgery or amputation on the psyche came from Christ, who carried out a study on the psychosocial adaptation of 45 long-term survivors (average 7 years from diagnosis) of bone cancer diagnosed in adolescence [14]. Structured, in-person, open-ended interviews were collected, and standardized instruments and closed-ended questionnaires were also completed by the patients. There was no difference between the psychopathology of osteosarcoma survivors and the normal population.

They then compared the three treatment groups of initial amputation, limb sparing with good outcome, and limb sparing with compromised outcome. The initial amputees were more likely to feel under employed, less likely to be married, and had poorer coping skills. Gender, age at diagnosis, and treatment type were not predictive of psychosocial distress. Better coping did not protect the initial amputees from higher distress. Those whose limbs were spared were protected from higher distress by better coping; however, with poorer coping they experienced even higher distress scores than the initial amputees.

Review of limb function studies

Important contributions to the literature pertaining to limb function following treatment of extremity soft tissue sarcoma have been made from Toronto, the

National Cancer Institute (NCI) in the United States, and the Royal Marsden Hospital in London among others.

U.S. experience

In 1984 Lampert reported a study of the limb function and quality of life in 40 patients with soft tissue sarcoma of the head and neck, trunk, or upper and lower extremities [15]. Most of their patients had also received chemotherapy. They concluded that patients with lower limb tumors had the greatest functional impairment. They then carried out a prospective study with serial assessments performed before and after treatment in a group of patients who were participants in randomized studies evaluating the efficacy of postoperative radiotherapy. They designed a battery of measurements to evaluate functional and psychosocial change in patients with extremity sarcoma undergoing limb-sparing therapy. All these patients received postoperative adjuvant chemotherapy.

Eighty-eight patients were evaluated over a $3\frac{1}{2}$ year period. Those with high-grade sarcoma grades 2 and 3 received five cycles of postoperative chemotherapy with doxorubicin and cyclophosphamide starting 3–4 weeks after surgery. When radiotherapy was given postoperatively, it was delivered to the areas of greatest risk between the joints proximal and distal to the primary lesion and including all involved muscle groups. Daily treatment of 1.8–2 Gy to a total dose of 45–50 Gy was given with a boost to 60–65 Gy. All patients were evaluated prior to the definitive surgery, and physiotherapy was continued after hospital discharge and during radiotherapy. Two thirds of the tumors were in the lower extremity, and approximately half of the patients had radiotherapy. The questionnaires and evaluations were completed prior to definitive surgical resection and at 6-month intervals postoperatively.

The impact of treatment on economic status, sexual activity, pain, and global quality of life were studied using a battery of psychosocial functional assessment tests. They were particularly interested in economic status, sexual activity, and pain. Economic assessment consisted of five questions regarding employment status, occupation, average number of working hours per week, average income per month, and percent of family income contributed by the patient. Sexual activity was documented by nine questions on marital status, frequency of sex, interest, pleasure, percentage of orgasms, importance of sexual activity, relationships, feelings of femininity and masculinity, feelings of desirability, and extent to which the frequency of sexual relations matched patient preferences.

Pain was measured by the McGill Pain Questionnaire and a visual analogue scale (VAS). The study used a total score of the pain questionnaire to reflect pain intensity. They also documented how much the pain interfered with daily activities and sleep, and the amount of pain medication. They used a Functional Living Index Cancer (FLIC) consisting of 22 questions to assess quality of life and Erdman's scale to assess independence [16]. They also evaluated limb function as described by Lampert et al. [15] and looked at joint contracture, early radiation effects, wound complications, and the need for support stockings and splints.

Results

The number of assessments carried out at 6 months post-therapy was 77 and at 12 months it was 65. After 18 and 24 months it dropped quite markedly to 57 and 53, respectively.

Employment. Thirty-six percent of employed patients had a decline in their employment status at 6 months, and none improved. This finding persisted at the 12-month assessment despite having finished all therapy.

Sexual activity. Several parameters of sexual activity declined significantly at 6 months. Forty-one percent of patients recorded a decrease in frequency of intercourse, and 13% had an increase. Significant numbers of patients reported a decline in their interest and pleasure from sex at 6 months. By 12 months a significant number of patients (48%) experienced a decrease in frequency. Interest at 12 months showed a similar decline. The decline in sexual activity was not confined to those who received chemotherapy.

Pain. There was no significant increase in pain over the period studied.

Global quality of life. There was an increase in FLIC scores by 12 months, but no change at 6 months, suggesting that the quality of life may have improved during this period.

Limb function. At 6 months a significant number of patients had evidence of decreased muscle strength and worsening of joint mobility and edema. The results were similar at 12 months, with significant number of patients experiencing an increase in edema and a decline in joint motion and muscle strength. However, performance of daily activity as assessed by the modified Erdman scale was not impaired in significant numbers of patients at 6 and 12 months. Although limb function was obviously impaired at both 6 and 12 months, there were inadequate numbers of patients to try to associate particular therapies with this problem. Joint contractures, mainly of the ankle, were only seen in 6 of 19 patients with high-grade sarcomas who received both radiation therapy and chemotherapy. The authors concluded that it was possible that a combination of chemotherapy and radiotherapy might be associated with an increased incidence of joint contractures.

Wound complications. There appeared to be a statistically significant association between the use of combination radiotherapy and adjuvant chemotherapy and the development of wound complications.

Conclusions

The authors confirmed a significant decline in limb function, sexual activity, and employment status at 12 months in the entire population. However, global quality of life measurements increased, indicating improved psychosocial/sociability status. Patients seemed to be able to compensate, perhaps because they felt they were cured. Decreased sexual function was clearly documented in the overall population, as also reported in previous work by Sugarbaker, which showed sexual function was more disturbed in those with limb conservation than in those who received amputation. It has been postulated that the combined effects of chemotherapy and the degree of radiation on testicular and ovarian dysfunction result in decreased sexual function. Alternatively, it could be that radiation fibrosis interferes with normal sexual activity, with doxorubicin sensitizing normal tissue to the effects of radiotherapy. The study did not confirm that radiotherapy was the cause of the changes. However, the numbers are rather small and we must remember that the use of subgroup analysis could result in the data being misinterpreted.

In 1991 Stinson reported the results of a large, long-term retrospective survey of the records of 152 patients who received limb-sparing surgery with radiotherapy at the NCI between 1975 and 1986 [17]. A detailed review of the radiotherapy delivered was carried out, including looking at field size, length of bone irradiated in phase 1 and 2, percentage diameter of the bone and extremity irradiated, details of the documented acute reaction, delays in treatment, and dose per fraction. Stinson et al. documented complications from treatment occurring later than 1 year postoperatively, including bone fractures, contractures, edema, pain, ulceration, tissue induration, and skin changes. The presence or absence of decreased range of motion and decreased muscle power, and the need for splints or walking devices, was also noted. Their results indicated that the degree of early skin reaction was exacerbated by the use of adjuvant chemotherapy, computerized planning, and inclusion of more than 50% of the diameter of the extremity in the field. Despite the author's explanation, it is difficult to understand why the use of computerized planning should be related to an increased acute reaction.

Chronic changes occurring over one year after treatment included contractures, which were associated with irradiation of the joint and treatment before 1980 (when computerized dosimetry was introduced). Chronic pain necessitating narcotic analgesia was associated with doses in excess of 1760 cGy, as was moderate or severe edema, muscle weakness, and decreased range of motion. Field length in excess of 35 cm was associated with increased lymphedema and loss of muscle power. Treatment of the lower limb was associated with more edema or loss of range of motion than other sites, and more chronic infection and ulceration was seen in the lower limb, where more than 75% of the diameter of the limb was irradiated. Moderate to severe tissue induration was associated with increased field length and lower extremity site.

The use of chemotherapy did not seem to be associated with increased late complications.

Their conclusions were that attention to various aspects of the radiotherapy technique would result in improved long-term function in patients treated for extremity soft tissue sarcoma. They felt that joint irradiation should only be done when absolutely necessary and that doses in excess of 65 Gy are not likely to be necessary and may result in more pain and edema, decreased strength and range of motion, and skin telangiectasia. They felt that the length and diameter of the extremity irradiated should be limited as much as possible, consistent with adequate tumor coverage, and that computerized treatment planning and the use of beam modifiers can be most helpful. Although bone fractures related to radiotherapy in this series were rare, they advised avoiding irradiation of large lengths or full diameters of bone where possible. Although chemotherapy increases the acute complications of treatment, they found that it appears to have no association with late sequelae.

Princess Margaret Hospital experience

The authors from this Toronto center reported the functional outcome of the treatment of 88 patients with soft tissue sarcoma or aggressive fibromatosis who were managed with a combination of surgery and radiotherapy [18]. Radiotherapy consisted of a total dose of 60–66 Gy for high-grade sarcomas and 50–60 Gy for low-grade sarcomas or fibromatoses. Postoperatively the entire surgical wound with a 5 cm margin was treated with 50 Gy, with a shrinking field technique used to complete the total dose. Preoperatively 50 Gy was given, and the remainder was administered after wound healing. None of the patients received adjuvant chemotherapy. Patients were assessed at 3-month intervals using Enneking's regional assessment of functional status. A global score was calculated by awarding five points for excellent, three for good, one for fair, and zero for poor in each of the seven Enneking functional attributes (motion, pain, stability, deformity, strength, psychological acceptance, and ability). In addition, information about employment status, activity level, and edema of the extremity was obtained.

The variables analyzed for association with functional outcome included patient age; tumor grade, size, and location; need to sacrifice a major motor nerve; development of local postoperative complications; and timing of radiation. Local complications were defined as those requiring repeat surgery for wound dehiscence or vascular occlusion. Neural sacrifice was defined as the resection of a major motor nerve that was functional at presentation.

Eighty-eight patients were assessed at 12 months, and 44 were reassessed at 24 months. The mean functional scores for the 6 anatomical regions ranged from 23 for the proximal thigh to 31 for the forearm (maximum possible, 35). Only the proximal thigh had significantly lower values than other sites. Seventy-three percent were classified as excellent or good, and 27% as fair or poor. Neural sacrifice, wound complications, and tumor size ≥15 cm were associated with functional scores lower than 21, with size and neural sacrifice being the only significant variables on multivariate analysis. Investigation of the interaction among these three variables suggested that the risk of a poor functional outcome was increased when two or more of the three factors were present.

Detailed analysis of the reasons for poor function in the 20 patients with a score <21 was also carried out. Nine of these patients had lesions arising in the proximal thigh, six of whom had major complications arising from surgery and three of whom required sacrifice of the sciatic or femoral nerve. Of the remaining 11 patients with a poor outcome, 5 had lesions of the shoulder, and 4 of these required a shoulder girdle resection and scored poorly with respect to motion, strength, and stability. Three other patients suffered fractures in the high-dose volume. Pain was not a problem in this study because only nine patients in this study had a fair result with respect to pain and one had a poor result. At 12 months 50% had returned to full employment and activities, 25% had modified their employment or activities in a minor way, and 19% had significant limitation of their pretreatment activities. Seven patients had stopped working because of their functional results, and three found themselves disabled for all activity. Twenty-seven percent had moderate or severe edema in the affected extremity. Comparison of scores at 12 and 24 months failed to demonstrate any change in limb function over this time period.

Conclusions

Despite the large and difficult types of tumors studied, 68 of 88 (77%) patients had acceptable functional results and 61 (69%) returned to full employment and activity or had minor limitations. Location of the tumor did not appear to be an independently significant variable for predicting poor functional outcome. The poor functional results seen in patients with proximal thigh or shoulder lesions seemed to be due to their having large tumors, increased problems with wound complications, or tumors requiring neural sacrifice to achieve an adequate margin. Other authors have also noted an association between wound complications and poor functional outcome [6]. How could these results be improved? The size of the tumor cannot be changed, and the three patients with local recurrence all had microscopic residual disease along major nerves, suggesting that a more conservative surgical approach is not appropriate. However, measures to improve wound healing do improve functional outcome, particularly in thigh tumors. Problems with late fractures can be prevented by prophylactic stabilization of the weakened bone segment in those patients who have undergone an open cortical resection.

Clearly new treatment methods are required for those patients in the high-risk groups identified in their study. One of these methods may involve the use of interstitial radioactive implants, as described by Zelefsky et al. [19] in 45 patients who had locally advanced lesions extending to or involving major neurovascular structures. For 70% of these patients this was the primary treatment, and 30% were treated for recurrent disease. A median dose of 40 Gy was delivered at 42 cGy per hour, with those patients having gross residual disease, multiple positive/close margins, or suboptimal dose or dosimetry delivered by the implant also receiving external-beam radiotherapy. Five-year actuarial local control and in-field local control rates were 70% and 79%, respectively. Eighty-four percent maintained functional extremities without evidence of recurrence, with only those receiving doses in excess of 90 Gy (9%) developing a neuritis.

European experience

At the Royal Marsden Hospital in London, a study of limb function and quality of life in patients with pelvic girdle or lower limb sarcoma treated by limb conservation was carried out on a group of patients who were disease-free 2 or more years after treatment. Fifty-four patients attending the Sarcoma Clinic with a median time since treatment of 50 months (range 24–152) were studied. Although most patients who received radiotherapy had conventional 2 Gy per day fractionation, seven patients in this study were treated with a hypofractionated, once-a-week schedule [8] and three with a twice-daily hyperfractionated schedule [7]. Chemotherapy was not routinely employed.

An assessment of lower limb function and patient quality of life was developed. This included an evaluation of range of movement, muscle power, gait, need for walking aids, lymphedema, and radiation fibrosis. The second part of the assessment was a questionnaire evaluating the patients' perceived quality of life, including pain, using a modified Erdman scale, which assessed locomotion and the ability to climb stairs, to dress/groom oneself, and to manage around the home [20,21]. Changes in vocational and leisure activities were also documented.

Results

Only 15 patients had normal range of movement in all evaluated joints. As in Chang's study, tumors of the lower leg were particularly unfavorable in that all these patients had problems in the ankle or foot (six of seven were moderate or severe). Only 12 patients had normal power in all muscle groups (6 patients treated by surgery alone and 6 given radiotherapy as well). Once again, there was a difference between those patients with tumors of the lower leg, all of whom had a moderate or severe reduction in muscle power, and the three patients with tumors around the knee, one of whom had mild weakness only.

Ten patients reported pain at the time of assessment, but only six patients required regular analgesia. Fifty percent of patients had normal functional scores, but the median functional score of those receiving a dose >60 Gy was 12.5 compared with 9 (i.e., normal) for those receiving 60 Gy or less (p <

0.0001, Mann-Whitney U test). Two thirds (45 of 68) of the abnormal replies represented only a mild loss of function, with most serious functional losses being in leisure and vocational activities.

Chi-squared testing suggests a significant trend for the use of conventional radiotherapy to be associated with a more severe restriction of the range of movement ($p < 0.005$) and a worse overall functional score ($p < 0.01$) than surgery alone. High dose/hypofractionated radiotherapy was also associated with poorer muscle power than the use of surgery alone $p < 0.005$) and with the presence of pain ($p < 0.05$), and significantly more patients in the high-dose radiotherapy group had an abnormal gait compared with the other groups.

The only significant independent prognostic factors for poor limb function in the conventionally treated group were increasing age ($p < 0.002$) and the use of radiotherapy ($p < 0.025$). The functional score was predominantly determined by gait ($p < 0.001$), with muscle power and range of movement (clearly interrelated) also being important ($p < 0.001$).

Overall gait remained the major factor determining the functional score ($p < 0.001$). The dose (2 Gy equivalent) of radiotherapy used was the only other important factor ($p < 0.02$) if gait was included in the model. The probability that this effect might be causal is increased by the confirmation of a significant relationship between dose ($p < 0.001$) and field length ($p < 0.05$) and the degree of fibrosis.

The use of radiotherapy ($p < 0.005$) and increasing tumor size ($p < 0.02$) were risk factors for the development of a reduced range of movement, with the degree of radiation fibrosis ($p < 0.001$) and the extent of lymphedema ($p < 0.025$) being the other related factors. Only radiation fibrosis ($p < 0.01$) was significantly associated with poor muscle power. The use of physiotherapy was favorable ($p < 0.01$).

Initial statistical evaluation suggested that patients receiving radiotherapy had a worse functional outcome. However, multivariate analysis indicates that a number of factors are interrelated in determining the overall functional outcome. When all 54 patients are included the degree of radiation fibrosis, influenced by the dose of radiotherapy, is an important factor in the development of both a poor range of movement and poor muscle power. The latter is important in the development of an abnormal gait, which (along with radiation dose) is the most important factor in determining functional outcome.

Another analysis was based on the 41 patients treated with conventional radiotherapy. In this analysis, female sex, increasing patient age, and the use of radiotherapy were demonstrated to be significant adverse prognostic factors for gait and limb function. None of the surgical variables entered into the analysis were found to be independent prognostic factors, although there was an association between extent of surgery and range of movement on univariate analysis. This may due to the major effect of radiotherapy on limb function or, more likely, that the small number of patients in this study does not permit a definitive assessment of all factors determining functional outcome. It is apparent that in this study, as in others reported in this chapter, the majority of these patients compensate for the significant restrictions in range of movement and muscle power seen on objective testing, and thereby retain excellent lower limb function.

In another study reporting the results of treatment of 156 patients who had been treated at the Netherlands Cancer Institute in Amsterdam, Keus reported that 69% of assessable patients had a normal functioning limb, in 23% there was mild loss of motion, while in 7% severe impairment of function developed [22]. The most frequently scored complication was mild fibrosis (40%). Severe fibrosis with marked induration or contracture occurred in 16% of the patients. In 7% ulceration or a fistula in the treated area developed. Other severe complications were lymphoedema in 4% and vascular complications in 2% of the patients.

Functional results from treatment of lesions of hand and foot

Hand and wrist are rare sites of presentation for soft tissue sarcomas, and therefore there have been few published data on the results of conservative treatment [23–25]. A series of 17 cases was reported by Okunieff in 1986 [24]. Careful use was made of the shrinking field technique to minimize the volumes that received doses in excess of 60 Gy. Local control was achieved in 82% of patients, and of the 12 patients with local and distant control, 10 had less than a 25% decrease in limb function and had no pain or edema associated with normal use of their hands. The authors highlighted the importance of physiotherapy following treatment. They noted that patients often considered the treated limb to be normal but that they needed reminding that following treatment it was much more vulnerable to damage. They were instructed not to use their treated hands in heavy work or to expose them to a major risk of injury, work, or sports and to wear gloves as necessary.

Talbert reported 78 cases with soft tissue sarcomas arising in the wrist, hand, ankle, or foot treated with a combination of surgery and radiotherapy [25]. Overall 40 patients (51%) had normal function; however, 8 of these 40 had some complication that eventually resolved. Thirteen had mild to moderate dysfunction, and all of these had pain. Four had decreased range of motion, one had mild edema, one had recurrent muscle spasm and decreased joint mobility, one had a temporary ulcer, one had persistent lymphedema after dissection for nodal recurrence, one had neuropathy, and one suffered decreased bone growth. Severe dysfunction occurred in six (8%), usually with persistent soft tissue ulceration and pain. Six patients (8%) underwent amputation for complications, and 13 (17%) required amputation for recurrence. Overall 68% retained a normal or fairly normal extremity, and 16% had severe dysfunction or needed amputation for complications. Early in the series patients were treated using a hypoxic tourniquet technique, which was associated with increased late complications compared with conventional treatment. If these were omitted from the analysis, 55% of patients had normal functional status, 16% had mild to moderate dysfunction, 7% had severe dysfunction, only 3 underwent amputation for complications, and 18 underwent amputation for disease. The complication rate was significantly higher for patients with lesions of the lower extremity than those with upper extremity lesions: in the upper extremity 23% of patients suffered some complications of treatment, in the lower 56%.

Selch reported 20 patients with soft tissue sarcomas of the foot managed at the University of California at Los Angeles (UCLA) by limb salvage between 1974 and 1988 [26]. Sixteen (80%) were treated with the intraarterial doxorubicin and hypofractionated radiotherapy (35 cGy in 10 fractions), and the other 4 underwent attempted wide excision without preoperative treatment. Functional status was evaluated using a modified Enneking system. Fourteen of these 20 patients alive with local control were eligible for functional assessment. The overall rating was excellent in 5, good in 7, and fair in 2.

It is clear from these studies that with care it is possible to achieve extremity preservation with acceptable function in the majority of patients with soft tissue sarcomas of the hand, wrist, ankle, or foot.

Treatment factors determining outcome

Extent of surgery

Intuitively there should be an association between the extent of surgical resection and functional outcome. However, there have been few successful attempts to associate them in the literature. Usually the association described is between the extent of resection and wound complications. The extent of surgery was not an independent prognostic factor for limb function in the prospective study by Robinson et al. in 1991 [9]. A further report from the Royal Marsden Soft Tissue Sarcoma Unit detailed their experience with functional compartmental resections in 37 patients with intracompartmental tumors of the quadriceps or buttock [27]. As with almost all previous studies of lower limb function, they noted that, despite objective limitation of movement and muscle power, the level of function of these patients was either normal or only mildly impaired. Eight of nine who had undergone a functional compartmental resection preserving some innervated muscle within the compartment had returned to their previous employment.

Wound complications

As has been described previously, a number of authors have associated wound complication rate with functional outcome. Peat et al. looked at the risk factors associated with major wound healing complications in 180 patients undergoing limb-salvage surgery for soft tissue sarcoma [28]. In univariate analysis the cross-sectional area of tumor resection, the use of preoperative irradiation, the width of the skin excision, a history of smoking, and a history of diabetes and/or vascular disease were associated with wound failure. Multivariate analysis revealed that preoperative irradiation and resection diameter accounted for the risk of complications. Patients treated with distant vascularized tissue transfers following preoperative irradiation had a lower complication rate.

It is important to note that wound complications are not just a function of the adjuvant therapy used. Saddegh and Baner [29] reported the overall incidence of wound complication was 40% (16 infections, 13 necroses, and 12 hematomas) in 103 patients treated without adjuvant therapies. A significantly lower complication rate was seen in the upper extremity (17%) compared with the trunk and lower extremity (45%). Wound complications for deep tumors were significantly related to large tumor size, old age, long operating time, and excessive blood loss. They suggest that these results could be improved by taking into account the risk factors associated with wound complications, better preoperative planning, and close cooperation with plastic surgeons for adequate wound coverage.

Radiotherapy technique

The type (external or brachytherapy), timing, volume, dose, and fraction size all influence the late effects of radiotherapy and thus subsequent limb function. Brachytherapy was extensively evaluated at the Memorial Sloan-Kettering Cancer Center [30]. Its use can significantly increase the complication rate of the surgical procedure. However, if care is taken this can be minimized and subsequent limb function is very acceptable.

An interesting study by Nielsen et al. [31] compared the field sizes that would have been used for preoperative and postoperative radiotherapy in 26 patients. The preoperative field size was significantly smaller than the postoperative field size. This difference was only significant for tumors of the lower extremity, although there were a few patients with tumors of the groin and upper extremity. The number of joints involved in the field were significantly smaller in the preoperative group than in the postoperative group. This study provides quantitative data to confirm the commonly held view that the volume of normal tissue irradiated is less when irradiation is given preoperatively versus postoperatively, although this is not invariably so. This may well lead to a reduced complication rate.

Karasek et al. looked at 41 patients treated for lower extremity (25), upper extremity (8), and truncal (8) sarcomas [32]. They found a positive correlation between the volume irradiated to $\geq$55 Gy and functional score, strength, fibrosis, and skin changes. Total dose independent of volume was significantly associated with skin changes. An increase in peak dose was associated with fibrosis and skin changes. As the volume of the peak dose increased, more fibrosis developed. Neither range of motion nor total functional score was correlated with joint dose. Edema and functional score were not related to either volume or percent of limb circumference spared (receiving less than 50 Gy).

In the study by Robinson et al. the issue of radiotherapy dose and fractionation was addressed [9]. The results of the multivariate analysis are shown in Table 1. The only significant independent prognostic factors for poor limb function in the conventionally treated group were increasing age ($p < 0.002$) and the use of radiotherapy ($p < 0.025$). Overall gait remained the major factor determining the functional score ($p < 0.001$). The dose (2 Gy equivalent) of radiotherapy used was the only other important factor ($p < 0.02$) if gait was included in the model. The probability that this effect might be causal is increased by the confirmation of a significant relationship between dose ($p < 0.001$) and field length ($p < 0.05$) and the degree of fibrosis. None of the surgical variables entered into the analysis were found to be independent prognostic factors, although there was an association between extent of surgery and range of movement on univariate analysis.

Chemotherapy

The limited evidence available suggests that conventional chemotherapy in the absence of radiotherapy does not appear to influence the late sequelae of

Table 1. Independent prognostic factors for development of poor range of joint movement, muscle power, gait, fibrosis, and functional score determined by multivariate analysis of all 54 patients and by a separate analysis of 41 patients treated conventionally at the Royal Marsden Hospital

		Significant independent factors	
Endpoint		Prognostic	Associated
Function			
All	Dose RT	$p < 0.002$	Gait ($p < 0.001$)
Conventional	Age	$p < 0.002$	Gait ($p < 0.001$)
	Use of RT	$p < 0.0025$	Muscle power ($p < 0.001$)
Gait			
All	None		Muscle power ($p < 0.02$)
Conventional	Female	$p < 0.001$	Muscle power ($p < 0.001$)
	Age	$p < 0.02$	ROM ($p < 0.001$)
Muscle power			
All	Physiotherapy	$p < 0.01$	Fibrosis ($p < 0.01$)
Conventional	Use of RT	$p < 0.001$	None
Range of movement			
All	Use of RT	$p < 0.005$	Fibrosis ($p < 0.001$)
	Size	$p < 0.02$	Lymphedema
	Physiotherapy	$p < 0.05$	
Conventional	Use of RT	$p < 0.02$	None
Fibrosis			
All	Dose RT	$p < 0.001$	None
	Field length	$p < 0.05$	

RT = radiotherapy; ROM = range of motion.

limb-conservation treatment [10]. However, used intraarterially particularly in combination with hypofractionated radiotherapy, there is an unacceptable complication rate. This is likely to impact on consequent limb function. Chemotherapy may also impact on quality of life in different ways by affecting sex drive and cardiac function [33].

Physiotherapy

Lampert et al. reviewed the rehabilitation of patients with sarcoma, including soft tissue sarcoma and pediatric sarcomas [34]. Multiple problems can be expected as sequelae to the treatment, for example, osteoporosis or fractures may result from radiation therapy. It is for important to emphasize the need caution with patients involved in risk-taking activities. Swimming, golf, and tennis are acceptable, but contact supports should be avoided. Edema due to inelasticity or excision of lymphatic channels is not uncommon. Therapists may suggest intermittent compression machines, support garments, and elevation of the limb. In the past the main barrier to optimal rehabilitation of patients with soft tissue sarcoma has been failure to identify the problems amenable to rehabilitative intervention. It is particularly important that continuous assessment and intervention be provided, especially in children. In general, physiotherapy should continue for at least one year after surgery in the adult population.

Conclusions

The careful choice of surgical options can optimize functional outcome. Incisional biopsy should be restricted to that minority of patients in whom histology cannot be assessed with a Tru-cut biopsy needle [35]. When incisional biopsy is performed, the site of incision must be carefully chosen so as not to interfere with the definitive operation, which should be performed by a surgeon familiar with limb-preservation surgery. Wound complications compromise functional outcome, and every effort must be made to minimize them.

Radiotherapy is an important adjuvant treatment in the management of soft tissue sarcomas. Surgery alone is associated with a high local recurrence rate unless a radical resection is performed. This can rarely be achieved without amputation [36]. Preoperative or postoperative radiotherapy with more conservative surgery reduces the local failure rate to 10–15% [2,4–7]. However, the use of radiotherapy increases the risk of impairment of limb function. The results can be optimized by following simple guidelines. When radiotherapy is indicated, it is important to avoid irradiating the full circumference of the limb and to spare joints where at all possible. This often requires the use of an immobilization device [37] and may be facilitated by the use of CT planning. The optimum dose is not known, but at least 60 Gy is required to control residual disease, and a small dose per fraction should be used. Higher doses increase the risk of fibrosis, with subsequent limitation of joint movement.

Routine high-quality physiotherapy is essential. The majority of patients with extremity soft tissue sarcoma have excellent limb function following conservation therapy. New techniques, such as TNF-α and melphalan limb perfusion, are required to improve the prospects for the more difficult cases [38].

References

1. Aaronson NK, Bullinger M, Ahmedzai S. A modular approach to quality-of-life assessment in cancer clinical trials. Recent Results Cancer Res 111:231–249, 1988.
2. Abbatucci JS, Boulier N, De Ranieri J, Mandard AM, Tanguy A, Busson A. Radiotherapy as an integrated part of the treatment of soft tissue sarcomas. Radiother Oncol 2:115–121, 1984.
3. Eilber FR, Giuliano AE, Huth JF, Morton DL. A randomized prospective trial using post-operative adjuvant chemotherapy (Adriamycin) in high-grade extremity soft-tissue sarcoma. Am J Clin Oncol 11:39–45, 1988.
4. Potter DA, Kinsella T, Glatstein E, Wesley R, White DE, Seipp CA, Chang AE, Lack EE, Costa J, Rosenberg SA. High-grade soft tissue sarcomas of the extremities. Cancer 58:190–205, 1986.
5. Barkley HT, Jr., Martin RG, Romsdahl MM, Lindberg R, Zagars GK. Treatment of soft tissue sarcomas by preoperative irradiation and conservative surgical resection. Int J Radiat Oncol Biol Phys 14:693–699, 1988.
6. Suit HD, Mankin HJ, Wood WC, Gebhardt MC, Harman DC, Rosenberg A, Tepper JE, Rosenthal D. Treatment of the patient with stage Mo soft tissue sarcoma. J Clin Oncol 6:854–862, 1988.
7. Robinson M, Barr L, Fisher C, Fryatt I, Stotter A, Harmer C, Wiltshaw E, Westbury G. Treatment of extremity soft tissue sarcomas with surgery and radiotherapy. Radiother Oncol 18:221–233, 1990.
8. Ashby MA, Ago CT, Harmer CL. Hypofractionated radiotherapy for sarcomas. Int J Radiat Oncol Biol Phys 12:13–17, 1986.
9. Robinson MH, Spruce L, Eeles R, Fryatt I, Harmer CL, Thomas JM, Westbury G. Limb function following conservation treatment of adult soft tissue sarcoma. Eur J Cancer 27:1567–1574, 1991.
10. Chang AE, Steinberg SM, Culnane M, Lampert MH, Reggia AJ, Simpson CG, Hicks JE, White DE, Yang JJ, Glatstein E, Rosenberg SA. Functional and psychosocial effects of multimodality limb-sparing therapy in patients with soft tissue sarcomas. J Clin Oncol 7:1217–1228, 1989.
11. Sugarbaker PH, Barofsky I, Rosenberg SA, Gianola FJ. Quality of life assessment of patients in extremity sarcoma clinical trials. Surgery 91:17–23, 1982.
12. Pittam et al. Personal Communication.
13. Postma A, Kingma A, De-Ruiter JH, Koops HS, Veth RPH, Goeken LNH, Kamps WA, Karakousis CP. Quality of life in bone tumour patients comparing limb salvage and amputation of lower extremity. J Surg Oncol 51:47–51, 1992.
14. Christ GC. The psychosocial adaptation to bone cancer diagnsoed during adolescence: A long-term follow-up study. Diss Abstract Int A 53:2545, 1993.
15. Lampert MH, Gerber LH, Glatstein E, Rosenberg SA, Danoff JV. Soft tissue sarcoma: Functional outcome after wide local excision and radiation therapy. Arch Phys Med Rehabil 65:477–480, 1984.

16. Schipper H, Clinch J, McMurray A. Measuring the quality of life of cancer patients: The Functional Living Index-Cancer: Development and validation. J Clin Oncol 2:472–483, 1984.
17. Stinson SF, DeLaney TF, Greenberg J, Yang JC, Lampert MH, Hicks JE, Venzon D, White DE, Rosenberg SA, Glatstein EJ. Acute and long term effects on limb function of combined modality limb sparing therapy for extremity soft tissue sarcoma. Int J Radiat Oncol Biol Phys 21:1493–1499, 1991.
18. Bell RS, O'Sullivan B, Davis A, Langer F, Cummings B, Fornasier VL. Functional outcome in patients treated with surgery and irradiation for soft tissue tumours. J Surg Oncol 48:224–231, 1991.
19. Zelefsky MJ, Nori D, Shiu MH, Brennan MF. Limb salvage and soft tissue sarcomas involving neurovascular structures using combined surgical resection and brachytherapy. Int J Radiat Oncol Biol Phys 19:913–918, 1990.
20. Convery FR, Minteer MA, Amiel D, Connett KL. Polyarticular disability: Functional assessment. Arch Phys Med Rehabil 58:494–499, 1977.
21. Scranton J, Fogel ML, Erdman WR. II: Evaluation of functional levels of patients during and following rehabilitation. Arch Phys Med Rehabil 51:1–21, 1970.
22. Keus RB, Rutgers EJT, Ho GH, Gortzak E, Albus-Lutter CE, Hart AAM. Limb sparing therapy of extremity soft tissue sarcomas: Treatment outcome and long-term functional results. Eur J Cancer 30A:10:1459–1463, 1994.
23. Johnstone PA, Wexler LH, Venzon DJ, Jacobson J, Yang JC, Horowitz ME, DeLaney TF. Sarcomas of the hand and foot: Analysis of local control and functional result with combined modality therapy in extremity preservation. Int J Radiat Oncol Biol Phys 29:735–745, 1994.
24. Okunieff P, Suit HT, Proppe KH. Extremity preservation by combined modality treatment of sarcomas of the hand and wrist. Int J Oncol Biol Phys 12:1923–1929, 1986.
25. Talbert ML, Zagars GK, Sherman NE, Romsdahl MM. Conservative surgery and radiation therapy for soft tissue sarcoma of the wrist, hand, ankle, and foot. Cancer 66:2482–2491, 1990.
26. Selch MT, Kopald KH, Ferreiro GA, Mirra JM, Parker RG, Eilber FR. Limb salvage therapy for soft tissue sarcomas of the foot. Int J Radiat Oncol Biol Phys 19(Suppl 1):124, 1990.
27. Pitcher ME, Thomas JM. Functional compartmental resection for soft tissue sarcomas. Eur J Surg Oncol 20:441–445, 1994.
28. Peat BG, Bell RS, Davis A, O'Sullivan B, Mahoney J, Manktelow RT, Bowen V, Catton C, Fornasier VL, Langer F. Wound-healing complications after soft-tissue sarcoma surgery. Plast Reconstr Surg 93:980–987, 1994.
29. Saddegh MK, Bauer HC. Wound complication in surgery of soft tissue sarcoma. Analysis of 103 consecutive patients managed without adjuvant therapy. Clin Orthopaed 289:247–253, 1993.
30. Arbeit JM, Lees DE, Corsey R, Brennan MF. Resting energy expenditure in controls and cancer patients with localized and diffuse disease. Ann Surg 199:292–298, 1984.
31. Nielsen OS, Cummings B, O'Sullivan B, Catton C, Bell RS, Fornasier VL. Preoperative and postoperative irradiation of soft tissue sarcomas: Effect on radiation field size. Int J Radiat Oncol Biol Phys 21:1595–1599, 1991.
32. Karasek K, Constine LS, Rosier R. Sarcoma therapy: Functional outcome and relationship to treatment parameters. Int J Radiat Oncol Biol Phys 24:651–656, 1992.
33. Weddington WW. Psychological outcomes in survivors of extremity sarcomas following amputation or limb-sparing surgery. Cancer Treat Res 56:53–60, 1991.
34. Lampert MH, Gahagen C. Physical therapy for the cancer patient. In CL McGarvey, ed. Rehabilitation of the Sarcoma Patient. Clinics in Physical Therapy. New York: Churchill Livingstone, 1990:111–135.
35. Ball ABS, Fisher C, Pittam M, Watkins RM, Westbury G. Diagnosis of soft tissue tumours by Tru-Cut[R] biopsy. Br J Surg 77:756–758, 1990.
36. Stotter AT, A'Hern RP, Fisher C, Mott AF, Fallowfield ME, Westbury G. The influence of local recurrence of extremity soft tissue sarcoma on metastasis and survival. Cancer 66:1119–1129, 1990.

37. Light KL. Immobilisation and treatment of patients receiving radiation therapy for extremity soft tissue sarcoma. Med Dosim 17:135–139, 1992.
38. Schraffordt-Koops H, Lienard D, Eggermont AM, Hoekstra HJ, VanGeel BN, Lejeune FJ. Isolated limb perfusion with high-dose TNF-alpha, gamma-IFN, and mephalan in patients with unresectable soft tissue sarcomas: A highly effective limb-sparing procedure. Society of Surgical Oncology, 46th Annual Cancer Symposium in Conjunction with Society of Head and Neck Surgeons March, 1993, Los Angeles, CA, p 1.

7. Benign and low-grade tumors of the soft tissues: Role for radiation therapy

Herman D. Suit, Ira J. Spiro, and Matthew Spear

Introduction

There is a misconception in some oncology circles that low-grade tumors are not likely to be controlled by clinically feasible radiation doses. This is so despite the abundant data that radiation alone achieves a high probability of permanent and complete responses of basal cell carcinomas of the skin, well-differentiated squamous cell carcinoma of the glottis, etc. Patients are not as concerned about the rate of response as about the probability that the response will ultimately be complete and permanent. The evidence available is that the low-grade soft tissue sarcomas respond as well as the high-grade ones. However, the difference between the low- and the high-grade sarcomas is that for low-grade sarcomas the time to achieve an observable response may be long. In this chapter we consider the response of fibromatosis and dermatofibrosarcoma protuberans (DFSP) to radiation alone or combined with surgery.

Fibromatosis

Clinical features

Fibromatoses are benign neoplasms comprised of fibroblastic cells and an extensive collagen matrix. They arise in the superficial fascia and the musculo-aponeurotic tissues at all body sites. There are four classes of superficial fibromatoses. These have a relatively benign natural history. They include lesions that arise in association with Dupuytren's contracture, superficial plantar fibromatosis, knuckle pads, and Peyronie's disease. Our interest in this chapter is the fibromatoses arising in the aponeurotic tissues and deep fascial tissues, which used to be called desmoid tumors. In this chapter, consideration is given only to these more aggressive and more deeply sited lesions.

The initial description of the deep-seated fibromatoses was in 1832 by Macfarlane, and the name was given in 1856 by Muller [1]. These are infrequent tumors, with an incidence in Scandinavian populations of ~2–4 cases/

J. Verweij, H.M. Pinedo, and H.D. Suit (eds). SOFT TISSUE SARCOMAS: PRESENT ACHIEVEMENTS AND FUTURE PROSPECTS.

year/million persons [2]. The most frequent sites of involvement by these fibromatoses are the torso and extremities. Trauma is a factor in the generation of occasional cases. They infrequently appear in the surgical bed and may be confused with a regrowth of the primary lesion. We have seen one such patient with fibromatosis developing at the site of a radical mastectomy. Another unusual feature of patients with fibromatosis in an extremity is that, despite multiple lesions, the repeat tumors are, with few exceptions, confined to the initially affected extremity. There is a genetic component to a small fraction of these deeply sited fibromatoses; namely, they are one of the components of Gardner's syndrome, although only a proportion of Gardner's syndrome patients (~10%) manifest fibromatosis. Among 71 families and 168 individuals in the Finnish Polyposis Registry, there were 19 persons who were known to have fibromatosis [3].

Clinical malignancy

Pathologists vary in their views on the most appropriate designation of fibromatosis: benign or malignant. The Soft-Tissue Task Force in 1977 classified fibromatosis as fibrosarcoma grade I (desmoid type) [4]. Posner et al. of the Memorial Sloan-Kettering Cancer Center ranked these tumors as low-grade malignancies, principally due to the property of local invasiveness [5]. These neoplasms are currently classed as benign by the WHO International Classification of Tumours [6]. Their natural history includes local infiltration and destruction, and essentially a zero probability of establishing metastases. They often recur after resection and may progress locally and cause death. Thus, although classified as benign, they do result in death due to local destruction in a small but important fraction of patients. As supporting evidence of their benign nature, the frequency of local control in patients whose surgical resection yielded specimens with microscopically positive margins or even minimal gross residual disease is not negligible [6]. Spontaneous regression has been reported. Extremely large lesions, for example, ≥20 cm, have been reported to be controlled locally following doses of ≤40 Gy [7]. Additionally, complete and sustained responses have been reported after hormonal manipulation or *low*-dose chemotherapy, which is essentially unknown for malignant neoplasms of the mesenchymal tissues. Whatever designation is applied to fibromatoses, they do not have a natural history or response to the various therapies that is comparable with that of the unquestioned sarcomas.

A report by Posner et al. [5] from the Memorial Sloan-Kettering Cancer Center indicated a fatal outcome in 11 of 131 patients. The anatomic sites were head/neck, two; chest wall, one; and abdominal wall/retroperitoneum, eight. In their analysis, the poor outcomes tended to be associated with age between 18 and 30 years, recurrent disease, and absence of postoperative radiation treatment. For most of the published data, deaths attributed to the fibromatosis are rare. There are few reports of transformation of a fibromatosis into a well- to moderately differentiated spindle cell sarcoma during the progress of the disease through one or several local recurrences. In those patients the accuracy of the initial diagnosis is usually questioned in terms of the validity of pathologic interpretation or the adequacy of tissue sampling.

Surgical treatment

Treatment of the patient with a fibromatosis is surgical resection, if this can be accomplished, and retain for the patient a 'reasonable' functional and cosmetic result. Planning of the resection should be based on the achievement of negative margins. However, an interesting fact pertaining to local control of fibromatosis by surgery is that regrowth is not certain, even though the surgical margins were microscopically positive or removal of all gross disease was not accomplished. This pertains especially to primary fibromatoses. However, the composite published experience indicates that there is a definite advantage to securing negative margins.

Posner et al. observed local regrowths in approximately 50% and 75% of patients after wide or partial resections, respectively. Radiation applied postoperatively reduced the local failure frequency. This was especially true for gross residual disease [5]. Rock et al. from the University of Minnesota likewise observed a correlation between the extent of resection and the failure rate [8]. This was likewise found in pediatric subjects [9]. Such an effect of surgical margins has not been uniformly observed. For example, Catton et al. found no significant difference in relapse rates according to margin status [10]. Reitamo et al. [11] reported the opposite result, that is, 17% and 24% relapse rates after incomplete and complete resections, respectively. Karakousis et al. [12] reported control rates of 69% (11 in 16) following surgery alone. The recently analyzed Massachusetts General Hospital (MGH) experience is that local failure was observed in 5 of 6 patients with gross residual and 5 of 12 patients with microscopic residual disease after surgery alone [13]. For patients with microscopically clear margins, there were 6 in 23 local failures (26%). For the entire group of 51 patients treated with surgery alone (including 10 patients for whom the margin status was not defined), the 5-year actuarial tumor-free rates were 77% and 48% for primary and recurrent lesion, respectively.

Radiation

Table 1 presents a summary of the recent published results of local control of fibromatosis by radiation alone and combined with surgery.

Radiation alone

McCollough et al. [7] found that radiation for grossly evident fibromatosis at the University of Florida yielded local control in 6 of 6 primary and 8 of 10 recurrent fibromatoses. That local control was realized in two patients whose

Table 1. Local control of desmoid tumors treated by radiation ± surgery

Center	Local control	Reference
JCRT	8/9	Greenberg et al., 1981 [31]
UCSF	13/19	Leibel et al., 1983 [32]
Amsterdam	19/21	Keus and Bartelink, 1986 [14]
Westminister Hospital	28/38	Stockdale et al., 1988 [33]
Institut Curie	12/16	Bataini et al., 1988 [34]
University of Florida	25/30	McCollough et al., 1991 [13]
Massachusetts General Hospital	43/51	Spear et al., 1994 (unpublished data)

fibromatoses were 20 × 22 cm and 20 × 25 cm following doses of 40 and 35 Gy is worth special note. This result could not be expected for a true malignant tumor of the mesenchymal soft tissues. Local control has been achieved at the MGH for each of the 5 primary tumors treated by radiation alone and for 9 of the 10 recurrent tumors, a total of 14 in 15. The 5-year actuarial local control rate for these 15 tumors is 92% [13].

Radiation and surgery

For treatment of microscopic residual disease at the University of Florida [7], local control was obtained in 3 of 4 primary and in 8 of 10 recurrent lesions (11 in 14), respectively. In their combined experience, only two failures were within the original radiation fields. Following surgery + radiation, local control was reported by Karakousis et al. [12] in 11 of 11 patients. Local control was obtained in 12 of 13 patients at the Netherlands Cancer Institute, as reported by Keus and Bartelink [14] in 1986. At the MGH, combined modality management was employed in 41 patients. At 5 years, the actuarial local control results were 79% and 67% for primary and recurrent lesions, respectively; this difference was not significant [12]. An analysis of the topography of the nine local failures showed that two were beyond the margins of the radiation fields (at 5 cm and 20 cm from the edge). Three of the failures were at the field margins.

Our interpretation of the published data is that 55–60 Gy given over 6–8 weeks achieves permanent control of fibromatosis in ~80% of patients. Furthermore, the outcome does not appear to have a definite dependence on tumor volume. This is implied by the observation that the results of radiation alone are apparently equivalent to radiation combined with surgery. There is a local control advantage for treatment of the primary compared with the recurrent fibromatosis by surgery, radiation, or the two combined.

Chemotherapy

Despite the pathological features of a very low-grade fibroblastic process, characterized predominately by collagen fibers and few cells, there have been reports of complete responses to moderate-dose chemotherapy [15]. Similarly, antiestrogen therapy has had some successes, especially tamoxifen [16]. A variety of other agents have been reported to yield an occasional complete response, for example, indomethacin [17].

Discussion

The experience from several institutions described earlier, provides ample evidence for the efficacy of radiation as a therapeutic modality for fibromatoses. This is true for radiation administered alone or in combination with surgery. Local control data on radiation alone of primary tumors is particularly impressive. This is despite the fact that fibromatosis is a benign fibroblastic lesion. Were the concept that low-grade tumors are radiation resistant valid, then fibromatoses would be particularly resistant. Another aspect of the published data relevant to this point is the documentation of good responses by fibromatoses to modest dose levels of chemotherapy and also of antiestrogen medication.

Despite these well-documented successes with nonsurgical methods, for the present our judgment is that the preferred treatment is resection. For primary lesions that have been resected but with microscopically positive margins, we would observe. The point is to avoid further surgery or radiation when there is a clinically useful probability of there being no subsequent regrowth and when the patient is not at risk of distant metastasis.

As to the priority that should be placed on using surgery for initial treatment, our opinion is that the degree of functional impairment that has been considered as reasonable may need some downward revision in view of the demonstrated high local control rates achieved using radiation alone. This is especially true in the management of lesions in the head/neck region, where good surgical margins are difficult to achieve. When radiation is employed, we use total dose levels of 50–60 Gy, administered at 1.8–2.0 Gy/fraction and 5 fractions/week. The actual dose used is a function of the magnitude of the treatment volume, conditions of the normal tissues, and the severity and nature of comorbidities. If judged reasonable, our dose is 60 Gy and is reduced to allow for important clinical concerns. Furthermore, there is now more than one option, that is, chemotherapy and hormonal manipulation.

For the patient who exhibits multifocal disease, that is, fibromatoses developing at several sites within an extremity, the role of chemotherapy could be evaluated by prospective clinical studies.

Dermatofibrosarcoma protuberans

Taylor was the first, in 1890, to record a gross description of a dermatofibrosarcoma protuberans. Darier and Ferrand defined the histological features in 1924, and in 1925 the name *dermatofibrosarcoma protuberans* (DFSP) was proposed by Hoffman [18].

Clinical features

These tumors are uncommon, that is, they make up <0.1% of all malignancies [18]. Of the 853 patients in the AFIP series, 47% were sited in the torso, 20% in the lower extremity, 18% in the upper extremity, and 14%, in the head/neck [19]. DFSP appears in the dermis as a slowly growing nodular mass. In our experience and that of the centers that have reported in the past decade, the lesion tends to be rather small, with the great majority being ≤5 cm [20]. They are generally painless in this small size range, unless impinging on neurovascular bundles. The male-to-female ratio is ~1.25–1.5:1. A rare variety of DFSP is Bednar tumor, in which there is melanin deposition. The gross appearance and clinical behavior are similar to those of 'standard' DFSP, except for the black/dark coloration.

Clinical malignancy

This group of histiocytic tumors borders between true malignancy and benign status. Regional or distant metastases are virtually unknown in patients who achieve local control of their primary DFSP. There are reports of occasional patients who do develop metastatic disease who have had multiple surgeries for repeated recurrences. In a review of the literature, Rutgers et al. [20] found a total of 37 patients who had developed metastatic disease; in 36 of these patients there had been ≥1 local regrowths of tumor. In the 37th patient, information was not given on this point. Most of the small number of patients who develop distant metastases have foci of fibrosarcoma in the predominately dermatofibrosarcoma protuberans. These are designated as DFSP-FS [21]. Thus, the propensity for these tumors to spread beyond the local lesion is extremely low for simple DFSP and is not very high for those lesions designated DFSP-FS. Hence, a successful treatment outcome depends almost entirely on the achievement of local control.

Pathology

Dermatofibrosarcoma protuberans are low-/intermediate-grade cutaneous sarcomas. Their microscopic appearance is fibrohistiocytic and is characterized as whorled and/or cartwheel. There usually is infiltration of the adjacent normal tissues [19]. Cytogenetic studies of the DFSP have shown that a relatively frequent abnormality is formation of ring 22 chromosomes [22]. These special findings are not known to have prognostic significance. There have been no studies that have demonstrated a relationship between the cytogenetic alterations and clinical behavior. Allan et al. [23] interpreted their cytogenetic findings as consistent with a monoclonal origin of DFSP.

There is a variant of DFSP that is characterized by the presence of fibrosarcomatous foci/regions in an otherwise standard dermatofibrosarcoma protuberans. Connelly and Evans described their experience with 30 DFSP patients and 6 patients whose tumor had fibrosarcomatous areas (DFSP-FS) [21]. They reported that the margins of the DFSP components were infiltrative, while the margins of the FS regions were rather circumscribed. Treatment was by surgery alone. The local control results were essentially the same for the two groups of tumors. There were two deaths, but these were in the DFSP-FS group.

Histopathological assessment of the status of the surgical margins is a critical part of planning the overall management strategy, that is, additional resection versus radiation. There may be an advantage in the assessment of margin status by staining for anti-CD-34 [24]. Goldblum [25] employed CD-34 staining and found that the stain was strongly positive in all portions of the 30 DFSP lesions examined. In comparison, seven lesions were classified as DFSP-FS; the stain was absent in the DFSP-FS components but present in the typical DFSP regions.

Surgical treatment

In medically intact patients, the recommended treatment for DFSP patients is wide surgical resection, that is, margins of ≥3–5 cm beyond the gross disease and negative margins on pathological study. The clinical advantage of obtaining such wide margins has been repeatedly stressed [20,21,26,27].

Approximately half of all patients experience local regrowth when their surgical procedure has not involved wide margins [20]. In the review of a total of 264 patients, a failure rate of ~13% was realized by the use of wide margin resection. They also noted that wide resections with clear margins were quite effective against recurrent lesions.

This was corroborated by Smola et al. [26], who reported local failures in 6 of 7 patients whose margins were ≤1 cm and 0 of 11 failures for margins of 1.5–3 cm. Bendix-Hansen et al. [27] observed no local failures in seven patients whose margins were ≥3 cm. They had eight local failures after local excision; these eight achieved local control of their recurrent disease with wide margin resection. Parker and Zitelli [28] evaluated the outcome of Mohs micrographic surgery in 20 patients. To achieve clearance, a margin of 2.5 cm was essential, except for tumors of ≤2 cm diameter, a 1.5 cm margin appeared effective. These 20 patients had local control at 3–105 months. Rutgers et al. [20] reported local control in 6 of 6 patients treated by wide resection for primary DFSP.

Radiation treatment

Today, a wide resection that is shown to have obtained negative margins is clearly an effective treatment method for DFSP. There are virtually no clinical data on the response of dermatofibrosarcoma protuberans to radiation, and the data are only a few case reports. Earlier radiation was thought to be of little efficacy, but there were no data on local regrowth rates as functions of dose and observation times. For example, Mark et al. [29], in their review of their experience with DFSP patients, mentioned a medically inoperable patient with a DFSP of the scalp who was treated with 64 Gy. This individual had local control for 3 years and died of intercurrent disease. The efficacy of radiation in achieving local control in patients whose surgical resection specimen has positive margins is demonstrated by a report from the Ontario Cancer Institute to the 1995 meeting of American Society of Therapeutic Radiology and Oncology [30]. They treated 19 such patients and local control was achieved in 17.

Experience of the Massachusetts General Hospital

We have treated 18 patients using radiation alone or radiation combined with surgery at the Massachusetts General Hospital. The outcome in these patients is presented here. Three patients were treated for their DFSP using radiation alone and 15 with radiation combined with surgery. These patients had disease located at the following sites: head/neck, 10; chest wall/shoulder, 5; upper extremity, 2; and lower extremity, 1. The male-to-female ratio was 11:7; patient ages were in the range of 24–67 years (median, 46 years). Most of these tumors were small, that is, ≤5 cm, in 14. Eight tumors were recurrent.

Two of the 18 tumors were grade II. Fifteen tumors were resected, and positive margins were found in 12 of the specimen (cells at the inked margins). Of the three negative margins, cells were present at ≤1 mm and at 3 mm. For the third, the first surgical procedure was for a 15-cm lesion, and margins were positive. A re-resection for local regrowth also had positive margins. The tumor bed was given 50 Gy and was then resected for a third time. This specimen had no recognizable tumor cells.

The radiation-treatment techniques were based on external photon or electron beams alone or combined with brachytherapy. The total doses used were 67–75 Gy for radiation alone; 60–78 Gy for radiation combined with resection and positive margins; and 50, 50, and 64 Gy for the three patients with negative margins.

Treatment results

The 10-year actuarial local control rate for the 18 patients was 88%. There were three local failures, and surgical salvage was successful in all three. Radiation was the sole treatment in three patients (one primary and two recurrent lesions). Sustained local control has been obtained in each of these patients, for example, no evident tumor at 85, 106, and 108 months. Cosmetic results are quite good in two patients; there is moderate atrophy and telangectesia in the third. Due to the paucity of clinical outcome data for this tumor, we present a brief clinical synopsis of these three patients.

Case reports

Patient 1. This 31-year-old female was seen for a postsurgical recurrent DFSP. The lesion was a nodular mobile 8.5 × 4.5 cm and overlaid the manubrium and right upper anterior chest wall. Treatment was 66.7 Gy by electron beam plus brachytherapy. The patient remains free of evident tumor at 9 years.

Patient 2. This 24-year-old male was seen for a primary 5 × 5 cm nodular nonfixed DFSP sited immediately behind the right frontal hairline. Treatment was 70 Gy given by electron beam plus brachytherapy. The patient is well with no evidence of tumor at 9 years.

Patient 3. This 55-year-old female presented with a 4 × 3 cm recurrent DFSP located over the right corner of her mouth and the lateral aspect of her chin. Her treatment was also by electron beam plus brachytherapy to 74 Gy. There has been near-complete regression of the nodularity with an excellent cosmetic result at 10 years.

Fifteen patients have been managed by combining radiation and surgery. There have been 3 local failures among the 15 patients. These occurred at 46, 132, and 17 months. The actuarial 10-year local control is 84%. These developed among the 12 patients whose surgical specimen had positive margins.

Each of the 3 local failures have had a locally successful surgical salvage. Fourteen patients are alive and are free of tumor and significant treatment-related morbidity. These results are based on a median observation time of 79 months. One patient died from intercurrent disease at 72 months post surgical salvage.

Discussion

The data presented here from the Ontario Cancer Institute and the Massachusetts General Hospital demonstrate that there is an effective alternate to radical surgery, which would result in major functional and/or cosmetic loss to the patient. Additionally, for the occasional patient who is not medically or technically operable or for whom surgery is not acceptable, radiation alone appears to provide a serious potential for long-term control with good cosmetic and functional outcomes.

The material presented in this review demonstrates a high level of efficacy of radiation against two categories of low-grade mesenchymal soft tissue neoplasms. We found no data to indicate a lesser effectiveness for the low-grade than for the high-grade disease. If there were a difference, the gain would appear to lie with treatment of low-grade lesions.

Acknowledgments

The authors wish to thank Claire Hunt, Cindy Triau, and Bill Daly for their excellent assistance with preparation of the manuscript, data collection, and data analysis.

References

1. McAnena OJ, Daly JM. Desmoid fibrosarcoma; Gardner's syndrome. In JH Raaf, ed. Soft Tissue Sarcomas. Diagnosis and Treatment. St. Louis, MO: CV Mosby, 1993:151.
2. McAnena OJ, Daly JM. Desmoid fibrosarcoma; Gardner's syndrome. In JH Raaf, ed. Soft Tissue Sarcomas. Diagnosis and Treatment. St. Louis, MO: CV Mosby, 1993:153.
3. Jarvinen HJ. Desmoid disease as a part of the familial adenomatous polyposis coli. Acta Chir Scand 153:379–383, 1987.
4. Russell WO, Cohen J, Enzinger F, Hajdu SI, Heise H, Martin RG, Meissner W, Miller WT, Schmitz RL, Suit HD. A clinical and pathological staging system for soft tissue sarcomas. Cancer 40:1562–1570, 1977.
5. Posner MC, Shiu MH, Newsome JL, Hajdu SI, Gaynor JJ, Brennan MF. The fibromatoses. Arch Surg 124:191–196, 1989.
6. Weiss SW. Histological Typing of Soft Tissue Tumours, 2nd ed. Berlin: Springer-Verlag, 1994.
7. McCollough WM, Parsons JT, van der Griend R, Enneking WF, Heare T. Radiation therapy for aggressive fibromatosis: The experience at the University of Florida. J Bone Joint Surg 73A:717–725.
8. Rock MG, Pritchard DJ, Reiman HM, Soule EH, Brewster RC. Extra-abdominal fibromatosis. J Bone Joint Surg 66A:1369–1374, 1984.
9. Faulkner LB, Hajdu SI, Kher U, LaQuaglia M, Exelby PR, Heller G, Wollner N. Pediatric desmoid tumor: Retrospective analysis of 63 cases. J Clin Oncol 13:2813–2818, 1995.
10. Catton CN, O'Sullivan B, Bell R, Cummings B, Fornasier V, Panzarella T. Aggressive fibromatosis: Optimisation of local management with a retrospective failure analysis. Radiother Oncol 34:17–22, 1995.
11. Reitamo JJ, Scheinin TM, Hayry P. The fibromatosis syndrome: New aspects in the cause, pathogenesis and treatment of the fibromatosis. Am J Surg 151:230–237, 1986.
12. Karakousis CP, Mayordomo J, Zografos GC, Driscoll DL. Desmoid tumors of the trunk and extremity. Cancer 72:1637–1641, 1993.
13. Spear M, Jennings LC, Efird JT, Mankin HJ, Springfield DS, Gebhardt MC, Spiro IJ, Rosenberg AE, Suit HD. Radiation therapy and surgery in the treatment of fibromatosis. Unpublished data.
14. Keus R, Bartelink H. The role of radiotherapy in the treatment of fibromatosis. Radiother Oncol 7:1–5, 1986.
15. Patel SR, Evans HL, Benjamin RS. Combination chemotherapy in adult desmoid tumors. Cancer 72:3244–3247, 1993.
16. Kinzbrunner B, Ritter S, Domingo J, Rosenthal CJ. Remission of rapidly growing desmoid tumors after tamoxifen therapy. Cancer 52:2201–2204, 1983.
17. Waddell WR, Gerner RE, Reich MP. Non-sterioid anti-inflammatory drugs and tamoxifen for desmoid tumors and carcinoma of the stomach. J Surg Oncol 22:197–211, 1983.
18. Gaskill HV, Aust JB. Dermatofibrosarcoma protuberans; fibromatosis of the hands and feet; pseudosarcomatous lesions. In JH Raaf, ed. Soft Tissue Sarcomas. Diagnosis and Treatment. St. Louis, MO: CV Mosby, 1993:101.
19. Enzinger FM, Weiss SW. Soft Tissue Tumors, 2nd ed. St. Louis, MO: CV Mosby, 1988:252.
20. Rutgers EJG, Kroon BBR, Albus-Lutter CE, Gortzak E. Dermatofibrosarcoma protuberans: Treatment and prognosis. Eur J Surg Oncol 18:241–248, 1992.

21. Connelly JH, Evans HL. Dermatofibrosarcoma protuberans. A clinicopathologic review with emphasis on fibrosarcomatous areas. Am J Surg Pathol 161:921–925, 1992.
22. Pedeutour F, Simon MP, Minoletti F, Sozzi G, Pierotti MA, Hecht F, Turc-Carel C. Ring 22 chromosomes in dermatofibro-sarcoma protuberans are low-level amplifiers of chromosome 17 and 22 sequences. Cancer Res 55:2400–2403, 1995.
23. Allan AE, Tsou HC, Harrington A, Stasko T, Lee X, Si SP, Grande DJ, Peacocke M. Clonal origin of dermatofibrosarcoma protuberans. J Invest Dermatol 100:99–102, 1993.
24. Jimenez FJ, Grichnik JM, Buchanan MD, Clark RE. Immunohistochemical margin control applied to Mohs micrographic surgical excision of dermatofibrosarcoma protuberans. J Dermatol Surg Oncol 20:687–689, 1994.
25. Goldblum JR. CD34 positivity in fibrosarcomas which arise in dematofibrosarcoma protuberans. Arch Pathol Lab Med 119:238–241, 1995.
26. Smola MG, Soyer HP, Scharnagl E. Surgical treatment of dermatofibrosarcoma protuberans. A retrospective study of 20 cases with review of literature. Eur J Surg Oncol 17:447–453, 1991.
27. Bendix-Hansen K, Myhre-Jensen O, Kaae S. Dermatofibro-sarcoma Protuberans. A clinicopathological study of nineteen cases and review of world literature. Scand J Plast Reconstr Surg 17:247–252, 1983.
28. Parker TL, Zitelli JA. Surgical margins for excision of dermatofibrosarcoma protuberans. J Am Acad Dermatol 32:233–236, 1995.
29. Mark RJ, Bailet JW, Tran LM, Poen J, Fu YS, Calcaterra TC. Dermatofibrosarcoma protuberans of the head and neck. Arch Otolaryngol Head Neck Surg 119:891–896, 1993.
30. O'Sullivan G, Catton C, Bell R, Fornasier V, Gullane P, Cummings B, Quirt I, Wunder J. Treatment outcome in dermatofibrosarcoma protuberans referred to a radiation oncology practice. Int J Radiat Oncol Biol Phys 32(S1):289, 1995.
31. Greenberg HM, Goebel R, Weischselbaum RR, Greenberger JS, Chaffey JT, Cassady JR. Radiation therapy in the treatment of aggressive fibromatoses. Int J Radiat Oncol Biol Phys 7:305–310, 1981.
32. Leibel SA, Wara WM, Hill DR, et al. Desmoid tumors: Local control and patterns of relapse following radiation therapy. Int J Radiat Oncol Biol Phys 9:1167–1171, 1983.
33. Stockdale AD, Cassoni AM, Coe MA, et al. Radiotherapy and conservative surgery in the management of musculo-aponeurotic fibromatosis. Int J Radiat Oncol Biol Phys 15:851–857, 1988.
34. Bataini JP, Belloir C, Mazabraud A, Pilleron PP, Cartigny A, Jaulerry C, Ghossein NA. Desmoid tumors in adults: The role of radiotherapy in their management. Am J Surg 155:754–760, 1988.

8. Brachytherapy for soft tissue sarcomas

Phillip M. Devlin and Louis B. Harrison

Introduction

In this chapter we focus on the use of brachytherapy for soft tissue sarcoma. It is recognized that external-beam radiation therapy has been the traditional radiation approach to these tumors. However, emerging retrospective and prospective data have shown the value of the brachytherapy approach. We review soft tissue sarcoma of the extremity and superficial trunk, and also of the retroperitoneum. We also review the implant technique, retrospective data, our prospective trial, and our current practice at the Memorial Sloan-Kettering Cancer Center (MSKCC).

Concept of brachytherapy

Brachytherapy consists of the placement of placing radioactive isotopes in close proximity to or directly into tumors. This allows for high doses of radiation to be delivered to the tumor or tumor bed with minimal doses to surrounding normal tissue. The therapeutic advantages of this approach are obvious. Whereas early experience was gained with radium, contemporary practice focuses overwhelmingly on iridium-192 and iodine-125. Cesium-137 still has a role in gynecological and other intracavitary applications. Iridium-192 emits gamma rays with average energy of 380 keV, has a half-life of 74.2 days, and has a half value layer in lead of 2.5 mm. Iodine mainly emits x-rays in the diagnostic range, with an average energy of 28 keV, a half-life of 60.2 days, and a half value layer of 0.025 mm in lead.

How brachytherapy differs from external-beam radiation therapy

The traditional radiation approach to sarcomas has involved adjuvant external-beam radiation therapy (EBRT). This treatment begins 4–8 weeks after surgery or is given as preoperative treatment. The radiation field sizes have been quite generous, with greater than or equal to a 5 cm margin around

J. Verweij. H.M. Pinedo. and H.D. Suit (eds). SOFT TISSUE SARCOMAS: PRESENT ACHIEVEMENTS AND FUTURE PROSPECTS.

Table 1. Comparison of different techniques for adjuvant sarcoma irradiation: brachytherapy versus external-beam radiation therapy

	Brachytherapy	External-beam radiation therapy
Time required	10–14 days	7–8 weeks
Volume irradiated	Tumor plus 1.5–2 cm	Tumor plus large margin (5 cm) with shrinking field
Scar irradiated?	No	Yes
Drain site irradiated?	No	Yes
Compartment irradiated?	No	Yes
Patient leaves hospital completing all therapy?	Yes	No

Reproduced with permission of author from [28].

Table 2. Differences in radiation treatment–related charges for preoperative external-beam irradiation and interstitial radiotherapy[a]

Charges	EB	IR	Difference[b]
Professional charges	\$4390	\$3240	\$1150
Hospital-based charges	\$6515	\$6600	\$85
Total	\$10,905	\$9840	\$1065

[a] Hospital-based charges are based on an average implant size of 80 cm of iridium wire, which represents the average length of an implant and includes an additional \$2550 of hospital-based charges for IR accounting for operating room time and 5 extra hospital room days.
[b] The difference was significant at $p < 0.0001$.
EB = external-beam irradiation; IR = interstitial therapy.
Reproduced with permission from Lippincott-Raven Publishers, Philadelphia PA [2].

the tumor bed and a shrinking field technique. Preoperative doses of 5000 cGy over 5 weeks and postoperative doses of 6000–7000 cGy over 6–8 weeks are typically used. Those patients receiving preoperative radiotherapy (RT) frequently receive a boost using brachytherapy or intraoperative radiation [1].

The brachytherapy approach is much different. It involves perioperative implantation of radioactive sources and delivery of approximately 4500 cGy over 4–6 days. The technical details are reviewed later. The margins of treatment are significantly less than those for EBRT (Table 1). Therefore, in the early years of this approach, the treatment validity needed to be proven. These early experiences are highlighted in the data presented in this chapter.

Another major difference in these techniques involves the cost of treatment. Janjan et al. [2], in an elegant analysis of the charges related to radiotherapy for soft tissue sarcomas treated preoperatively with EBRT versus interstitial implantation, showed significantly lower charges were used for patients undergoing the implantation (Table 2). The cost savings are even greater when the logistical savings are considered. The fact that patients can return to work immediately, without going for 6–8 weeks of outpatient radiation, and that they do not have to arrange care for their children, rides to the hospital, parking for their car, transportation costs, etc., all yield a real cost savings for the brachytherapy patient.

Technique

Every patient is seen in consultation by the surgeon and radiation oncologist so that proper planning for the procedure can take place. The surgery is jointly attended by the radiation oncologist and the surgeon. After the surgeon completes a resection, the radiation oncologist performs the brachytherapy implant. The target volume is marked with surgical clips. This area includes the tumor bed plus a 1.5–2.0 cm margin in all directions. Blind-ended plastic brachytherapy catheters are passed through the skin through a trocar and sutured to the tumor bed with chromic catgut. Where possible, the catheters may be embedded in the muscle of the tumor bed to give increased stability and dose coverage to the muscle. A surgical drain is usually placed, the skin is closed, and the catheters are affixed to the skin with buttons, crimps, and nylon suture. The extruding catheters are bound together with a large Penrose drain and are included in the sterile bandage for safety and ease during transport (Fig. 1).

Early in the postoperative period, localization films are taken for purposes of dosimetry calculations. Patients are routinely visited and examined at least twice per day to make sure that the catheters remain intact. Depending on the anatomical location, an immobilization dressing or a sling is often helpful in keeping the involved area minimally disturbed. The wound is frequently examined for signs of infection.

The localization process is fairly simple and is done on a simulator. The catheters we use are preassembled with dummy seed strands to simplify the procedure. The patient is brought to our department, the wound is undressed, and a skin grid is placed for the calculation of the dose to wound. Two films are taken at least 20 degrees apart. These films are subsequently digitized for three-dimensional (3D) computer localization and optimization. A best-fit–least-squares algorithm is employed to provide the best coverage of the target with a minimum dose to the skin flaps. The computer plan is approved by the physician before the radionuclides are ordered by overnight courier.

The loading is done on the fifth or sixth postoperative day. Occasionally, because of wound healing issues, the loading may be delayed by 1–2 additional

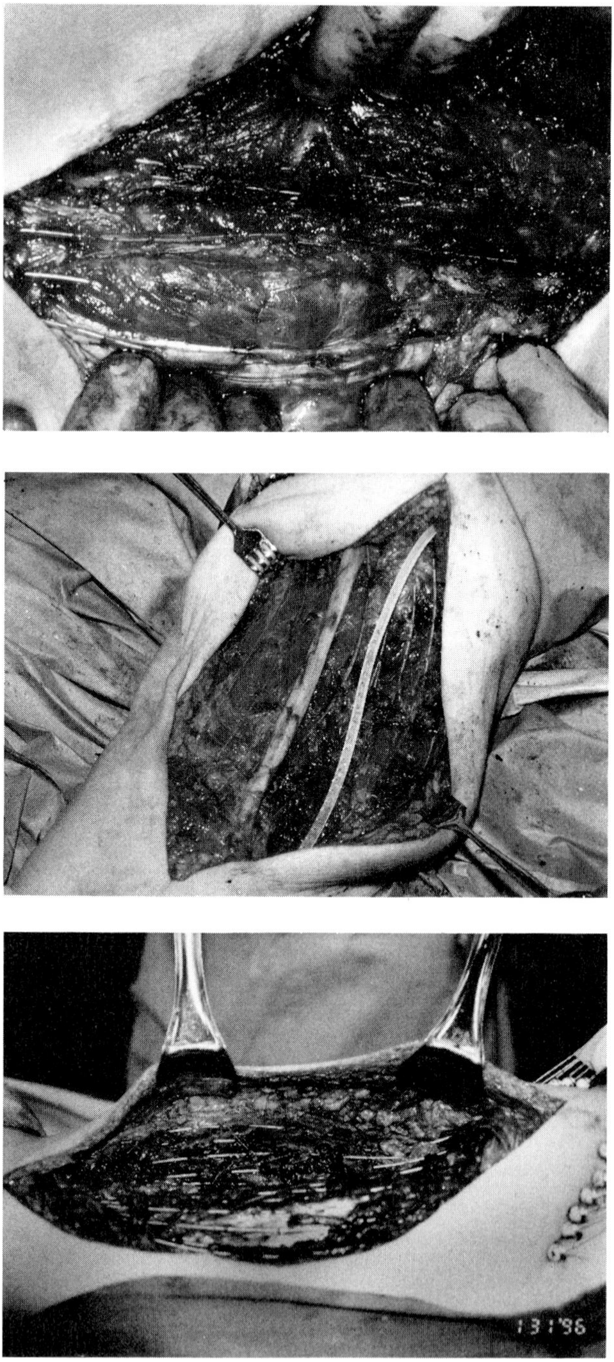

Figure 1. Blind-ended brachytherapy catheters in tumor bed of patient with thigh sarcoma. The femoral nerve has been preserved.

days. Further delays are usually discouraged. If the wound situation does not permit loading, the catheters are removed and an external beam is employed. Sterile technique and instruments minimize the risk of procedure-related infection. Appropriate shielding is arranged by our dedicated radiation safety officers before the loading. These integral members of our clinical team also educate patients, family, and nursing staff on radiation exposure issues. A most gratifying addition is their skill in fashioning custom, lead-vinyl drapes, boots, and other shielding that allows essentially no radiation exposure to others when I-125 is employed. The loading, monitoring of the loaded patient, unloading, and removal of catheters require extra attention from the clinical staff. For the entire time, physicians, physicists, and radiation safety staff must be available.

The prescription dose for the brachytherapy procedure is 4500 cGy over 4–6 days. The prescription isodose line is chosen as the line that adequately encompasses the target volume. The typical plan delivers 900–1000 cGy/day to this volume. For patients in whom the implant is used as a boost, to be followed by an external beam, the typical doses are 1500–2000 cGy with the implant and 4500–5000 cGy with the external beam. This latter approach is reserved for patients with positive margins, concern about the geometry of the implant at the edge of the target volume, or other biological/physical circumstances that require a wider volume of irradiation that the implant alone can provide. This issue is discussed later in the chapter.

At the end of the implantation the sources must be promptly and safely removed and stored. Sterile technique is used to withdraw the catheters. The surgical drain is not removed until after the unloading to avoid disturbing its geometry. There may be some advantageous geometric sparing of the wound caused by the presence of the drain.

Retrospective data

In 1985 Hilaris et al. [3] reported the initial MSKCC experience in which 17 previously untreated patients with primary soft tissue sarcoma of the extremities were managed with conservative, limb-sparing surgery plus postoperative brachytherapy to the tumor bed. Six of the patients would have traditionally required amputation to resect all disease. Thirteen had high-grade histology, and 15 had involved margins of resection. All received iridium-192 implants via afterloading catheters with a median dose of 40 Gy over 4–5 days. The margin of coverage was 1.5 cm on the tumor bed as outlined by both the surgeon and radiation oncologist at the time of surgery. No local recurrences were seen at a median follow-up of 34 months. This initial experience strongly supported the efficacy of adjuvant brachytherapy in the local eradication of traditionally poor prognosis soft tissue sarcoma.

Shiu et al. [4] reported on 33 patients with locally advanced soft tissue sarcoma of the extremity treated with function-saving resection and brachytherapy. This series included the 17 previously untreated patients reported by Hilaris as well as 16 patients who presented with a local recurrence after prior treatment. More than half of these patients were advised to have amputation at other institutions prior to referral. Twenty-three had high-grade lesions and 10 had low-grade lesions. Although gross resections were done and all wounds could be primarily closed, these operations were not oncologically optimal. The proximity of the tumor to major neurovascular structures and to bone resulted in microscopic and even small macroscopic residual disease in most cases. Most patients received brachytherapy alone, with a median dose of 4000 cGy over 4–5 days (range 2500–6000 cGy). Five patients also received supplemental external-beam irradiation (2000–2400 cGy over 2–3 weeks). Despite the unfavorable nature of this patient population, local control was quite encouraging, with a median follow-up of 3 years; all 17 previously untreated patients achieved local control and 10 of the 16 (62.5%) recurrent disease patients achieved local control. The difference in local control between primary and recurrent cases was significant (Fig. 2).

Eleven of 33 patients developed wound complications in the series. Two lost the affected limb as a result of treatment complications. Analysis of the complications group led to the conclusion that in two patients better tissue coverage at the time of surgery would have avoided the problem. Five of the patients had undergone iridium-192 loading on the first postoperative day and three on the second. A further discussion of complications and how to avoid

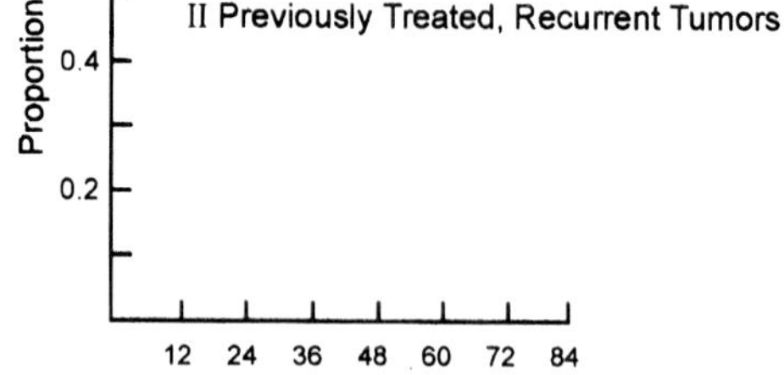

Figure 2. Probability of local tumor control after treatment. Group I: Previously untreated tumors. Group II: Previously treated, recurrent tumors. Limb disease-free intervals were plotted using the Kaplan–Meir method. The log-rank test was used for statistical comparison of the difference between the two groups. Reproduced with permission of Wiley-hiss, Inc. a subsidiary of John Wiley & Sons, Inc. from [4].

them is presented later. Most (64%) of these tumors were greater than 5 cm in diameter (12 of 17 and 9 of 16), 70% (12 of 17 and 11 of 16) were high grade, 61% (6 of 17 and 14 of 16) involved major neurovascular or skeletal structures, and 94% (15 of 17 and 16 of 16) had inadequate or microscopically positive margins. Despite these adverse features, the limb and its function were mostly preserved. The theory that high-dose brachytherapy alone after conservative surgical resection of high-grade sarcoma could adequately treat the tumor bed to prevent local recurrence was supported.

The initial pilot study described by Shiu in 1984 was updated in 1991 [5] to include 45 patients treated with conservative surgery and perioperative brachytherapy. Because two of these patients underwent retreatment, 47 treatments were evaluable. Sixty-four percent of tumors were greater than 10 cm, 68% were high grade, and 30% were locally recurrent after a previous nonbrachytherapy treatment. Gross or microscopic disease was left at or close to the margin in 69% of the patients. Twenty-seven percent had pathologic evidence of invasion of a neurovascular structure. The median tumor bed implant dose was 4400 cGy over approximately 5 days. Treatment was initiated 5 days postsurgery.

The 5-year disease-free survival (DFS) was 66%. Local control was obtained in 70% of the 47 treated sites. There were 14 local recurrences, 9 of which were infield recurrences. It was noted in 3 of the 9 recurrences that supplementary EBRT was not given after excision of a high-grade tumor with multiple positive margins. In two the implant dosimetry was inadequate. Seven of 45 patients required amputation for control of recurrent tumor, and the remaining 38 (84%) achieved functional preservation without limb recurrence.

While the MSKCC group utilized adjuvant brachytherapy alone, others have combined a brachytherapy boost with supplemental external-beam radiation. Schray et al. [6] reported the Mayo Clinic experience integrating brachytherapy with conservative surgery and EBRT. Between 1981 and 1988, 63 patients were treated for soft tissue sarcoma and underwent conservative surgery. Fifty-nine patients also received either preoperative or postoperative EBRT. A 4% local failure was seen in the brachytherapy group, with a median follow-up of 20 months. Only a single patient in this group failed within the treated volume. Preoperative EBRT was associated with a 25% wound complication rate as compared with 5% for the postoperative EBRT group. Of 53 patients with extremity, shoulder, or pelvic girdle tumors, 51 (96%) had functional extremities at the time of evaluation. There were two patients who required salvage amputation for recurrence. Four patients had isolated local failure, one had combined local and distant failure, and six had distant metastases alone. All local recurrences and distant metastases were in the setting of high-grade tumors. Local recurrence was not related to tumor size. Their brachytherapy technique involved the placement of nylon afterloading catheters to cover the tumor bed volume with a 2–4 cm margin in a plane that was perpendicular to the long axis of the tumor, often perpendicular to the skin incision. The tubes were primarily affixed by positioning and only rarely were sutured to tissue. The implant was reviewed with orthogonal films using dummy seeds, and the dosimetry was completed on a computer. Approximately one third of the implants used more that one plane. The average prescription dose to the target was 48.6 cGy/h delivered with iridium-192 over an average of 44.2 hours, giving an average absorbed dose at the target of 2052 cGy. The average skin dose was 1188 cGy or 58% of the target dose. See other retrospective brachytherapy reviews for more details [7–13].

Prospective data

Memorial Sloan-Kettering Cancer Center trial

Although the retrospective series of Hilaris and Shiu suggested an excellent outcome with adjuvant brachytherapy, there were still several questions to be addressed, which include the following: Which patients require adjuvant radiation to improve local control? Because the treatment volume and technique for brachytherapy differs so much from the traditionally used EBRT, is the brachytherapy approach appropriate? (See Figure 3).

The initial [14] and long-term results [15,16] have been published. Between 1982 and 1987, 126 patients with soft tissue sarcoma were entered into a prospective randomized trial. Preoperative signed informed consent was obtained. All patients were either previously untreated or presented to us with local recurrence, having received no prior radiation or chemotherapy. The distribution of clinical characteristics is shown in Tables 3 and 4. All under-

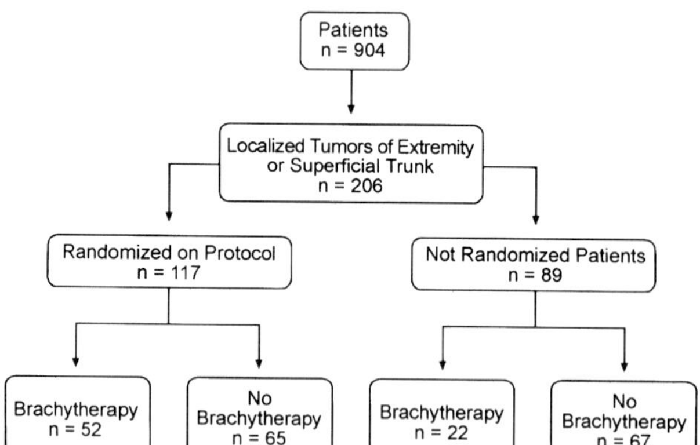

Figure 3. Soft tissue sarcoma of extremity or superficial trunk. Randomization and treatment profile from July 1, 1982 to December 31, 1986. Adapted from [14] with permission of the author.

Table 3. Distribution of clinical characteristics by randomization arm: Brachytherapy versus no brachytherapy

	BRT (n = 55)		No BRT (n = 70)	
Characteristic	No.	(%)	No.	(%)
Age				
<60 years	36	(65)	42	(60)
≥60 years	19	(35)	28	(40)
Sex				
Male	30	(45)	46	(66)
Female	25	(46)	24	(34)
Presentation status				
Primary	50	(91)	59	(84)
Recurrent	5	(9)	11	(16)
Location				
Proximal	49	(89)	59	(84)
Distal	6	(11)	11	(16)
Site				
Lower extremity	39	(71)	49	(70)
Upper extremity	9	(16)	16	(23)
Superficial trunk	7	(13)	5	(7)
Depth				
Superficial	21	(38)	18	(26)
Deep	34	(62)	52	(74)

BRT = brachytherapy.
Adapted from [14] with permission of the author.

went a grossly complete resection with a limb-sparing operation. Resection was accomplished without violating the tumor, and without resection of bone or vascular structures. Intraoperatively, after the resection was completed the patients were randomized to receive either adjuvant radiation therapy in the form of brachytherapy or no adjuvant therapy. The brachytherapy consisted of an interstitial implant via afterloading catheters using iridium-192. The tumor bed was jointly evaluated by the surgeon and a radiation oncologist. A target area was defined by adding a 2-cm margin in the interior and superior dimension, and a 1.5- to 2.0-cm margin in the medial and lateral dimensions. The radiation oncologist then implanted this target area with an array of afterloading catheters, placed percutaneously, spaced at approximately 1-cm increments in the long axis of the tumor bed. The catheters were sutured in place with chromic catgut sutures, and fixed to the skin with buttons and silk sutures. A surgical drain was placed over the catheters and tumor bed. The wound was then closed in layers. No special effort was made to treat the surgical scar, the drain site, or the wide margins that are typically included in EBRT.

Table 4. Distribution of histological and other tumor-related characteristics by randomization arm

	BRT		No BRT	
	No.	(%)	No.	(%)
Histologic grade				
Low	11	(20)	18	(26)
High	44	(80)	52	(74)
Histologic type				
Liposarcoma	21	(38)	28	(40)
MFH	13	(24)	17	(24)
MPNT	6	(11)	3	(4)
Fibrosarcoma	5	(9)	3	(4)
Leiomyosarcoma	4	(7)	6	(9)
Synovial sarcoma	4	(7)	4	(6)
(Extraskeletal) osteosarcoma	1	(2)	1	(1)
Rhabdomyosarcoma	1	(2)	4	(6)
Chondrosarcoma	0	(0)	2	(3)
Angiosarcoma	0	(0)	2	(3)
Size				
<5 cm	19	(35)	21	(30)
≥5 cm	36	(65)	49	(70)
Margins of resection				
Positive	11	(20)	11	(16)
Negative	44	(80)	59	(84)

BRT = brachytherapy; MFH = malignant fibrous histiocytoma; MPNT = malignant peripheral nerve tumor.
Adapted from [15] with permission of the author.

Results

The median follow-up time is 76 months. Table 5 gives 5-year actuarial control rates. Local control was significantly improved in the group of patients receiving adjuvant brachytherapy. However, when broken down by grade, the local control advantage was limited to patients with high-grade lesions. The 5-year actuarial local control was 89% for the brachytherapy-treated group versus 66% for the patients with high-grade tumors who received surgery alone, as shown in Figures 4 and 5. This level of local control compares favorably with other retrospective series in which wider field external radiation therapy was utilized.

There are several issues that are worth noting. The brachytherapy treatment only takes 4–6 days. This compares very favorably with the 6–8 weeks needed for external-beam therapy. The patient can leave the hospital postoperatively with the entire treatment completed. The patients return to active life quickly and conveniently without protracted daily visits to the hospital. Less normal tissue is irradiated, which can only improve the functional outcome, as presented later. In this present era of heightened awareness of the

Table 5. Five-year actuarial control rates

	Brachytherapy	No brachytherapy	p
LC—all patients	82%	69%	0.04
LC—high grade	89%	66%	0.0025
Freedom from DM	83%	76%	0.60
DSS—all patients	84%	81%	0.65

LC = local control; DSS = disease specific survival; DM = distant metastases.

Adapted from [16] with permission of W. B. Saunders Publishing, Orlando FL.

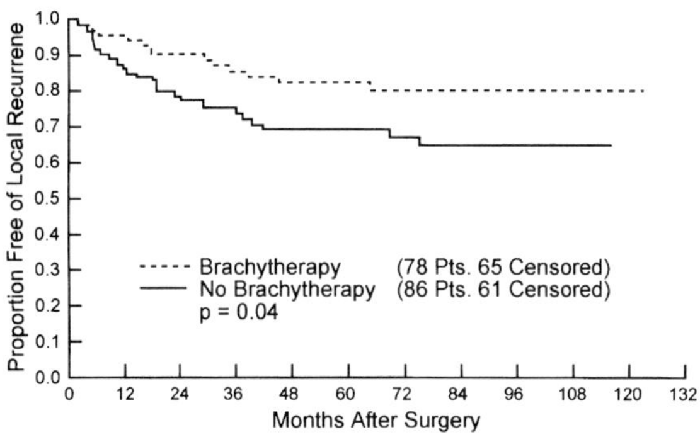

Figure 4. Actuarial plot of freedom from local recurrence for the entire study group. Adapted from [16] with permission of W. B. Saunders Publishing, Orlando FL.

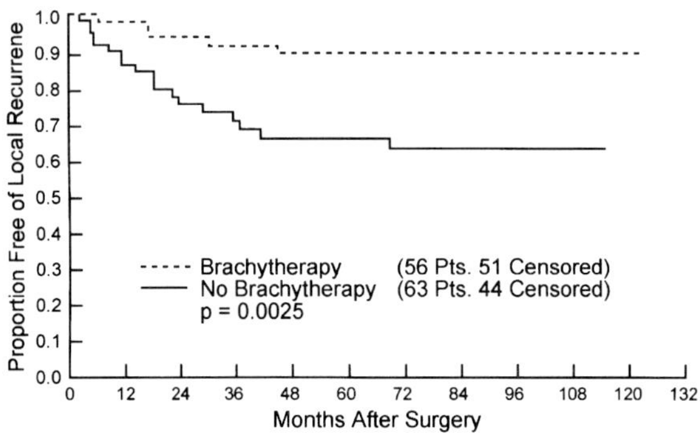

Figure 5. Actuarial plot of freedom from local recurrence for the 119 patients with histopathologic high-grade lesions. Adapted from [16] with permission of W. B. Saunders Publishing, Orlando FL.

costs of therapy, the ability to provide an equivalent chance of cure with less overall costs, both medical and societal, is increasingly attractive. The lack of benefit of brachytherapy in low-grade sarcomas is further supported by the follow-up study of Pisters et al. [17]. External-beam RT remains the adjuvant choice for these lesions.

Functional outcome data

Thirty-eight of 82 long-term survivors of the MSKCC randomized trial were put through objective functional and psychological testing to evaluate the outcome. Level walking was tested with the Footswitch Analyzer, in which patients ambulated at free speed to determine velocity, cadence, stride length, single-limb stance, and symmetry. Maximum isometric muscle torques were measured on the LIDO Active Rehabilitation System. Abductors, adductors, flexors, and extensors were all evaluated. Additionally, all patients completed the Arthritis Impact Measurement Scale (AIMS) to assess the psychofunctional impact of brachytherapy. The results showed no significant differences in the functional parameters of isometric muscle torque, gait velocity, cadence, stride length, single-limb stance test, or symmetry between those who did and did not receive brachytherapy. The psychological portion of the AIMS showed a significantly higher level of anxiety, depression, and appreciation of illness in the brachytherapy group, although no adverse perceived functional effects from brachytherapy were found [18].

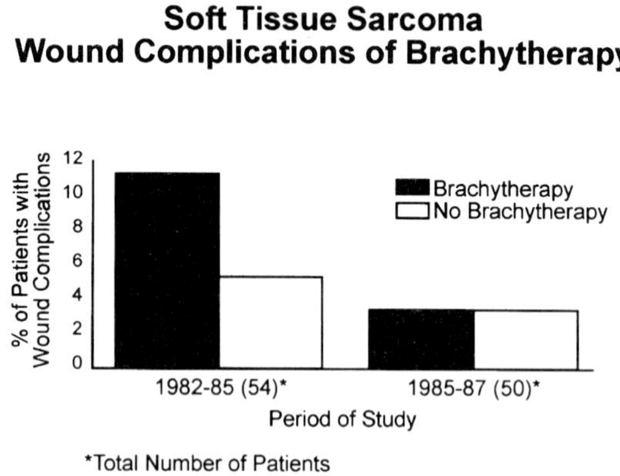

Figure 6. Major and moderate wound complications with brachytherapy in soft tissue sarcoma. Reproduced with permission of Lippincott Raven Publishers, Philadelphia, PA from [21].

Complications

Shiu et al. [19] and Arbeit et al. [20] have reported on the moderate and major wound complications for patients undergoing surgery alone compared with the surgery plus brachytherapy. It was found that 44% of brachytherapy wounds had complications versus only 14% in the surgery-alone series ($p = 0.0006$) Arbeit showed a correlation between time of loading and wound breakdown. Loading in the first 5 postoperative days led to a significantly higher incidence of wound breakdown. This has been related to fibroblast proliferation. Since 1985 we have had the policy of not loading patients until at least the fifth postoperative day. Ormsby et al. [21] reported that during the first 2 years after this policy was instituted, the moderate and major wound complication rate for brachytherapy wounds was 14% versus 10% for surgery alone (not statistically significantly different; Fig. 6). This policy continues at the present time.

Special situations

Locally advanced tumors involving major neurovascular structures

Zelefsky et al. [24] reported 45 patients with locally advanced soft tissue sarcomas that extended to or involved major neurovascular structures. These patients were treated using a limb-sparing technique. An en-bloc resection was undertaken, but the tumor was dissected off the major nerves and vessels. In 69% either gross disease remained or there was a close margin (within 5 cm of the cut and inked margin of resection), 64% of the tumors were 10 cm or greater, 68% had a high-grade histology, and 28% were pathologically proved to invade neurovascular structures. These were treated with brachytherapy catheters, which had been placed directly onto the neurovascular structures. The median dose was 44 Gy with iridium-192 over 4–5 days. The 5-year actuarial local control was 70%. True infield local recurrence was 21%, with the remainder failing at the periphery of the field. The 5-year distant metastasis-free survival was 69%. These patients compare favorably with the stage IIIB patients of the Massachusetts General Hospital reported by Suit et al. [25], suggesting that this is a useful approach for these lesions (Table 6).

The main complication was radiation-induced injury to the treated peripheral nerve seen in 4 patients between 6 and 20 months after treatment. The total doses received by these patients was between 91 and 148 Gy. No patient treated with a total dose of less than 90 Gy experienced toxicity. All of these patients were able to resolve their nerve deficits with vigorous physical therapy and a scar release procedure in one patient. This experience suggested that tumor-bed brachytherapy after conservative excision of high-grade sarcoma involving a major neurovascular structure was a useful alternative to amputation and set a upper limit of 90 Gy to avoid neurotoxicity.

Table 6. Treatment results Stage IIIB soft tissue sarcomas

Study	No. of cases	5-year actuarial local control (%)	5-year actuarial survival (%)
MGH preoperative radiation	35	83	48
MGH postoperative radiation	26	68	41
MSKCC adjuvant brachytherapy	47	79	66

MGH = Massachusetts General Hospital; MKSCC = Memorial Sloan-Kettering Cancer Center.
Adapted from [34] with permission of author.

Free flaps and brachytherapy

Hidalgo and Carrasquillo [22] reported three MSKCC cases of locally recurrent high-grade sarcoma that were treated by wide excision, brachytherapy, and free-flap reconstruction. All the flaps survived and wounds healed uneventfully with the addition of 45 Gy in the immediate postoperative period. Operative and follow-up views are shown in Figure 7. Panchal et al. [23] studied whether reconstruction with a microvascular free flap reduced the incidence of wound breakdown in the presence of early postoperative brachytherapy following wide excision of three soft tissue sarcomas of the extremity and seven head-and-neck carcinomas. Nine of the 10 patients had no wound breakdown, demonstrating that brachytherapy can be delivered in this manner without an increase in the frequency of wound breakdown.

Locally recurrent sarcoma

Although amputation is the most common recommendation for locally recurrent extremity sarcoma, the limb-sparing approach was also attempted in this group. Nori et al. [26] reported 40 patients who all had failed surgery and radiation therapy. The same limb-sparing regime was utilized with a median dose of 4500 cGy (range, 3000–4800 cGy) with brachytherapy. The local control was 69%. Survival in this review, was found to depend on the number of prior recurrences. For two or less recurrences, the 5-year actuarial overall survival was 85% versus 55% for those with three or more recurrences. The overall wound complication rate was 12.5%. Thus the vast majority of this poor prognosis group were provided with adequate limb salvage.

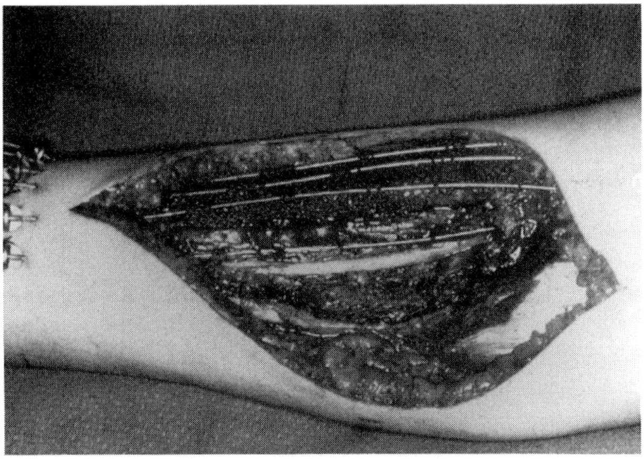

A

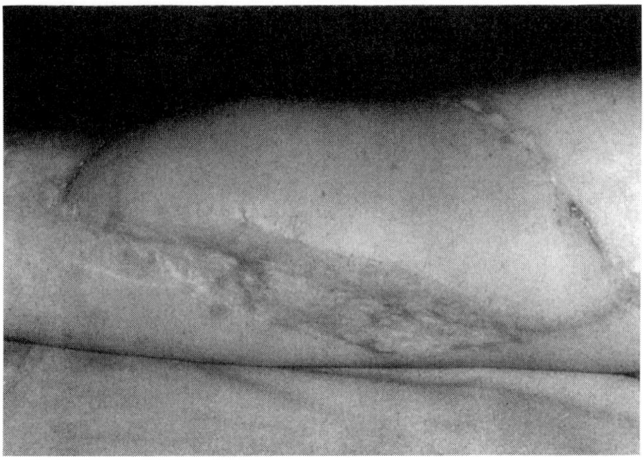

B

Figure 7. **A:** Case 3. A large excision for recurrent epithelioid sarcoma of the middle third of the leg is shown. Most of the soleus has been resected. A fine Dacron mesh has been placed over the tibia to allow the catheters to be anchored close to the bone. **B:** The healed wound is shown 8 months after postoperative administration of 4500 cGy through the catheters. Reproduced from [22] with permission of Waverly Publishing, Baltimore MD.

Young patients: Iodine-125 Versus Iridium-192

Another potential problem to consider when irradiating sarcoma patients is the dose delivered to the reproductive organs or organs in which radiation-induced alterations in reproductive function or radiation-induced cancers are of increasing concern. This is of special interest in sarcoma patients because these patients are often younger in age. The dose to the surrounding normal tissue is minimized by the use of a temporary iodine-125 implant instead of iridium-192. Because these catheters have to be individually constructed by the physicist and the iodine-125 seeds are significantly more expensive, the use of this radionuclide is more difficult. However, there may be a significant therapeutic gain [27].

Table 7 compares these isotopes in the same patient, a 17 year old with a posterior thigh tumor implant. In both instances the absorbed dose to the target is the desired 10 Gy per day. The comparison of doses delivered to the ovaries, breast, and thyroid are shown. There is a clear advantage to iodine-125 in this situation. Additionally, the dose to the skin wound is also significantly diminished. It is our current policy to use temporary iodine-125 for all pediatric implants and other patients in whom there is a major dosimetric gain in favor of iodine. For patients outside the reproductive years, or for anatomical locations away from radiosensitive vital organs, iridium-192 is still preferred [28].

The treatment energy for iodine-125 is 28 keV compared with 380 keV for iridium-192. This energy differential provides many attractive characteristics. The potential for radiation exposure to clinical staff, family, and other patients is minimized. Isolation of the patient is rarely required. Almost total shielding of the isotopes can be achieved by fashioning overdrape garments for the treatment area from lightweight lead-vinyl polymer. (The half-value layer of iodine-125 is 0.025 mm lead vs. 2.5 mm lead for iridium-192). Advantage can also be taken of the predominant manner of absorption of the emitted rays. Whereas the iridium gamma ray is absorbed by Compton effect and is independent of the atomic number of the absorbing tissue, the iodine x-ray (in the diagnostic range) is absorbed by the photoelectric effect and is attenuated proportional to the third power of the atomic number of the absorbing material. This allows for closer implantation to radiosensitive structures encased in bone, such as the spinal cord, without the fear of dosing the spinal cord.

Significant components of pediatric case reviews for brachytherapy discuss patients with soft tissue sarcoma. Fontanesi et al. [29] reported on a heteroge-

Table 7. Comparison of iridium-192 and high-activity iodine-125 in 17 year old with desmoid in the right posterior thigh

	Iridium-192	Iodine-125
Target dose	Homogeneous	Homogeneous
Skin average	262 cGy/day (60 cm^2)	68 cGy/day (60 cm^2)
Skin maximum dose	422 cGy/day	210 cGy/day
Right ovary	151 cGy/day	17 cGy/day
Left ovary	43 cGy/day	1 cGy/day
Breasts	11 cGy/day	0 cGy/day
Thyroid	8 cGy/day	0 cGy/day

Reproduced with permission of author from [28].

neous group of pediatric patients in whom brachytherapy was used. In total, 4 of 4 patients with soft tissue (nonrhabdomyo) sarcoma survived without disease as well as 5 of 5 rhabdomyosarcoma patients. Three of four nonrhabdomyo-sarcomas were controlled when brachytherapy was used as a boost in addition to external-beam radiotherapy. Twelve of 14 (85.7%) patients with non-ocular disease were controlled within the implant volume.

Gerbaulet et al. [30] reported a large pediatric cancer series from the Institut Gustav Roussy, with local control in 33 of 45 patients using doses between 36 and 75 Gy. This is confirmed by the reports of Cherlow et al. [31] and Martinez et al. [32]. Even with the use of iridium-192, these series testify to the applicability of brachytherapy in the pediatric population. Curran et al. [33] reported the University of Pennsylvania's experience, supporting both the efficacy and minimal toxicity of brachytherapy in children with sarcoma in the primary and salvage modes.

Desmoid tumors

In 1991 Zelefsky et al. [34] reported on the cumulative MSKCC experience with locally advanced and recurrent desmoid tumors treated with surgery and radiation therapy, mainly brachytherapy. Seventy-five percent had multiple prior recurrences, 50% with tumors greater than 8 cm, 16% with gross residual disease, and 79% with tumor at or close to the surgical margin of resection. Sixty-six percent of these cases were locally controlled with brachytherapy (median dose 40 Gy) alone, as previously described. One third of the local failures were at the periphery of the implanted volume. Combining low-grade histology, diffuse tumor margins, and presumed slow cell-cycle time, this study concluded that when implants are used, they should only be used as a boost (20–25 Gy) supplemented by external beam (45–50 Gy) to a more generous volume for desmoid tumors. Of course, postoperative external beam alone is also an excellent option.

Positive margins

Alekhteyar et al. [35] reviewed the impact of brachytherapy plus EBRT on local control in a subset of patients in whom the margins of resection were positive. The combination of modalities produced increased local control compared with the use of brachytherapy alone (90% vs. 59% at 2 years; $p = 0.08$). The overall wound complication rate was 26% for brachytherapy alone versus 38% for brachytherapy plus external beam ($p = 0.31$). The combined major and moderate wound complication rare was 16% for brachytherapy alone versus 27% for combined brachytherapy and EBRT ($p = 0.39$). From an oncologic viewpoint, a positive margin patient requires a wider field of radiation therapy than the implant alone can provide, and a higher dose than external beam alone can provide. The combination of brachytherapy (15–

20 Gy) and EBRT (45–50 Gy) gives a very high dose to the involved and appropriate area.

Retroperitoneal sarcoma

Retroperitoneal sarcomas present a challenging clinical problem. These tumors are usually large and often require resection of major abdominal organs. Despite complete resection, local recurrence occurs in at least 50% of cases [36], thus demonstrating the need for further local therapy. There is the clear need to add adequate radiation therapy in an effort to improve local control. However, the presence of nearby structures, such as the small bowel, colon, kidney, liver, etc., make the delivery of therapeutic doses of external-beam radiation (>6000 cGy) virtually impossible.

For this reason, there has been a growing interest in combining resection with intraoperative radiation therapy (IORT) and external beam [37]. Indeed, a prospective randomized trial from the National Cancer Institute (NCI) demonstrated improved local control for patients treated with IORT [38]. Additional information is available [39,40].

At our institution we have used a unique form of IORT that is the product of our brachytherapy experience. It involves the use of an intraoperative high-dose-rate (HDR) remote afterloader and an intraoperative applicator. The applicator is a multichannel flexible pad that can be applied to the surface of the tumor bed. The channels that emanate from this applicator are connected to the HDR machine via special connecting tubes. The HDR machine is then programmed to deliver a customized radiation dose distribution to the tumor bed, with normal organs retracted out of the field. Figure 8 shows a clinical example. We have previously described the detailed techniques of this approach [41], which requires a special operating room that is shielded for the delivery of radiation therapy.

Our program started in November 1992 and involved surgical resection, HDR-IORT (1500 cGy), followed by EBRT (4500 cGy). Between November 1992 and October 1995, 26 patients have been enrolled in this study, including 17 males and 9 females with an age range of 24–79 years (median, 58 years). Patient characteristics include 11 primary and 15 recurrent lesions, and 17 had high-grade histology and 9 had low-grade lesions. The follow-up ranges from 1 to 33 months, with a median of 11 months. Preliminary results reveal crude local control of 85% for all patients, with 91% local control for primary cases and 80% for recurrent cases. A longer follow-up is needed to assess the true efficacy of this approach, but early data are encouraging. Total complications have been in the 30–40% range, which appears consistent with the aggressive surgical and radiotherapeutic approach.

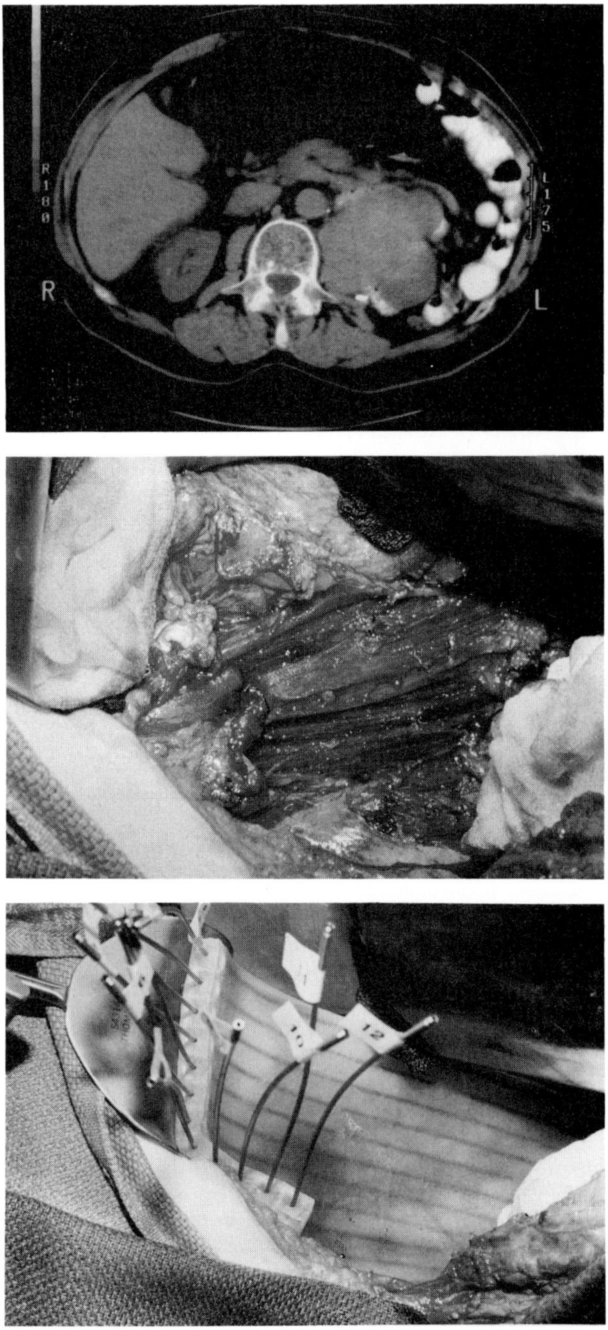

A

B

C

Figure 8. **A:** CT scan of high-grade sarcoma in the left renal fossa. **B:** Intraoperative view of left renal fossa after en-bloc resection of tumor and kidney. Surgical clips denote the margin of resection to be covered by intraoperative radiation therapy. The small intestine is packed away from the target area. **C:** Harrison-Anderson-Mick (HAM) high dose-rate intraoperative applicator in position with catheters ready to be attached to the high dose-rate afterloader.

Current practice guidelines

It is our current practice with extremity sarcoma to treat high-grade tumors with negative margins with adjuvant brachytherapy alone (4500 cGy over 4–6 days). High-grade tumors with positive margins are boosted with brachytherapy of 15–20 Gy and then will go on to receive 45–50 Gy external-beam therapy as an outpatient beginning 2–3 weeks postoperatively, depending on wound healing. Low-grade lesions are treated with adjuvant external beam (6000–6600 cGy) over 6–7 weeks. lesions less than 5 cm are managed with surgery alone, unless there is concern about the margins. This often is true for lesions of the hands, feel, head and neck, etc. In these situations, adjuvant brachytherapy or external beam, or both combined, is given, depending on the circumstances. For retroperitoneal sarcomas we are continuing our current approach of surgery, HDR-IORT, followed by external-beam radiation.

References

1. Suit HD, Mankin HJ, Wood WC, et al. Treatment of the patient with stage Mo soft tissue sarcoma. J Clin Oncol 6:854–862, 1988.
2. Janjan NA, Yasko AW, Reece GP, et al. Comparison of charges related to radiotherapy for soft tissue sarcomas treated by preoperative external beam irradiation versus interstitial implantation. Ann Surg Oncol 5:415–422, 1994.
3. Hilaris BS, Shiu MH, Nori D, et al. Limb-sparing therapy for locally advanced soft-tissue sarcoma. Endocurietherapy/Hyperthermia Oncol 1:17–24, 1985.
4. Shiu MH, Turnbull AD, Nori D, et al. Control of locally advanced extremity soft tissue sarcomas by function-saving resection and brachytherapy. Cancer 53:1385–1392, 1984.
5. Shiu MH, Hilaris BS, Harrison LB, et al. Brachytherapy and function-saving resection of soft tissue sarcoma arising in the limb. Int J Radiat Oncol Biol Phys 21:1485–1492, 1991.
6. Schray MF, Gunderson LL, Sim FH, et al. Soft tissue sarcoma: Integration of brachytherapy, resection and external irradiation. Cancer 66:451–456, 1990.
7. Gemer LS, Trowbridge DR, Neff J, et al. Local recurrence of soft tissue sarcoma following brachytherapy. Int J Radiat Oncol Biol Phys 20:587–592, 1991.
8. Herbert SH, Corn BW, Solin LJ. Limb-preserving treatment for soft tissue sarcomas of the extremities — the significance of surgical margins. Cancer 72:1230–1238, 1993.
9. Fein D, et al. Sarcomas of soft tissues: Radiation sensitivity, treatment field margins, pathological margins and dose. Int J Radiat Oncol Biol Phys 32:969–976, 1995.
10. Habrand JL, Gerabaulet A, Pejovic MH, et al. Twenty years experience of interstitial iridium brachytherapy in the management of soft tissue sarcomas. Int J Radiat Oncol Biol Phys 20:405–411, 1991.
11. Mills EED, Hering ER. Management of soft tissue tumors by limited surgery combined with tumor bed irradiation using brachytherapy and supplementary teletherapy. Br J Radiol 54:312–317, 1981.
12. Collins JE, Paine CH, Ellis F. Treatment of connective tissue sarcomas by local excision followed by radioactive implant. Clin Radiol 27:39–41, 1976.
13. Cionini L, Marzano S, Olmi P. Soft tissue sarcomas: Experience with intraoperative brachytherapy in the conservative management. Ann Oncol 3 (Suppl 2):S63–S66, 1992.
14. Brennan MF, Hilaris BS, Shiu MH, et al. Local recurrence in adult soft tissue sarcoma — a randomized trial of brachytherapy. Arch Surg 122:1289–1293, 1987.

15. Harrison LB, Franzese F, Gaynor JF, Brennan MF. Long term results of a prospective randomized trial of adjuvant brachytherapy in the management of completely resected soft tissue sarcomas of the extremity and superficial trunk. Int J Radiat Oncol Biol Phys 27:259–265, 1993.
16. Pisters PWT, Harrison LB, Leung DHY, et al. Long term results of a prospective randomized trial of adjuvant brachytherapy in soft tissues sarcoma. J Clin Oncol 14:859–868, 1996.
17. Pisters PWT, Harrison LB, Woodruff JM, et al. A prospective randomized trial of adjuvant brachytherapy in the management of low-grade soft tissue sarcomas of the extremity and superficial trunk. J Clin Oncol 12:1150–1155, 1994.
18. Schupak KD, Lane JM, Weilepp AE, et al. Functional assessment of surgery plus brachytherapy for soft tissue sarcoma. In press.
19. Shiu M, Hilaris B, Harrison LB, et al. Brachytherapy and function-saving resection of soft tissue sarcoma arising in the limb. Int J Radiat Oncol Biol Phys 21:1485–1492, 1991.
20. Arbeit J, Hilaris B, Brennan MF. Wound complications in the multimodality treatment of extremity and superficial truncal sarcomas. J Clin Oncol 5:480–488, 1987.
21. Ormsby M, Hilaris BS, Nori D, et al. Wound complications of adjuvant radiation therapy in patients with soft tissue sarcomas. Ann Surg 210:93–99, 1989.
22. Hidalgo DA, Carrasquillo IM. The treatment of lower extremity sarcomas with wide excision, radiotherapy and free-flap reconstruction. Plastic Reconstr Surg 89:96–101, 1991.
23. Panchal JI, Agrawal NR, McLean NR, Dawes PJ. Early postoperative brachytherapy following free flap reconstruction. Br J Plast Surg 46:511–515, 1993.
24. Zelefsky M, Nori D, Shiu M, et al. Limb salvage and soft tissue sarcomas involving neurovascular structures using combined surgical resection and brachytherapy. Int J Radiat Oncol Biol Phys 19:913–918, 1990.
25. Suit H, Mankin H, Wood W, et al. Treatment of patients with stage M0 soft tissue sarcoma. J Clin Oncol 6:854–862, 1988.
26. Nori D, Schupak K, Shiu M, Brennan MF. Role of brachytherapy in recurrent extremity sarcoma in patients treated with prior surgery and irradiation. Int J Radiat Oncol Biol Phys 20:1229–1233, 1991.
27. Genest P, et al. Iodine-125 as a substitute for iridium-192 in temporary interstitial implants. Endocuriether Hyperther Oncol 1:223–228, 1985.
28. Harrison LB. Brachytherapy for sarcomas. Presented at 36th Annual Meeting, American Society for Therapeutic Radiology and Oncology, San Francisco, CA, October 1994.
29. Fontanesi J, Rao BN, Fleming MD, et al. Pediatric brachytherapy — The St. Jude Children's Research Hospital experience. Cancer 74:733–739, 1994.
30. Gerbaulet A, Panis X, Flamant F, Chassagne D. Iridium afterloading curietherapy in the treatment of pediatric malignancies — The Institut Gustav Roussy experience. Cancer 56:1274–1279, 1985.
31. Cherlow JM, Syed AM, Puthawala A, et al. Endocurietherapy in the treatment of pediatric tumors. Pro. Am Soc Clin Oncol 7:259, 1988.
32. Martinez A, Goffinet DR, Donaldson SS, Palso B. The use of interstitial therapy in pediatric malignancies. From Radiat Oncol 12:91–100, 1978.
33. Curran WJ, Litman P, Raney RB. Interstitial radiation therapy in the treatment of childhood soft tissue sarcomas. Int J Radiat Oncol Biol Phys 14:169–174, 1988.
34. Zelefsky M, Harrison LB, Shiu MH, et al. Combined surgical resection and iridium-192 implantation for locally advanced and recurrent desmoid tumors. Cancer 67:380–384, 1991.
35. Alekhteyar KM, Leung DM, Brennan MF, Harrison LB. The effect of combined external beam radiotherapy and brachytherapy on local control and wound complications in patients with high-grade soft tissue sarcomas of the extremity with positive microscopic margin. Int J Radiat Oncol Biol Phys 36:321–324, 1996.
36. Jaques DP, Coit DG, Hajdu SI, Brennan MF. Management of primary and recurrent soft tissue sarcoma of the retroperitoneum. Ann Surg 212:51–59, 1990.
37. Tepper JR, Suit HD, Wood WC, et al. Radiation therapy of retroperitoneal soft tissue sarcomas. Int J Radiat Oncol Biol Phys 10:825–830, 1984.

38. Sindelar WF, Kinsella TJ, Chen PW, et al. Intraoperative radiotherapy in retroperitoneal sarcomas: Final results of a prospective, randomized, clinical trial. Arch Surg 128:402–410, 1993.
39. Willet CG, Suit HD, Tepper JE, et al. Intraoperative electron beam radiation therapy for retroperitoneal soft tissue sarcoma. Cancer 68:278–283, 1991.
40. Gunderson LL, Nagorney DM, McIlrath DC, et al. External beam and intraoperative electron irradiation for locally advanced soft tissue sarcomas. Int J Radiat Oncol Biol Phys 25:647–656, 1993.
41. Gunderson LL, Willett CG, Harrison LB. Intraoperative radiotherapy, current status — 1994. Presented at 36th Annual Meeting, American Society for Therapeutic Radiology and Oncology, San Francisco, CA, October 1994.

9. Three-dimensional planning and conformal radiotherapy

Clive Harmer and Margaret Bidmead

Introduction

The value of three-dimensional (3D) planning and conformal radiotherapy in the treatment of soft tissue sarcoma has already been established [1]. In a previous volume on soft tissue sarcomas in this series (Cancer Treatment and Research), Suit and Willett succinctly described the sequential steps required for optimal radiation therapy [2]. Alternatives to external-beam radiotherapy, including intraoperative brachytherapy and proton beam therapy, were highlighted, although such techniques are applicable in only a minority of situations. Fast neutron therapy offers no proven advantage and may lead to excessive morbidity [3].

The ideal dose of radiation is that which reliably eradicates all tumor but does not result in unacceptable normal tissue damage [4]. For any given tissue, the volume irradiated is the single most important factor leading to normal tissue morbidity and will limit the total dose that can be applied; this, in turn, relates to the probability of local control, because a dose-response relationship has been established [5]. The target volume varies according to whether the treatment is being given preoperatively or postoperatively, and according to the size, site, and grade of the primary tumor. A shrinking field technique is invariably recommended in order to minimize the highest dose volume. This volume is most critical when treating sarcomas arising in the head and neck [6], tumors arising in the retroperitoneum [7], and soft tissue sarcomas of children [8]. It is also particularly crucial when re-irradiation is contemplated [9].

A preoperative magnetic resonance (MR) scan is the most valuable investigation to assist with definition of the target volume. A computed tomograph (CT) scan may provide almost as much information but all too often neither is available because the original operation was undertaken without the diagnosis of sarcoma having been considered. In all cases, assessment of the extent of tumor is of paramount importance and should be discussed with the surgeon. A written copy of the operative procedure must be obtained, together with the histopathology report describing the macroscopic and microscopic appearances, including the margins of resection (a wider re-excision may be recommended). Postoperatively a diagnostic CT scan may be necessary to confirm

J. Verweij, H.M. Pinedo, and H.D. Suit (eds). SOFT TISSUE SARCOMAS: PRESENT ACHIEVEMENTS AND FUTURE PROSPECTS.

complete excision of tumor or the extent of residual tumor; MRI may be difficult to interpret postoperatively if edema or seroma is present. A therapy CT planning scan will be required in all cases requiring radiotherapy for accurate dosimetry.

Not to be underestimated in the definition of the optimal target volume is the anatomical position of the part of the body to be treated. For example, when treating the forearm, consideration must be given to whether the position should be prone or supine, depending on the site and extent of the tumor, together with the directions of the potential extension. Careful patient positioning is also valuable in ensuring a corridor of normal tissue sparing as well as maximal exclusion from the treatment volume of adjacent joints. An example is inclusion of a surgical scar in the region of the elbow: If this is either medially or laterally placed, then the arm is preferably treated with the elbow fully extended. Whereas if the scar runs centrally over the antecubital fossa, then it is preferable to treat with the elbow flexed at 90° and the hand on the hip to spare the region around the olecranon. All these anatomical considerations need to be made and the optimum patient position decided on prior to acquisition of the therapy CT scan.

Reproducible patient immobilization is a further prerequisite for conformal radiotherapy and must also be devised prior to the therapy CT scan. If a perspex shell is used, care should be taken to avoid treatment fields passing through the shell, unless a high dose is required to be administered to the skin. A careful decision needs to be made as to the optimal method of immobilization, which will vary with the anatomical site.

Extremely long fields are frequently necessary, but it is preferable to treat at an extended distance than to match isocentric fields, even if these are matched at the isocenter at an area not grossly involved with tumor, as suggested by Dusenbery et al. [10]. In order to shield adjacent normal tissues, simple beam blocking is adequate in some situations. Frequently, however, complex shaping of the volume will demand conformal treatment, and 3D planning is the best method for achieving this. The multileaf collimator is the ultimate method of achieving elegant beam shaping in a quick, accurate, and reproducible manner. Together with the use of a dynamic wedge, it may also reduce the incidence of cumulative trauma disorder in radiation therapists/radiographers [11].

Advantages of three-dimensional planning

The objective of three-dimensional planning and conformal radiotherapy is precise and reproducible treatment of the defined target volume with maximal avoidance of adjacent normal tissue. Its major advantage is in avoiding or at least minimizing normal tissue damage, both acute and, more importantly, late normal tissue damage. Historically, relatively little attention has been given to the technique for treatment of soft tissue sarcomas, partly because the volumes treated are so large. For extremity sarcomas, the degree of late normal tissue damage from radiotherapy is related to limb function, being correlated with both field length and dose [5]. The literature also suggests that the slope of the dose-response curve for normal tissue damage is steep over the dose range commonly used in curative treatment [12]. Three-dimensional planning has shown potential benefit in other sites, such as the pelvis [13].

For treatment of soft tissue sarcomas, local control is dependent on dose. This is true when radiation is used alone [14], when given preoperatively [5], and when given as adjuvant postoperative irradiation [15]. Dose escalation therefore offers the greatest potential benefit of conformal treatment, offering the possibility of improved local control. Studies in this area are in progress, but no randomized phase 3 trial has been reported to date. Several algorithms using clinical data in conjunction with dose-volume histograms (DVH) have been developed that allow biological estimation of tumor control probability (TCP) and normal tissue complication probabilities (NTCP) in order to quantify and compare clinical data [16].

Disadvantages of three-dimensional planning

The greatest disadvantage of 3D planning and conformal radiotherapy is the possibility that the tumor volume will be inadequately covered, which may result in local recurrence. Such a marginal miss may be amenable to further conservation surgery but clearly defeats the objective. Considerable care with reference to the relevant anatomy, together with knowledge of the directions and extent of potential spread of the disease, are required. Soft tissue sarcomas present the clinician with a challenge in this respect, being much more difficult to predict than tumors arising from other organs, such as the prostate, where the relevant anatomy is both simple and predictable.

The other major disadvantages of conformal radiotherapy are its high cost and the considerable time it demands. However, computer software is now commercially available and is becoming more 'user friendly' for trained operators when used with state-of-the-art linear accelerator technology. A financial cost-benefit analysis is clearly required, although it will be difficult to quantify the benefits of improved local control and reduced morbidity. In addition, a comparative analysis of the time input required by physicians and physicists in contrast with the time required for conventional two-dimensional planning should be undertaken.

Three-dimensional planning technique

One of the most important prerequisites for 3D treatment planning is reliable patient immobilization. Currently the use of a treatment shell and/or a patient support system (e.g. Vacfix) provides efficient immobilization, which may be further improved by a stereotactic fixation device such as a pelvic frame. Diagnostic CT or MR scans are used to identify the gross tumor volume (GTV) and clinical target volume (CTV). Developments in fusion software techniques that use MRI diagnostic information together with CT patient contours and heterogeneity information improve accuracy. Once the CTV has been defined, the patient can be screened and marked up for relocation on a simulator so that the exact therapy position is defined before the therapy CT scan is made.

The CT scan is made in the treatment position to obtain contour and heterogeneity information for accurate dosimetry calculations. The CT data are then imported into the 3D treatment planning system. Three-dimensional treatment planning dosimetry involves the following stages:

1. Definition of the CTV on multiple transverse slices to determine the volume in three dimensions.
2. Selection of the radiation field direction in order to treat the target volume while minimizing the dose to the surrounding organs.
3. Optimization of the treatment plan by using appropriate beam modifiers (such as wedges and compensators) and adjusting the relative weighting of one field to the others in order to ensure the most suitable distribution.
4. Production and use of beams eye views (BEVs), which allow visualization of the reconstructed volume from the chosen beam direction in order to define the conformal planning target margin.
5. Calculation of the DVHs that are used to evaluate different treatment plans in order to identify the plan that gives the lowest dose to the smallest volume of surrounding normal tissues. DVHs are calculated for surrounding muscle, bone, and other critical structures.
6. Application of NTCPs and TCPs to these DVH data in order to evaluate the radiation treatment and to relate it quantitatively to the clinical endpoints.
7. Production of conformal shielding blocks or multileaf collimator patterns to provide accurate and reproducible shielding for each fraction of the treatment.

Once the optimal three-dimensional plan has been produced, verification is required on a treatment simulator. BEVs from the treatment planning computer and digitally reconstructed radiographs (DRRs) from CT scan data are compared with simulator films of the proposed treatment field in order to verify the patient setup and radiation field positions in relation to patient anatomy. Record and verify systems that link the treatment planning computer to the simulator and treatment machine via a computer network are valuable to ensure the reproducibility and integrity of data. They can also be used to set the field, gantry, collimator, and couch parameters automatically. This speeds up the treatment process considerably and, in turn, reduces the potential for patient movement during treatment.

The final stage in the treatment process is verification of the radiation fields on the treatment unit, ideally achieved by megavoltage imaging. An imaging device is attached to the treatment accelerator so that the image is taken exactly perpendicular to the radiation field and is optimal for 3D verification. The image should be obtainable during a short period of radiation delivery so that real-time comparison with simulator film, BEV, and DRRs is possible, with intervention if necessary. Verification of the treatment field and patient positional information is then possible for each fraction of the radiation treatment [17].

At the Royal Marsden, conformal 3D planning is achieved on Target I (I.G.E.) and Cadplan (Varian/Dosetek). Patients are simulated on a Ximatron, with data imported over the Novel network of the RMS system, and treatment is given on a 2100C accelerator with a multileaf collimator. Verification is performed daily using the PortalVision system with a retractable arm (Varian Oncology Systems).

Illustrative examples

A 54-year-old midwifery teacher presented in 1989 with recurrent fibromatosis involving the right side of the root of her neck, causing narrowing and displacement of the trachea. It had previously been resected in 1984 and 1985 but had become inoperable, with fixity to major vessels and vertebral bodies. She also had sarcoid with pulmonary fibrosis. Figure 1 shows the therapy CT slice through the center of the tumor. She was 3D planned for a wedged pair of nearly parallel, oblique opposing portals to avoid the spinal cord, shoulders, and as much of the lung as possible. Phase 1 delivered a modal dose of 50 Gy, with a slightly foreshortened phase 2 volume going to a total of 60 Gy in 30

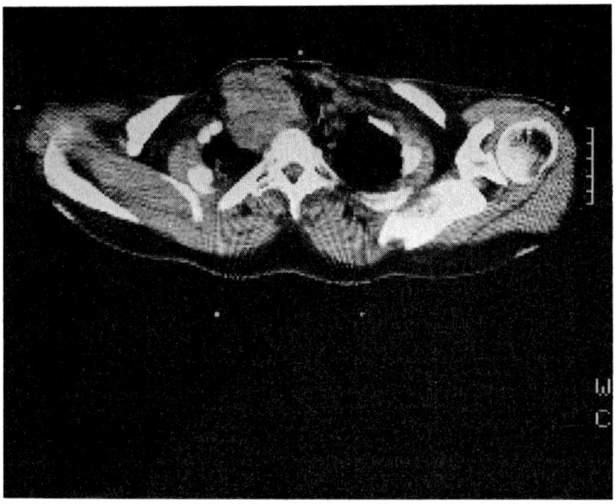

Figure 1. Therapy CT scan demonstrating tumor arising in the root of the right side of the neck, with centimeter scale and metal reference wires.

fractions over 6 weeks. Figure 2 shows the simulator check film; conformal lead could have been added. There was slight regression and no tumor regrowth at the time of death from pulmonary fibrosis 6 years later.

The second case example is of a 25-year-old diving instructor with a paraspinal soft-tissue Ewing's sarcoma. He achieved less than a partial response with chemotherapy and the residue was inoperable. Figure 3 illustrates one of the three conformally shaped fields used for treatment. The positions of the target volume, kidneys, spinal canal, and multileaf collimator are shown superimposed on the digitally reconstructed radiograph. Figure 4 illustrates the wire-frame outline set used for planning, with the shaded target volume encompassed by the isodose net (representing the 90% isodose level) and the geometric outline of the treatment fields.

The third case example is of a 50-year-old lady from Ghana who 6 years previously had a clear cell sarcoma excised from the right side of the vulva. She represented with metastatic groin and external iliac nodes, which were macroscopically excised. Figure 5 shows a simulator image of the anterior oblique treatment field with the positions of the MLC leaves identified, together with the outlined bony anatomy that was used for matching daily megavoltage portal images with the simulator (reference) image.

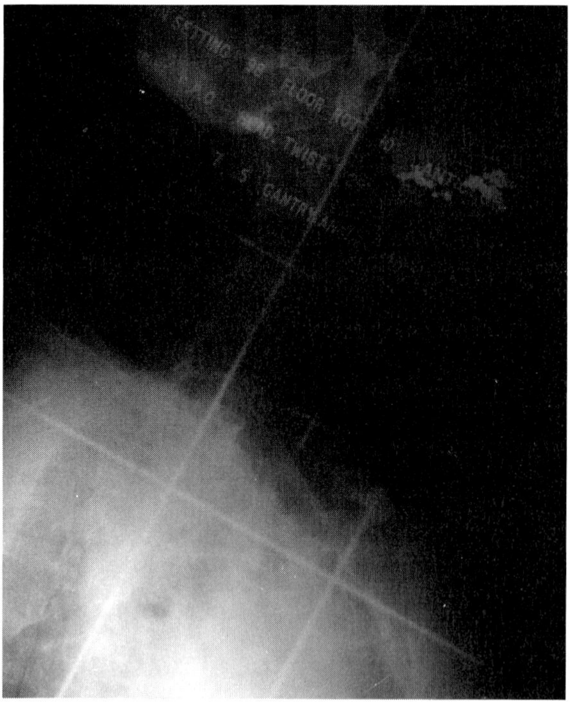

Figure 2. Simulator check film of right postero-oblique portal showing avoidance of the shoulder, spinal cord, and lung, with head twist and gantry angle.

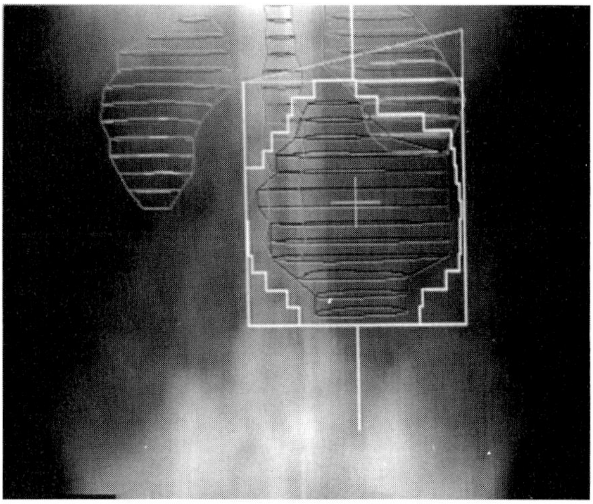

Figure 3. Digitally reconstructed radiograph with target volume and critical organs highlighted, showing the position of the MLC defining the conformational shielding from the direction of one treatment field.

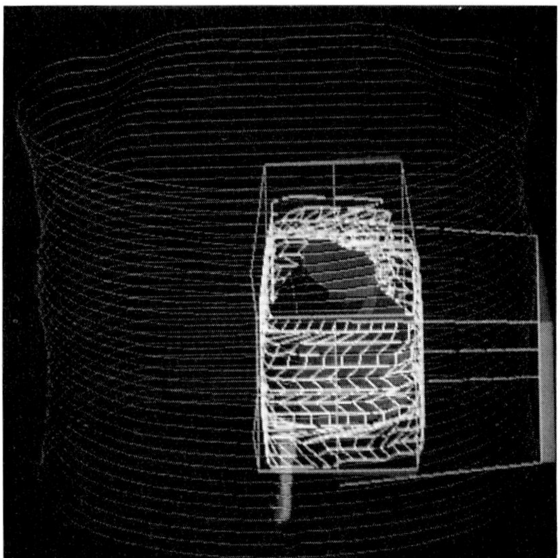

Figure 4. Wire frame display of the outline set showing a 90% isodose net encompassing the target volume.

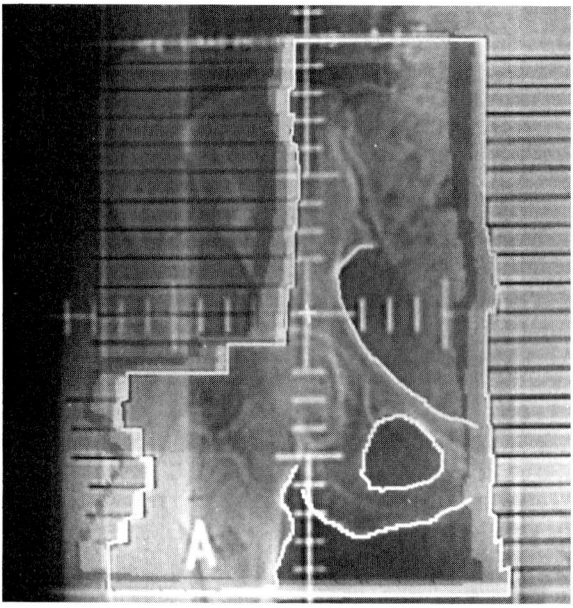

Figure 5. Simulator film of anterior oblique field showing the position of the MLC and anatomical structures used for matching megavoltage portal images.

Results of Royal Marsden Series

Both conformal and conventional planning were carried out for a group of 11 consecutive unselected patients with extremity soft tissue sarcoma who were to be treated with radical preoperative or postoperative radiotherapy during 1990 [18]. The most common site was the thigh, and the mean size of tumor was 11.3 cm (range 5–15 cm). The phase 1 field length varied from 28 to 45 cm. Two or more fields were treated either daily or twice daily. For each patient both conventional and conformal plans were devised, with 3D dose distributions calculated for use on a 5 MV linear accelerator. Oblique field arrangements with compensating wedges were used when necessary Cumulative dose-volume histograms (CDVH) were calculated for the tumor, target, muscle, bone, and other at-risk structures of both unblocked and blocked fields. Figure 6 shows the CDVHs for one patient for muscle and bone outside the target volume, demonstrating the effect of conformal blocking on the volume of normal tissue irradiated.

There was a greater than 20% reduction in the volume of tissue receiving 50% and 80% of the dose in all five patients with sarcoma of the thigh when conformal shielding was used, as shown in Figure 7. Isodose levels are expressed as a percentage of the dose to the isocenter for each treatment plan. The volume of specific structures receiving 90% of the dose provided a clini-

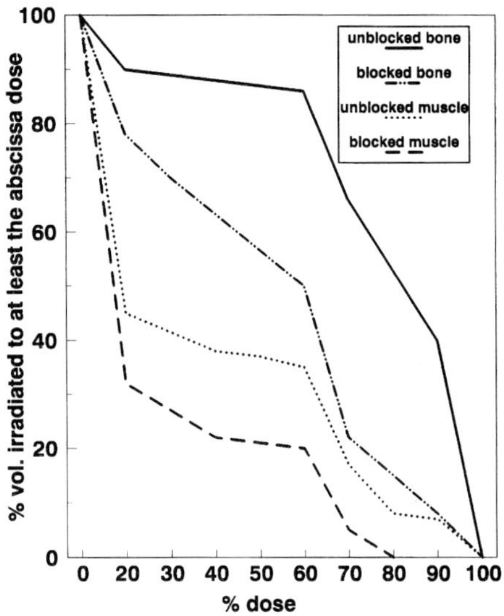

Figure 6. Cumulative dose volume histogram (CDVH) for one patient demonstrating the effect of customized beam blocking on the dose to bone and muscle outside the target volume.

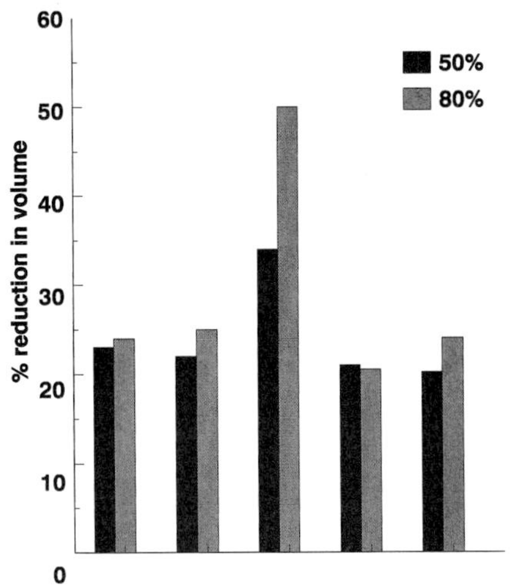

Figure 7. Effect of conformational shielding on the total volume receiving 50% and 80% of the dose to the isocenter in five patients with sarcoma of the thigh.

cally relevant reference for evaluation of normal tissue sparing. The normal tissues for which the effect of conformal blocking was studied are detailed in Table 1, including the average volume of each that was able to be spared by conformal blocking. Muscle comprised the largest volume of normal tissue irradiated in these patients. Figure 8 illustrates the effect of conformal plan-

Table 1. Average volumes of normal tissue (outside target volume) irradiated when no conformational shielding was used

	Patients	Mean volume (cm^3)	Range (cm^3)
Muscle	10	4166	908–9447
Bone	11	630	332–923
Pelvic contents	4	1171	126–2301
Spinal cord	2	26	15 & 37
Tendo-achilles	2	5	2 & 8
Patella	1	12	—

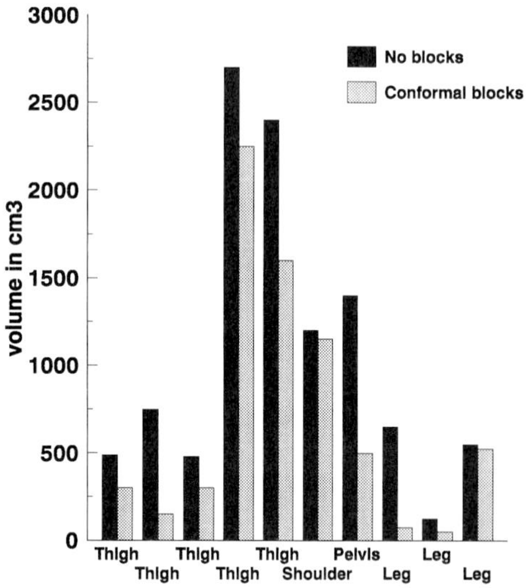

Figure 8. Volumes of muscle for 10 patients who received at least 90% of the dose to the isocenter with and without conformational blocks.

ning on the muscle volume that received at least 90% of the dose for 10 patients in the study.

Discussion

The Royal Marsden study described here has demonstrated that 3D conformal planning can result in a marked reduction of normal tissue volumes irradiated. The complexity of the actual treatment field arrangements with 3D planning was not increased, although the 3D planning process itself is much more complicated than 2D planning. Subsequent limb function correlates with both the phase 1 field length [19] and the dose of radiotherapy [20]. Less impairment of subsequent limb function is to be expected as a result of shielding large volumes of muscle. It is also important to reduce the dose to the long bones in order to minimize the possibility of subsequent fracture; it is difficult to achieve this without 3D planning because of the proximity of bone to the involved muscle compartment. A reduction in the dose to the viscera (particularly the gut, lung, spinal cord, and gonads) is also advantageous.

The Royal Marsden Soft Tissue Sarcoma Unit receives 200 new referral patients each year, about half of whom require radiotherapy. A minority need only simple palliative treatment, but most receive radical irradiation, either with curative intent or for high-dose palliation. All of these patients are CT planned because this is invariably helpful for accurate outlining, determination of heterogeneities, and the manufacture of compensators. Some patients with limb sarcomas are treated with simple lead blocking, but the majority are also conformally 3D planned despite the constraint of physician and physicist time. Patients with tumors of the head, neck, thorax, abdomen, or pelvis are selected as those for whom the benefit is likely to be greatest.

Quality control

The greater the precision of radiotherapy, the greater must be the quality control. Three-dimensional planning therefore demands a considerable degree of sophistication in this respect and is one reason why the Royal Marsden Radiotherapy Department is applying for the European Standard of Quality Control, ISO 9001. Every step in the treatment planning procedure must be carefully checked, and all machines, hardware, and software need to be subjected to rigorous scrutiny for accuracy.

Repeated portal imaging during therapy is the best way to confirm that the intended treatment is being delivered. In the absence of portal imaging as a routine procedure, in-vivo dosimetry with lithium fluoride or diode detectors and spot checks with conventional check films are invaluable. A small randomized trial of patient repositioning during radiotherapy using a megavoltage imaging system has been completed at the Royal Marsden, Sutton [21]. In 12 patients receiving pelvic radiotherapy, the mean field placement accuracy improved from 4.3 mm to 2 mm, and the proportion of treatments given with a field-placement error of 5 mm decreased from 69% to 7%. When on-line intervention was used, it was concluded that use of this system could allow a possible reduction in size of the margins needed around the target volume. Off-line image analysis can also be used to identify and reduce simulator to treatment errors.

Conclusions and future applications

The use of 3D planning and conformal radiotherapy is currently limited to phase 1 and 2 studies. Preliminary results have shown a reduction in acute side effects, which has led to dose-escalation studies, especially for carcinoma of the prostate. Carefully randomized phase 3 studies are necessary to assess not only late morbidity and local tumor control but also overall improvements in outcome and survival. While awaiting publication of such studies, it can be agreed that the concept of 3D conformal planning in the treatment of soft tissue sarcomas is attractive.

CT planning should be routinely employed if only to assist with accurate outlining and the manufacture of appropriate compensators. Simple blocking of radiation portals should be undertaken to exclude excessive volumes of adjacent normal tissue and can be performed in all departments, even without the use of 3D planning. At some sites, such a simple approach will prove adequate, but in the majority the additional time required for more sophisticated planning will almost certainly be of benefit to the patient. In the United Kingdom, the Medical Research Council has recently set up a group to look at technical advances in radiotherapy for the treatment of tumors at all sites. Subcommittees have been established to look specifically at both 3D planning and conformal therapy.

Attention should now be turned towards using portal measurements to compute the dose actually delivered to the patient [22]. Transit dosimetry is defined as the use of treatment-time portal images (megavoltage images) to determine the dose distribution delivered to the patient at the time of treatment [23]. Finally, it should be remembered that physical optimization of radiotherapy is only half the battle in achieving local tumor control. The other half is biological optimization, based primarily on dose and fractionation schedules [24]. These twin goals must be persued with equal enthusiasm.

Acknowledgments

It gives us great pleasure to thank all those surgeons who have been kind enough to refer patients for radiotherapy and, in particular, Mr. Meirion Thomas. We are most grateful to all of our colleagues in the Radiology, Radiotherapy, and Physics Departments. Special thanks go to Ms. Sandrine Leprêtre for typing this manuscript and to the Department of Photography at the Royal Marsden, London.

References

1. Robinson MH, Bidmead AM, Harmer CL. Value of conformal planning in the radiotherapy of soft tissue sarcoma. Clin Oncol 4:290–293, 1992.
2. Suit HD, Willett CG. Radiation therapy of sarcomas of the soft tissues. In Pinedo HM, Verweij J, Suit HD, eds. Soft Tissue Sarcomas. Cancer Treatment and Research Series. Kluwer Academic Publishers, Boston, MA 1991:64.
3. Glaholm J, Harmer CL. Soft-tissue sarcoma: Neutrons versus photons for post-operative irradiation. Br J Radiol 61:829–834, 1988.
4. Harmer CL, Frampton M, Wiltshaw E. Role of radiotherapy and chemotherapy in manage-

ment of soft tissue sarcomas. In Bloom HJG et al., eds. Head and Neck Oncology. New York: Raven Press, 1986:237–252.
5. Robinson MH, Ball ABS, Schofield J, Fisher C, Harmer CL, Thomas JM. Pre-operative radiotherapy for initially inoperable extremity soft tissue sarcomas. Clin Oncol 4:36–43, 1992.
6. Eeles RA, Fisher C, A'Hern RP, Robinson M, Rhys-Evans P, Henk JM, Archer D, Harmer CL. Head and neck sarcomas. Br J Cancer 68:201–207, 1993.
7. Fein DA, Corn BW, Lanciano RM, Herbert SH, Hoffman JP, Coia LR. Management of retroperitoneal sarcomas: Does dose escalation impact on locoregional control? Int J Radiat Oncol Biol Phys 31:129–134, 1995.
8. Harmer CL. Management of soft tissue sarcomas in adolescents. In Selby P, Clifford SB, eds. Cancer and the Adolescent. London: British Medical Association Publishing Group, 1996:69–89.
9. Graham JD, Robinson MH, Harmer CL. Re-irradiation of soft-tissue sarcoma. Br J Radiol 65:157–161, 1992.
10. Dusenbery KE, Thompson RC, Levitt SH. Extremity soft tissue sarcoma in adults. In Levitt SH, Khan FM, Potish RA, eds. Levitt and Tapley's Technological Basis of Radiation Therapy: Practical Clinical Applications. Philadelphia: Lea & Febiger, 1992:358.
11. Aribisala E. Cumulative trauma disorder: Occupational hazard of the '90s. Radiat Therap 2:27–29, 1993.
12. Duncan W, Williams JR, Kerr GR, Arnott SJ, Quilty PM, Rodger A. An analysis of the radiation related morbidity observed in a randomised trial of neutron therapy for bladder cancer. Int J Radiat Oncol Biol Phys 12:2085–2096, 1986.
13. Tait DM, Nahum AE. Conformal therapy. Eur J Cancer 26:750–753, 1990.
14. Tepper JE, Suit HD. Radiation therapy alone for sarcoma of soft tissue. Cancer 56:475–479, 1985.
15. Fein DA, Lee WR, Lanciano RM, Corn BW, Scott HH, Hanlon AL, Hoffman JP, Eisenberg BL, Coia LR. Management of extremity soft tissue sarcomas with limb-sparing surgery and postoperative irradiation: Do total dose, overall treatment time, and the surgery-radiotherapy interval impact on local control? Int J Radiat Oncol Biol Phys 32:969–976, 1995.
16. Kutcher GJ, Burman C, Brewster L, Goitein M, Mohan R. Histogram reduction method for calculating complication probabilities for three-dimensional treatment planning evaluations. Int J Radiat Oncol Biol Phys 21:137–146, 1991.
17. Mubata CD, Bidmead AM, Jones CH. Measurement of patients set-up variations using an electronic portal imaging system. Proceedings of 19th LH Gray Conference (BJR), 1995, in press.
18. Robinson MH. Soft tissue sarcoma: Prognostic factors and results of treatment, with special reference to the role of radiotherapy. M.D. Thesis, Cambridge University, 1992:268–276.
19. Robinson MH, Cassoni A, Harmer CL, Fisher C, Thomas JM, Westbury G. High dose hyperfractioned radiotherapy in the treatment of extremity soft tissue sarcomas. Radiother Oncol 22:118–126, 1991.
20. Stinson SF, Delaney TF, Yang J, Lampert M, Venzon D, Hicks J. Acute and long term effects on limb function of combined modality therapy in patients treated with limb sparing surgery for soft tissue sarcoma of the extremity. Int J Radiat Oncol Biol Phys 20:125, 1990.
21. Gildersleve J, Dearnaley DP, Evans PM, Law M, Rawlings C, Swindell W. A randomised trial of patient repositioning during radiotherapy using a megavoltage imaging system. Radiother Oncol 31:161–168, 1994.
22. Webb S. The Physics of Three-Dimensional Radiation Therapy. Medical Science Series. Bristol, UK: IOP Publishing, 1993:283.
23. The COVIRA Project. Therapy Plan Verification by Transit Dosimetry. COVIRA status report, 1995:21.
24. Harmer CL. Precision radiotherapy for the clinician. Varian Proceedings, Second Asian Users Meeting, Hong Kong, 1992:30.

10. Radiation-induced bone and soft tissue sarcomas: Clinical aspects and molecular biology

Ira J. Spiro and Herman D. Suit

Introduction

The development of treatment-induced cancer is one of the most devastating late complications of cancer therapy. Fortunately, these are quite uncommon in adult patients, that is, less than 1 in 200 at 20 years. In pediatric patients the risks are higher and may approach 1 in 5 at 20 years for patients with Ewing's sarcoma and retinoblastoma.

Patients who develop these second malignancies have usually been cured of their presenting cancers and have assumed that they will live cancer–free. Treatment of patients with radiation-induced cancers is often complicated by prior surgical and high-dose radiation treatment. Radiation is usually not a therapeutic option, even in combination with surgery. Also, active chemotherapeutic drugs such as doxorubicin may not be applicable if used as therapy for the presenting cancer due to the risk of cardiomyopathy. Surgical options may be limited due to the changes secondary to prior surgery and radiation. Therefore, patients are offered fewer options for the management of induced tumors. Despite the clinical problem that treatment-induced tumors present, little is known about the risk factors and molecular mechanism(s) of development. Furthermore, it is not clear whether some cancer patients are at a heightened risk or all patients carry the same risk. This review seeks to summarize the existing literature on radiation therapy–induced sarcoma in order to address some of these issues.

Clinical aspects of radiation-induced sarcomas

Nonfamilial sarcoma induction

Since the initial observation of induced tumors following radiotherapy, it was noted that a large proportion were bone or soft tissue sarcomas. Sarcomas are tumors of mesenchymal origin, usually arising in bone or soft tissue. Without a prior history of radiation exposure, primary sarcomas are quite rare, comprising only 0.7% of all cancers, with a yearly incidence in the United States of

J. Verweij, H.M. Pinedo, and H.D. Suit (eds). SOFT TISSUE SARCOMAS: PRESENT ACHIEVEMENTS AND FUTURE PROSPECTS.

approximately 5500 cases. In contrast, the Late Effects Study Group reported that sarcomas are the most common second malignancy and that 68% of these were associated with a prior course of radiation treatment [1]. Clearly, other tumor types are induced by radiation, but these are a minority of cases. Hence, the emphasis of this review is on radiation-induced sarcoma (RIS).

Radiation, and specifically radiation therapy, has long been recognized as capable of producing sarcomas. Cahan et al. [2] compiled one of the first comprehensive literature reviews on the subject in 1948. In this review, animal studies on RIS dated back to 1910 [3], with a human case occurring in 1922 [4]. A review by Laskin et al. [5] describes a sarcoma following the treatment of lupus [6]. Since the report of Cahan et al. [2], dozens of retrospective reviews on RIS have appeared in the scientific literature [5,7–19]. Many of these studies have approached the problem from the type of original presenting cancer (e.g., Hodgkin's disease or breast cancer), while others have looked at specific types of induced tumors (e.g., osteogenic sarcoma or soft tissue sarcoma).

In addition to the retrospective studies described earlier several studies exist that have looked at large numbers of irradiated patients in an attempt to assess the risk of RIS in specific cancer patient populations. In 1987, Tucker et al. [20], reported for The Late Effects Study Group on bone sarcomas in children, associated with radiotherapy and chemotherapy. In this study, 48 of 9170 patients surviving more than 2 years developed a bone cancer (relative risk, 133). Of interest, patients treated for retinoblastoma and Ewing's sarcoma carried the highest relative risks, 999 and 649, respectively. Relative risk was observed to increase with increasing radiation dose and with the use of alkylating agents. The cumulative risk at 20 years for the entire cohort was 2.8%, although this risk climbed to 5.5% at 30 years. The 20-year risks for retinoblastoma patients and Ewing's patients were 14.1% and 22.1%, respectively. Another cohort study, on adult women with breast cancer treated with radiotherapy, was reported by Taghian et al. [21]. Eleven sarcomas developed in 6919 patients, with a cumulative risk of 0.43% at 20 years and 0.78% at 30 years. The nearly eightfold difference in relative risk between the two studies may be due to a lower risk for adult patients in general and breast cancer patients in particular.

The criteria for RIS were first described by Cahan et al. [2]. These have been modified by other authors and generally include: (1) a prior history of a malignancy treated with radiation, (2) development of a histologically confirmed sarcoma within the field of irradiation used to treat the first tumor, and (3) a latency of several years between irradiation and sarcoma development. The latency period is arbitrary and has been set by various authors at 2–5 years.

Cancer syndromes

Bilateral retinoblastoma has served as a clinical paradigm for the two-hit Knudson hypothesis [22]. It has long been appreciated that patients with this disease are at high risk for osteosarcoma both within and outside of radiation fields [23–27]. In fact, patients with bilateral retinoblastoma show the highest relative risks of second cancers [28]. A recent review of a large cohort of retinoblastoma patients showed that 49 of 51 bone and soft tissue tumors occurred in irradiated patients, although it was yet to be determined whether these occurred infield [29]. This susceptibility to second nonocular tumors was presumed to arise from the same genetic defect that led to the retinoblastoma. The retinoblastoma (*Rb*) gene was eventually isolated, and the retinoblastoma phenotype was shown to be due to either inherited or new germinal mutations in this gene.

In addition to retinoblastoma, patients with the Li-Fraumeni syndrome are at high risk for developing second tumors, including bone and soft tissue sarcomas [30]. Patients with this syndrome are now known to carry germline mutation in the *p53* gene [31]. Malkin et al. have reported several cases of RIS in children with multiple malignancies in whom germline *p53* mutations were present [32]. As in the case of retinoblastoma, it is reasonable to presume, but unproved, that radiation injury to the wild-type *p53* allele played a role in the development of the radiation-induced sarcoma in these patients.

At least nine tumor suppresser genes have now been cloned, with the list expanding yearly [33,34]. In general, only small percentages of the overall cancer population carry germline mutations in these genes. It is unknown at present whether mutations in these genes play a role in RIS. For example, RIS following breast cancer is hypothesized to occur in patients with germline BRCA1 mutations. If this were in fact true, it would indicate that there are a small number of breast cancer patients with a very high risk of developing RIS, with the overall population of patients having a low risk. Currently, the risk of RIS is calculated as a function of the number of events divided by the total population at risk. If these events were occurring predominately in patients with germline mutations in a tumor suppresser gene, the risk of RIS in such patients would be grossly underestimated.

In addition to the tumor suppresser genes, other genes such as DNA repair genes may play a role in RIS. Patients with underlying DNA repair defects may accumulate DNA damage in genes that prevent or lead to neoplasia. One example is the ataxia-telangectasis (*AT*) gene. *AT* heterozygotes, which make up approximately 1% of the general population, are known to have elevated cancer risks [35]. This study also suggested that exposure to diagnostic ionizing radiation further increased the breast cancer risk. Whether such patients are at increased risk for RIS is not clear. The recent identification of the *AT* gene may elucidate this point [36].

Summary of risk factors

In addition to genetic factors, a number of other factors probably contribute to the risk of RIS [37]. These include both host and treatment-related factors (Table 1). Other factors possibly relating to the increased risk of RIS include younger age and gender. There are also treatment-related factors that contrib-

Table 1. Factors contributing to the risk of radiation-induced sarcoma

Host factors
Genetics
Age
Gender
Immunodeficiency
Tissue irradiated
Treatment-related factors
Radiation quality, dose, dose rate, dose per fraction
Radiation volume
Chemotherapy

ute to RIS. These include total radiation dose, dose per fraction, radiation quality, and volume of tissue exposed to radiation. In addition to radiation, chemotherapeutic agents have been associated with second cancers, usually acute myeloid leukemia (AML) [38–41]. In some of these studies, the risk of secondary AML is as high as 6–12% at 6 years after treatment. Chemotherapy has also been observed to increase the rate of radiation-induced cancers in general [42–44] and specifically of RIS [20]. There is great concern among oncologists that as cancer therapy becomes more aggressive, in terms of combining drugs and radiation and dose escalation, induced cancers may become more common. Because of the complexity of risk factors, it would be difficult to predict the absolute risk of RIS for an individual patient.

Clinical outcome of patients

Only a small number of studies have looked at the clinical outcome of patients with RIS. There are no convincing data to suggest that RIS has a different biology than sporadic sarcomas. Often patients with RIS cannot receive aggressive therapy because of prior experience with surgery, radiation, and chemotherapy in the treatment of their original presenting tumor. Also, RIS can arise in areas such as (1) the pelvis, where tumors can become quite large before being detected, and (2) and the spine, where, despite relatively early detection, en-bloc surgical resection is difficult or impossible. Weatherby et al. [45] noted that 23 of 24 patients with RIS of the spine, pelvis, or shoulder girdle were dead of disease, while 8 of 27 patients with extremity lesions survived 5 years or more. Wiklund et al. [46] showed that radically treated patients had a 5-year survival exceeding 40%, whereas non–radically treated patients had corresponding values of less than 20%. Other authors show a 5-year survival in the range of 11–17% [47,48].

Molecular biology of radiation-induced tumors

Currently, little is known regarding the mechanisms of radiation-induced tumor formation [34]. Specifically, the causative genetic lesions have not been identified. Furthermore, as discussed earlier, it is not understood whether these individuals have an underlying genetic abnormality that contributed to the formation of their first tumor and enhanced the likelihood of their development of a radiation-induced second tumor. It would be important to establish whether certain cancer patients were at higher risk for the development of treatment-induced cancers so that they could be informed of their risk and followed accordingly.

Retinoblastoma gene

Sporadic osteosarcoma and soft tissue sarcomas have also been shown to frequently involve the *Rb* gene [49–53]. Several cases of RIS in bilateral retinoblastoma patients have shown loss of the normal remaining allele in tumor DNA (D. Yandell, personal communication). It is tempting and reasonable to speculate that such a tumor arose as a result of the direct effect of radiation-associated damage on the normal allele, although this has not been proven.

p53 *gene*

It is attractive to hypothesize that the *p53* tumor suppressor gene is a target in RIS formation. Alterations in *p53* function can occur through discrete mutations, rearrangements, and gross deletions [54–56]. Therefore, altered gene function can occur following a variety of different lesions, rather than being a requirement for a specific mutation at a particular locus, as in the case of the *ras* family of genes. Consistent with this hypothesis, several studies have demonstrated *p53* alterations in radiation-induced murine osteosarcomas [57,58]. In a study of seven cell lines established from human radiation-induced tumors, two showed *p53* alterations, including one with an eight base-pair deletion [59]. Also, mice deficient in *p53* are susceptible to a variety of neoplasms, including bone and soft tissue sarcomas (see later) [60]. Irradiated transgenic mice harboring mutant *p53* alleles develop tumors more rapidly than their nonirradiated littermates [61]. Similarly, as discussed earlier, patients with the Li-Fraumeni syndrome, who carry germline *p53* mutations, develop sarcomas [31,62] and may be at higher risk for radiation-induced tumors [63]. There is also considerable evidence that *p53* alterations lead to the development of sporadic sarcomas [64–68]. Therefore, these data support the hypothesis that damage to the *p53* gene may be associated with or the causative factor for radiation-induced tumor formation.

The *p53* gene is also intriguing as a target for radiation-induced carcinogenesis since its function has been linked to DNA repair [69], apoptosis [70–72], and loss of senescence [73]. Loss of apoptotic function and senescence may allow clonal expansion of a radiation-transformed cell and the loss of repair capability may allow other genetic defects to accumulate in the process of multistage carcinogenesis. The *p53* protein is also interesting because it exists as a tetramer, formed from the gene products of each allele [74]. Mutant proteins can form complexes with wild-type proteins in the tetramer and can disrupt the normal function of the complex [75–79]. This influence of mutant forms of the *p53* protein on wild-type proteins has been referred to as *transdominance.* This property is unique to the *p53* gene.

Other carcinogens besides ionizing radiation have been linked to *p53*. Some of these studies indicate that there are 'signature' lesions in the *p53* gene attributable to specific carcinogens [80]. UV-induced mutations in *p53* in nonmelanoma human skin cancers indicate that damage is deposited in a carcinogen-specific fashion with the appearance of tandem CC to TT transitions [81]. Similar findings have been observed in UV-induced mouse skin cancers [82]. Radon-associated lung cancers frequently show G to T transversions at codon 249 [83]. Other examples include specific *p53* mutations in vinyl chloride–induced hepatic angiosarcomas [84] and endemic hepatocellular carcinoma associated with aflatoxin B_1 exposure or hepatitis B virus [85]. These studies indicate that for many carcinogens genetic damage is frequently deposited in a carcinogen-specific manner.

We have observed alterations in the *p53* gene in human RIS. In a sample of 16 tumors, 6 showed discrete *p53* alterations detected by single-strand conformational polymorphism analysis and direct genomic sequencing. Three of these six involved small deletions in the range of 6–12 base pairs, one was a tandem 2 base-pair change, and the two remaining alterations were point mutations (Table 2). The majority of *p53* mutations described in the literature involve single base changes, with less than 3.5% involving deletions of $\geq$2 base pairs [86]. Even among sporadic (i.e., non–radiation-induced) sarcomas that exhibit *p53* alterations, the majority (36 of 37) [combined data from 49,64,65,87) involve single base changes. Only 1 of these 37 patients showed a small (four base-pair) deletion [64]. Small deletions in the *p53* gene have been previously observed in association with radiation: a human mammary epithelial cell line transformed by radiation in vitro [88] and a cell line established from a RIS [59]. We hypothesize that these small microdeletions may be a signature lesion for prior radiation exposure. Of interest, we have detected no germline *p53* mutations among 23 patients with RIS. This second finding would indicate that *p53* germline mutations (i.e., the Li-Fraumeni syndrome) are not a predominant feature of RIS.

Radiation, unlike most carcinogens, can induce a broad spectrum of DNA damage, including point mutations, deletions, insertions, and gross structural alterations [89,90]. The DNA damage produced by ionizing radiation is mediated by the formation of hydroxyl radicals [90]. The heterogeneity of DNA damage induced by x-rays is well illustrated by studies of the human *hprt* gene. Alterations in this gene have been well characterized following in vitro radiation exposure and include point mutations, frame shifts, tandem base substitutions, and small deletions. In one study, small deletions (4–25 base pairs) were more commonly seen in radiation-induced mutants than in spontaneous mutants (20% vs. 5%) [91]. These small deletions were flanked by short sequence repeats. Others have also seen small deletions in the *hprt* gene following x-ray treatment. These deletions occurred at sites where flanking sequences showed direct repeats with deleted sequences [92], or at sites of possible hairpin structures [93]. Deletions at short regions of sequence homology have also been seen in *lacI* transgenic mice irradiated in vivo [94], further supporting the idea that small deletions are part of the spectrum of radiation-induced DNA damage.

Similar to the findings described earlier, the deletions and the tandem two base-pair change that we observed (Table 2) occurred at sites of repeat motifs in the *p53* gene (data not shown). Illegitimate nonhomologous recombination is seen after strand scission with restriction endonucleases at the human *aprt* locus [95]. In these studies, small deletions (1–36 base pairs) occurred at sites of 1–4 complimentary bases at the recombination junctions. These findings suggest that radiation may induce double-strand breaks in the *p53* gene, leading to small deletions following illegitimate recombination.

Transgenic and knockout mouse models

Genetically altered mice provide a unique opportunity to study radiation carcinogenesis. Mice, either lacking one or both alleles of a given tumor suppresser gene or carrying a mutant form of a human oncogene or tumor suppresser gene, can be readily produced. These animals also provide a model system for human disease states, characterized by genetic alterations that result in a phenotypic predisposition to tumor development. Lee et al. [96] showed that 10 of 26 mice carrying a mutant human *p53* transgene developed radiation-induced tumors by 10 weeks compared with 1 in 28 irradiated wild-type animals. Of interest, sarcomas were the most common radiation-induced tumor in these animals. Previous experiments have shown that non–radiation-induced tumors in these animals (occurring at 12–18 months) are more frequently lung adenocarcinomas or lymphomas [97]. Kemp et al. have shown

Table 2.

Presenting tumor site	Presenting tumor histology	Induced tumor site	Induced tumor histology	Interval to 2nd tumor	*p53* alteration	*p53* exon
Tongue	Squamous	Neck	MFH	2	T*GG* to T*AA*	5
Cervix	Squamous	Pelvic soft tissue	Extraskeletal osteosarcoma	26	Deletion	5
Skin	Squamous	Scalp	MFH	15	*C*CT to *G*CT	8
Pelvis	Lymphoma	Sacrum	MFH	5	Deletion	6
Leg	MFH	Femur	Osteosarcoma	8	G*A*C to G*T*C	7
Mediastinum	Hodgkin's	Scapula	Osteosarcoma	7	Deletion	4

that irradiated *p53* heterozygous adult mice (+/−) are more susceptible to tumor development (median time to tumor development 40 weeks) than untreated heterozygotes (median time to tumor development >70 weeks) [98]. Analysis of radiation-induced tumor DNA showed loss of the remaining allele in 96% of irradiated +/− animals. Null mice (−/−) also showed a greater frequency of radiation-induced tumors than untreated animals, although these animals had to be treated at an earlier age (2–6 days) for the effect to be seen. These studies underscore the importance of *p53* alterations in the development of RIS.

Other oncogenes

A number of other oncogenes have been implicated in radiation-induced tumors other than sarcomas in animal models or in humans. These include *ras* [99], *gsp* [99], c-*fos* [100], k-*ras* [101–103], *ret* [104], and c-*myc* [105–106]. c-*myc* has also been implicated in radiation-induced murine osteosarcomas [107].

Prospects for the future

Intensification of multimodal cancer therapy leading to improved survival, combined with more rigorous long-term cohort follow-up aided by the use of computerized databases, will most likely result in an increase in the observed rate of treatment-related malignancy. It may become possible through extended genetic screenings, able to examine multiple loci, to identify the majority of patients at higher risk for the development of RIS. Such patients could be appraised of their heightened risk and followed accordingly. In the meantime, until such molecular markers are available cancer clinicians should be wary of patients with remarkable personal or family cancer histories. In patients who have known genetic mutations in one of the genes for which screening is currently available (e.g., *Rb*, *p53*, *BRCA1*), the benefits and risks of treatment should be carefully weighed. Radiation oncologists should make every effort to utilize the benefits of conformal therapy and three-dimensional CT and MRI-based treatment planning to minimize the treatment of nontarget tissues. Reductions in the amount of irradiated normal tissue should result in a real reduction in the amount of RIS.

References

1. Meadows AT, Baum E, Fossati-Bellani F, et al. Second malignant neoplasms in children: An update from the late effects study group. J Clin Oncol 3:532–538, 1985.
2. Cahan WG, Woodard HQ, Higinbotham NL, et al. Sarcoma arising in irradiated bone. Cancer 1:3–29, 1948.
3. Marie P, Clunet J, Ravlot-LaPointe G. Contribution a l'etude du developement des tumeurs malignes sur le ulcers de roentgen. Bull Assoc Franc l'Etude Cancer 3:404–426, 1910.

4. Beck A. Zur Frage des Rontgensarkoms, zugleich ein Beitrag zur Pathogenese des Sarkoms. Munchen Med Wchnschr 69:623–624, 1922.
5. Laskin WB, Silverman TA, Enzinger FM. Postradiation soft tissue sarcomas. An analysis of 53 cases. Cancer 62:2330–2340, 1988.
6. Perthes G. Zur Frage der Roentgentherapie des Carcinomas. Archiv fur Klinische Chirurgie (Berlin) 74:400–405, 1904.
7. Robinson E, Neugut A, Wylie P. Clinical aspects of post-irradiation sarcomas. J Natl Cancer Inst 80:233–240, 1988.
8. Davidson T, Westbury G, Harmer CL. Radiation-induced soft tissue sarcoma. Br J Surg 73:308–309, 1986.
9. Kim JH, Chu FCH, Woodward HQ, Huvos A. Radiation induced sarcomas of bone following therapeutic radiation. Int J Radiat Oncol Biol Phys 9:107–110, 1983.
10. Mark RJ, Poen J, Tran LM, et al. Postirradiation sarcomas. Cancer 73:2653–2662.
11. Hatfield P, Schulz M. Postirradiation sarcoma. Radiology 96:593–602, 1970.
12. Mindell ER, Shah NK, Webster JH. Postradiation sarcoma of bone and soft tissues. Orthop Clin North Am 8:821–834, 1977.
13. Phillips TL, Sheline GE. Bone sarcomas following radiation therapy. Radiology 81:992–996, 1963.
14. Sim FH, Cupps RE, Dahlin DC, Ivins JC. Postradiation sarcoma of bone. J Bone Joint Surg 54A:1479–1489, 1972.
15. Tountas AA, Fornasier VL, Harwood AR, Leung PHK. Postirradiation sarcoma of bone. Cancer 43:182–187, 1979.
16. Senyszyn JJ, Johnston AD, Jacox HW, Chu FCH. Radiation-induced sarcoma after treatment of breast cancer. Cancer 26:394–403, 1970.
17. Sabanas AO, Dahlin DC, Childs DS, Ivins JC. Postradiation sarcoma of bone. Cancer 9:528–542, 1956.
18. Arlen M, Higinbotham NL, Huvos AG, et al. Radiation-induced sarcoma of bone. Cancer 28:1087–1099, 1971.
19. Huvos AG, Woodard HQ, Heilweil M. Postradiation malignant fibrous histiocytoma of bone. Am J Surg Pathol 10:9–18, 1986.
20. Tucker MA, D'Angio GJ, Boice JD, et al. Bone sarcomas linked to radiotherapy and chemotherapy in children. N Engl J Med 317:588–593, 1987.
21. Taghian A, De-Vathaire F, Terrier P, et al. Long-term risk of sarcoma following radiation treatment for breast cancer. Int J Radiat Oncol Biol Phys 21:361–367, 1991.
22. Knudson AG. Mutation and cancer: Statistical study of retinoblastoma. Proc Natl Acad Sci USA 68:820–3, 1971.
23. Roarty JD, McLean IW, Zimmerman LE. Incidence of second neoplasms in patients with bilateral retinobalstoma. Ophthalmology 91:1583–1587, 1988.
24. Winther J, Olsen JH, De-Nully Brown P. Risk of nonocular cancer among retinoblastoma patients and their parents. Cancer 62:1458–1462, 1988.
25. Der-Kindren DJ, Doten JW, Nagelkerke NJD, et al. Non-ocular cancer in patients with hereditary retinoblastoma and their relatives. Int J Cancer 41:499–504, 1988.
26. Abramson DA, Ellsworth RM, Kitchin FD, Tung G. Second nonocular tumors in retinoblastoma survivors. Ophthalmology 91:1351–1355, 1984.
27. Draper GJ, Sanders BM, Kingston JE. Second primary neoplasms in patients with retinoblastoma. Br J Cancer 53:661–671, 1986.
28. Tucker MA, D'Angio GJ, Boice JD, et al. Bone sarcomas linked to radiotherapy and chemotherapy in children. N Engl J Med 317:588–593, 1987.
29. Eng C, Li FP, Abramson DH, et al. Mortality from second tumors among long-term survivors of retinoblastoma. J Natl Cancer Inst 85:1121–1128, 1993.
30. Li FP, Fraumeni JF. Soft-tissue sarcomas, breast cancer, and other neoplasms. Ann Int Med 71:747–752, 1969.30.
31. Malkin D, Li FP, Strong LC, et al. Germ line p53 mutations in a familial syndrome of breast cancer, sarcomas, and other neoplasms. Science 250:1233–1238, 1990.

32. Malkin D, Jolly KW, Barbier N, et al. Germline mutations of the p53 tumor-suppressor gene in children and young adults with second malignant neoplasms. N Engl J Med 326:1309–1315, 1992.
33. Weinberg RA. Oncogenes and tumor suppressor genes [review]. CA Cancer J Clin 44:160–170, 1994.
34. Sankaranarayanan K, Chakraborty R. Cancer predisposition, radiosensitivity and the risk of radiation-induced cancers. I. Background. Radiat Res 143:121–143, 1995.
35. Swift M, Morrelll D, Massey RB, Chase CL. Incidence of cancer in 161 families affected by ataxia-telangiectasia. N Engl J Med 325:1831–1836, 1991.
36. Savitsky K, Bar-Shira A, Gilad S, et al. A single ataxia telangiectasia gene with a product similar to PI-3 kinase. Science 268:1749–1753, 1995.
37. Parker RG. Radiation-induced cancer as a factor in clinical decision making. Int J Radiat Oncol Biol Phys 18:993–1000, 1990.
38. Detourmignies L, Castaigne S, Stoppa AM, et al. Therapy-related acute promyelocytic leukemia: A report on 16 cases. J Clin Oncol 10:1430–1435, 1992.
39. Winick NJ, McKenna RW, Shuster JJ, et al. Secondary acute myeloid leukemia in children with acute lymphoblastic leukemia treated with etoposide. J Clin Oncol 11:209–217, 1993.
40. Pui CH, Ribeiro RC, Hancock ML, et al. Acute myeloid leukemia in children treated in epipodophyllotoxins for acute lymphoblastic leukemia. N Engl J Med 325:1682–1687, 1991.
41. Van Leeuwen FE, Chorus AMJ, Van den Belt-Dusebout AS, et al. Leukemia risk following Hodgkin's disease: Relation to cumulative dose of alkylating agents, treatment with teniposide combinations, number of episodes of chemotherapy, and bone marrow damage. J Clin Oncol 12:1063–1073, 1994.
42. Tucker MA, Coleman CN, Cox RS, et al. Risk of second cancers after treatment for Hodgkin's disease. N Engl J Med 318:76–81, 1988.
43. Lowsky R, Lipton J, Fyles G, et al. Secondary malignancies after bone marrow transplantation in adults. J Clin Oncol 12:2187–2192, 1994.
44. Cimino G, Papa G, Tura S, et al. Second primary cancer following Hodgkin's: Updated results of an Italian multicentric study. J Clin Oncol 9:432–437, 1991.
45. Weatherby RP, Dahlin DC, Ivins JC. Postradiation sarcoma of bone. Review of 78 Mayo Clinic cases. Mayo Clin Proc 56:294–306, 1981.
46. Wiklund TA, Blomqvist CP, Raty J, et al. Postirradiation sarcoma. Cancer 68:524–531, 1991.
47. Davidson T, Westbury G, Harmer CL. Radiation-induced soft-tissue sarcoma. Br J Surg 73:308–309, 1986.
48. Huvos AG, Woodard HQ, Cahan WG, et al. Postradiation osteogenic sarcoma of bone and soft tissues. Cancer 55:1244–1255, 1985.
49. Stratton MR, Moss S, Warren W, et al. Mutation of the p53 gene in human soft tissue sarcomas: Association with abnormalities of the RB1 gene. Oncogene 5:1297–1301, 1990.
50. Wunder JS, Czitrom AA, Kandel R, Andrulis IL. Analysis of alterations in the retinoblastoma gene and tumor grade in bone and soft-tissue sarcoma. J Natl Cancer Inst 83:194–200, 1991.
51. Toguchida J, Ishizaki K, Sasaki MS, et al. Chromosomal reorganization for the expression of recessive mutation of retinoblastoma susceptibility gene in the development of osteosarcoma. Cancer Res 48:3939–3943, 1988.
52. Reissmann PT, Simon MA, Lee WH, Slamon DJ. Studies of the retinoblastoma gene in human sarcomas. Oncogene 4:831–843, 1989.
53. Cance WG, Brennan MF, Dudas ME, et al. Altered expression of the retinoblastoma gene product in human sarcomas. N Engl J Med 323:1457–1462, 1990.
54. Hollstein M, Sidransky D, Vogelstein B, Harris CC. p53 mutations in human cancers. Science 253:49–53, 1991.
55. Frebourg T, Friend SH. The importance of p53 gene alterations in human cancer: Is there more than circumstantial evidence? J Natl Cancer Inst 85:1554–1557, 1993.

56. Levine AJ, Momand J, Finlay CA. The p53 tumour suppressor gene. Nature 35:453–456, 1991.
57. Chandar N, Billig B, McMaster J, Novak J. Inactivation of p53 gene in human and murine osteosarcoma cells. Br J Cancer 65:208–214, 1992.
58. Strauss PG, Mitreiter K, Zitzelsberger H, et al. Elevated p53 RNA expression correlates with incomplete osteogenic differentiation of radiation-induced murine osteosarcomas. Int J Cancer 50:252–258, 1992.
59. Brachman DG, Hallahan DE, Beckett MA, et al. p53 gene mutations and abnormal retinoblastoma protein in radiation-induced human sarcomas. Cancer Res 51:6393–6396, 1991.
60. Donehower LA, Harvey M, Slagle BL, et al. Mice deficient for p53 are developmentally normal but susceptible to spontaneous tumours. Nature 356:215–221, 1992.
61. Lee JM, Abrahamson JLA, Kandel R, et al. Susceptibility to radiation-carcinogenesis and accumulation of chromosomal breakage in p53 deficient mice. Oncogene 9:3731–3736, 1994.
62. Malkin D. p53 and the Li-Fraumeni syndrome. Cancer Genet Cytogenet 66:83–92, 1993.
63. Levine AJ. The p53 tumor-suppressor gene. N Engl J Med 326:1350–1352, 1992.
64. Toguchida J, Yamaguchi T, Ritchie B, et al. Mutation spectrum of the p53 gene in bone and soft tissue sarcomas. Cancer Res 52:6194–6199, 1992.
65. Andreassen A, Oyjord T, Hovig E, et al. p53 abnormalities in different subtypes of human sarcomas. Cancer Res 53:468–471, 1993.
66. Mulligan LM. Matlashewski GH, Scrable HJ, Cavenee WK. Mechanisms of p53 loss in human sarcomas. Proc Natl Acad Sci USA 87:5863–5867, 1990.
67. Masuda H, Miller C, Koeffler HP, et al. Rearrangement of the p53 gene in human osteogenic sarcomas. Proc Natl Acad Sci USA 84:7716–7719, 1987.
68. Miller CW, Aslo A, Tsay C, et al. Frequency and structure of p53 rearrangement in human osteosarcoma. Cancer Res 50:7950–7954, 1990.
69. Smith ML, Chen IT, Zhan Q, et al. Interaction of the p53-regulated protein Gadd 45 with proliferating cell nuclear antigen. Science 266:1376–1380, 1994.
70. Symonds H, Krall L, Remington L, et al. p53 dependent apoptosis suppresses tumor growth and progression in vivo. Cell 78:703–711, 1994.
71. Lowe SW, Schmitt EM, Smith SW, et al. p53 is required for radiation-induced apoptosis in mouse thymocytes. Nature 362:847–849, 1993.
72. Clarke AR, Purdie CA, Harrison DJ, et al. Thymocyte apoptosis induced by p53 dependent and independent pathways. Nature 362:849–852, 1993.
73. Bond JA, Wyllie FS, Wynfort-Thomas D. Escape from senescence in human diploid fibroblasts induced directly by mutant p53. Oncogene 9:1885–1889, 1994.
74. Friedman PH, Chen X, Bargonetti J, Prives C. The p53 protein is an unusualy shaped tetramer that binds directly to DNA. Proc Natl Acad Sci USA 90:3319–3323, 1993.
75. Srivastava S, Wang S, Tong YA, et al. Dominant negative effect of a germ-line mutant p53: A step fostering tumorigenesis. Cancer Res 53:4452–4455, 1993.
76. Milner J, Medcalf EA. Cotranslation of activated mutant p53 with wild type drives the wild-type p53 protein into the mutant conformation. Cell 65:765–774, 1991.
77. Unger T, Nau MM, Segal S, Minna JD. p53: A transdominant regulator of transcription whose function is abated by mutations occurring in human cancer. EMBO J 11:1383–1390, 1992.
78. Gerwin BI, Spillare E, Forrester K, et al. Mutant p53 can induce tumorigenic conversion of human bronchial epithelial cells and reduce their responsiveness to a negative growth factor, transforming growth factor β_1. Proc Natl Acad Sci USA 89:2759–2763, 1992.
79. Srivastava S, Wang S, Tong YA, et al. Several mutant p53 proteins detected in cancer-prone families with Li-Fraumeni syndrome exhibit transdominant effects on the biochemical properties of the wild-type 53. Oncogene 8:2449–2456, 1993.
80. Vogelstein B, Kinzier KW. Carcinogens leave fingerprints. Nature 355:209–210, 1992.

81. Brash DE, Rudolph JA, Simon JA, et al. A role for sunlight in skin cancer: UV-induced p53 mutations in squamous cell carcinoma. Proc Natl Acad Sci USA 88:10124–10128, 1991.
82. Kanjilal S, Pierceall WE, Cummings KK, et al. High frequency of p53 mutations in ultraviolet radiation-induced murine skin tumors: Evidence for strand bias and tumor heterogeneity. Cancer Res 53:2961–2964, 1993.
83. Taylor JA, Watson MA, Devereux TR, et al. p53 mutation hotspot in radon-associated lung cancer. Lancet 343:86–87, 1994.
84. Hollstein M, Marion MJ, Lehman T, et al. p53 mutations at A:T base pairs in angiosarcomas of vinyl chloride-exposed factory workers. Carcinogen 15:1–3, 1994.
85. Aguilar F, Hussain SP, Cerutti P. Aflatoxin B_1 induced the transversion of G→T in condon 249 of the p53 tumor suppressor gene in human hepatocytes. Proc Natl Acad Sci USA 90:8586–8590, 1993.
86. Jego M, Thomas G, Hamelin R. Short direct repeats flanking deletions, and duplicating insertions in p53 gene in human cancers. Oncogene 8:209–213, 1993.
87. Leach FS, Tokino T, Meltzer P, et al. p53 mutation and MDM2 amplification in human soft tissue sarcomas. Cancer Res 53:2231–2234, 1993.
88. Wazer DE, Chu Q, Liu XL, et al. Los of p53 protein during radiation transformation of primary human mammary epithelial cells. Mol Cell Biol 14:2468–2478, 1994.
89. Hutchinson F. Molecular biology of mutagenesis of mammalian cells by ionizing radiation. Semin Cancer Biol 4:85–92, 1993.
90. Breimer LH. Ionizing radiation-induced mutagenesis. Br J Cancer 57:6–18, 1988.
91. Nelson SL, Giver CR, Grosovsky AJ, Spectrum of X-ray – induced mutations in the human *hprt* gene. Carcinogen 15:495–502, 1994.
92. Okinaka RT, Anzick SL, Oller A, Thilly WG. Analysis of large X-ray–induced mutant populations by denaturing gradient gel electrophoresis. Radiat Res 135:212–221, 1993.
93. Denault CM, Skopek TR, Liber HL. The effects of hypoxia and cysteamine on x-ray mutagenesis in human cells. II. *hprt m*RNA expression and cDNA sequence analysis of induced mutants. Radiat Res 136:271–279, 1993.
94. Winegar RA, Lutze LH, Hamer JD, et al. Radiation-induced point mutations, deletions and micronuclei in lacI transgenic mice. Mut Res 307:479–487, 1994.
95. Phillips JW, Morgan WF. Illegitimate recombination induced by DNA double-strand breaks in a mammalian chromosone. Mol Cell Biol 14:5794,5803, 1994.
96. Lee JM, Abrahamson LA, Kandel R, et al. Susceptibility to radiation-carcinogenesis and accumulation of chromosomal breakage in p53 deficient mice. Oncogene 9:3731–3736, 1994.
97. Laviguer A, Maltby V, Mock D, et al. High incidence of lung, bone, and lymphoid tumors in transgenic mice overexpressing mutant alleles of the p53 oncogene. Mol Cell Biol 9:3982–3991, 1989.
98. Kemp CJ, Wheldon T, Balmain A. p53-deficient mice are extremely susceptible to radiation-induced tumorigenesis. Nature Genet 8:66–69, 1994.
99. Challeton C, Bounacer A, DuVillard JA, et al. Pattern of ras and gsp oncogene mutations in radiation-associated human thyroid tumors. Oncogene 11:601–603, 1995.
100. Ishihara H, Yoshida K, Nemoto K, et al. Constitutive overexpression of the c-fos gene in radiation-induced granulocytic leukemia in mice. Radiat Res 135:394–399, 1993.
101. Sloan SR, Newcomb EW, Pellicer A. Neutron radiation can activate K-ras via a point mutations in codon 146 and induces a different spectrum of ras mutations than does gamma radiation. Mol Cell Biol 10:405–408, 1990.
102. Wright PA, Williams ED, Lemoine NR, Wynford-Thomas D, Radiation-associated and 'spontaneous' human thyroid carcinomas show a different pattern of ras oncogene mutation. Oncogene 6:471–473, 1991.
103. Sawey MJ, Hood AT, Burns FJ, Garte SJ. Activation of c-myc and c-K-ras oncogenes in primary rat tumors induced by ionizing radiation. Mol Cell Biol 7:932–935, 1987.
104. Ito T, Seyama T, Iwamoto KS, et al. In vitro irradiation is able to cause RET oncogene rearrangement. Cancer Res 53:2940–2943, 1993.

105. Garte SJ, Burns FJ, Ashkenazi-Kimmel T, et al. Amplification of the c-myc oncogene during progression of radiation-induced rat toxin tumors. Cancer Res 50:3073–3077, 1990.
106. Felber M, Burns FJ, Garte SJ. Amplification of c-myc oncogene in radiation-induced rat skin tumors as a function of linear energy transfer and dose. Radiat Res 131:297–301, 1992.
107. Sturm SA, Strauss PG, Adolph S, et al. Amplification and rearrangement of c-myc radiation-induced murine osteosarcomas. Cancer Res 50:4146–4153, 1990.

11. Chemotherapy for metastatic soft tissue sarcomas

William P. Steward

Introduction

Once soft tissue sarcomas have become metastatic, or if local disease is too extensive for control with surgery and/or radiotherapy, chemotherapy may be considered as a possible treatment modality. Unfortunately adult soft tissue sarcomas are among the most chemoresistant of all malignancies, and it is important to know the limitations of its use as well as its potential value. This chapter summarizes our current knowledge of the activity of single-agent chemotherapy and of combination regimens, and reviews the potential value of high-dose and dose-intensive regimens. Given the limited value of conventional chemotherapy in this disease, future directions for research are discussed and the importance of treating patients within controlled clinical trials is emphasized.

Single-agent chemotherapy

There are only two commercially available single agents with greater than 20% reproducible activity against soft tissue sarcomas, doxorubicin and ifosfamide. Unfortunately, the experience with many agents is often inadequate to make clear statements about their value in this disease, particularly because many studies have included insufficient numbers of patients. This is a serious problem in any population of patients with soft tissue sarcomas, which will contain individuals with a wide variety of prognostic factors that may influence the likelihood of response. Such factors include performance status, prior chemotherapy, site and extent of disease, and histological type and grade of sarcoma. It is always essential to consider the patient characteristics when interpreting the results of studies in this disease. It is also important to note that the evaluation of response has become increasingly rigorous because CT imaging has frequently replaced plain radiography and quality control in cooperative groups has improved. This is almost certainly a factor in the widely observed reduction in response rates being seen in recent years for patients with soft tissue sarcomas included in trials.

J. Verweij, H.M. Pinedo, and H.D. Suit (eds). SOFT TISSUE SARCOMAS: PRESENT ACHIEVEMENTS AND FUTURE PROSPECTS.

Anthracyclines

Doxorubicin has been extensively examined in adult soft tissue sarcoma and is one of the most active single agents. The first phase II study was performed by the Southwest Oncology Group (SWOG) in 1973 [1] and demonstrated 2 complete responses (CRs) and 13 partial remissions (PRs) among 49 patients (overall response rate 31%). Subsequent studies by many cooperative groups revealed often widely varying activity, with a range of 9–70%. An overview of 619 previously untreated patients in trials that have included single-agent doxorubicin reveals an average response rate of 22% [2], a figure that is very similar to that seen in recently published, large, well-documented studies and one that probably accurately reflects the activity of doxorubicin in this disease.

Several groups have attempted to optimize the use of doxorubicin, by altering either the dose or schedule. A small number of randomized [3–6] and nonrandomized [7] studies have suggested that a dose-response relationship exists in sarcomas. The first such trial from the SWOG [3] divided patients into 'good' and 'poor' risk groups depending on a variety of factors, including whether or not the clinician felt they could tolerate three cycles at a dose of 50 mg/m^2. For the good-risk patients who were randomized to 75 mg/m^2, 60 mg/m^2, or 45 mg/m^2, the response rates were 37%, 20%, and 18%, respectively. The poor-risk patients received 50 mg/m^2 or 25 mg/m^2 and the respective response rates were 11% and 0%. Despite the obvious problems with this trial design, its results, taken in conjunction with those of the other similar trials, suggest that there is a dose-response relationship for doxorubicin and it appears to be important to achieve a dose intensity of at least 70 mg/m^2 every 3 weeks to obtain an optimal response rate. Much of the variability in the reported activity of doxorubicin for the different phase II studies could have resulted from different delivered dose intensities.

Unfortunately, increasing the dose of doxorubicin therapy is often limited by severe toxicity, particularly cumulative cardiotoxicity. Anthracycline analogues have been examined in an attempt to find an effective agent with less side effects, but the results have generally been disappointing. Carminomycin was initially reported to have comparable activity to doxorubicin (27% response rate) [8], but a subsequent study by the European Organization for Research and Treatment of Cancer (EORTC) revealed only 1 PR (3%) in 33 evaluable patients [9]. Epirubicin has been more extensively investigated, and an early randomized trial compared equimolar doses (75 mg/m^2) of doxorubicin and epirubicin in nonpretreated patients. The response rate was slightly higher for doxorubicin (25%) than epirubicin (18%), although the difference was not statistically significant [10]. At these dose levels, the myelosuppression of epirubicin was much lower and studies using equitoxic doses were thus performed. At 100–130 mg/m^2, myelosuppression increased but, unfortunately, activity was no greater (19% in 32 patients) [11]. A large randomized study has recently been completed by the EORTC Sarcoma Group comparing doxorubicin 75 mg/m^2 with epirubicin 150 mg/m^2 (given as a single bolus or fractionated over 3 days) [12]. In this study 334 non-pretreated patients were entered, and the overall response rate was 18%, with no difference among the three arms. There was significantly greater myelosuppression in both the epirubicin arms, and cardiotoxicity was seen at a similar incidence for both agents. There does not, therefore, appear to be any advantage to using the anthracycline analogues that are currently available over doxorubicin, at least in patients with previously untreated soft tissue sarcomas.

Alkylating agents

Interest in the use of alkylating agents in the treatment of soft tissue sarcomas was limited until ifosfamide became available. Cyclophosphamide showed overall single agent activity of only 8% in the 82 patients included in phase II studies [13]. Evidence of the activity of ifosfamide had been reported in the late 1970s and early 1980s, with one study that contained 18 patients demonstrating a 67% response rate [14]. The serious urothelial toxicity of the metabolites of ifosfamide prevented further trials until the development of the uroprotector, mesna, revived interest in this agent. One of the earliest formal phase II studies was performed at the Royal Marsden Hospital, and a promising 38% response rate was seen in 42 patients [15]. A subsequent important study by the EORTC randomized 171 patients to roughly equitoxic doses of cyclophosphamide (1.5 g/m^2) or ifosfamide (5 g/m^2), and allowed crossover to the other arm for patients who progressed [16]. The response rate to ifosfamide (overall, 18%; previously untreated patients 25%) was higher than for cyclophosphamide (overall, 8%; previously untreated patients, 13%). Four responses occurred among 33 patients crossed from cyclophosphamide to ifosfamide, whereas no activity was seen in patients crossed from ifosfamide to cyclophosphamide. Ifosfamide, therefore, appeared to be superior in terms of activity, and its choice for further study in combination regimens by the group was supported by its significantly lower associated myelosuppression.

Antimetabolites

Methotrexate has minimal activity in soft tissue sarcomas and 5-fluorouracil is inactive [17]. Several newer antimetabolites have been tested in phase II studies in recent years. Fludarabine phosphate was administered to 20 previously treated patients at a dose of 100–125 mg/m^2 every 3 weeks at Wayne State University but no activity was seen [18]. PALA (N-phosphonacetyl-L-aspartate), an inhibitor of pyrimidine biosynthesis, has been investigated in two studies. In the first, no activity was seen in 17 pretreated patients [19]. A subsequent study added dipyridamole in the hope that this would inhibit the transport of circulating uridine into the tumor cells and thus prevent rescue of the cells from the effects of PALA [20]. Only one partial remission (5%) was seen among 19 patients entered into the study, and side effects were severe, including diarrhea, vomiting, and headache.

Two analogues of methotrexate have been investigated, and modest activity has been reported. Trimetrexate was used in three trials at the Dana Farber Cancer Institute and the National Cancer Institute of Canada (NCIC). The first of these utilized a dose of 8 mg/m^2/day for 5 successive days every 3 weeks [21]. No responses were seen in 14 patients, and toxicity was severe, with myelosuppression and mucositis. The second study [22] varied the dose (8–12 mg/m^2) depending on the extent of prior therapy, and 4 partial responses were documented in 25 patients (16% response rate). The final study involved single bolus infusions (125 mg/m^2) repeated every 2 weeks [22]. Two partial remissions (8%) were seen in 25 patients. The results of all three studies combined indicate a 10% overall response rate, which, given the toxicity of the agent, is insufficient to warrant further development. The other analogue, edatrexate (10-EDAM), has theoretical benefits over methotrexate in that it is more effectively transported across cell membranes and more highly polyglutamated than the parent compound. A phase II study at the Memorial Sloan–Kettering Cancer Center [23], using a dose of 80 mg/m^2 weekly for 5 weeks followed by 2-weekly administration in 34 evaluable non-pretreated patients, resulted in five partial responders (14% response rate). Given the modest activity but lack of serious toxicity, edatrexate is being examined in combination with ifosfamide in soft tissue sarcomas.

Vinca alkaloids and taxoids

Vincristine is frequently incorporated into combination chemotherapy regimens, although formal phase II studies have never been performed in soft tissue sarcomas and anecdotal reports from larger single-agent studies have suggested a low response rate of only 5% [13]. A large randomized study by the Eastern Cooperative Oncology Group (ECOG) investigated the role of vindesine and randomized 298 patients to single-agent doxorubicin 70 mg/m^2 or to the same dose of doxorubicin with vindesine 3 mg/m^2 repeated every 3 weeks. Response rates were the same in both arms (17% and 18%, respectively), and there was no significant difference in time to progression and survival [24]. This study strongly suggests that vindesine is inactive in soft tissue sarcomas and simply adds to toxicity when used in combination.

Recent interest has focussed on the two taxoids, docetaxel (taxotere) and paclitaxel (taxol). The EORTC Sarcoma Group reported the results of a study using docetaxel 100 mg/m^2 every 3 weeks in 29 patients who had all received prior chemotherapy [25]. An encouraging response rate of 17% was seen — results similar to those with doxorubicin and DTIC in the relapse setting. Preliminary results from the NCIC using the same regimen in untreated patients have been reported and show a more disappointing response rate of only 11% [26]. Paclitaxel appears to be inactive, with no responses observed among 13 patients (9 with no prior chemotherapy) treated at a dose of 200 mg/m^2 at the University of Florida [27].

Other agents

Dacarbazine (DTIC) is frequently employed in the treatment of adult soft tissue sarcomas and has a remarkably consistent response rate of approximately 18% in phase II studies [28]. Unfortunately toxicity is substantial, with severe nausea and vomiting, myelosuppression, and pain at the injection site. A fractionated administration over 5 days has often been employed, but single-bolus delivery appears equally effective [29] and is more acceptable for the patient.

Cisplatin has been used in 103 patients in phase II studies [13] and has an overall response rate of 12%. Its activity appears to be limited to gynecological sarcomas [30], and it has no activity in other sites. Carboplatin has similar activity, with three complete and three partial remissions in 50 patients (overall response rate 12%) [31].

The topoisomerase I (topotecan and irinotecan) and II (etoposide) inhibitors have been widely studied in a variety of malignancies but limited information is available on their activity in soft tissue sarcomas. Topotecan 1.5 mg/m^2 was administered daily ×5 to 17 non-pretreated patients in a study of the NCIC and two partial responses (13%) were seen, suggesting only modest activity [32]. No studies with irinotecan have been reported, but collected experience in 52 patients treated with etoposide in three broad phase I/II studies reveal only one partial response [33–35]. This lack of activity was confirmed in a study of 19 evaluable patients who received ifosfamide 8 g/m^2 plus etoposide 100 mg/m^2 [36]. Only two partial responses were observed (response rate 10.5%), suggesting that etoposide did not enhance the activity of ifosfamide (although the dose of etoposide was suboptimal). A phase II study by the EORTC with single-agent etoposide is ongoing and should provide definitive information on the role of this agent in soft tissue sarcomas.

Combination chemotherapy

In an attempt to improve the results of treatment of advanced soft tissue sarcomas, several combination chemotherapy regimens have been used. Murine models with sarcoma 180 demonstrated greater tumor volume reduction with the combination of doxorubicin and dacarbazine than with either agent alone without significantly increased toxicity [37]. The first study was performed by the SWOG and was reported by Gottlieb et al. [38] in 1972. Doxorubicin 60 mg/m^2 on day 1 and DTIC 250 mg/m^2/day on days 1–5 were administered to 210 evaluable patients. Twenty-five complete responders (12%) and 67 partial responders (30%) were documented, with the encouraging observation of long-term survival (>3 years) for the majority of the CRs. A retrospective comparison with previous experience of the group using single-agent doxorubicin suggested that combination therapy was associated with a survival advantage, the median survival being increased from 8 to 15 months [39]. A subsequent study added vincristine to the doxorubicin/DTIC combination, and an identical response rate of 42% (10% CR) was obtained in 107 evaluable patients [40]. When the dose intensity of doxorubicin in this combination was reduced to 50 mg/m^2 every 5 weeks in a study of 54 patients at the Mayo Clinic, the results were inferior, with a response rate of only 11% (CR 2%) [41], supporting evidence for the importance of the dose intensity of anthracyclines in this disease.

Although cyclophosphamide was active in childhood sarcomas, its activity in adult disease is minimal. Despite this it was added to Adriamycin, vincristine, and DTIC in several studies in what is one of the most common regimens (CyVADIC) used to treat soft tissue sarcomas. The first report was from the M. D. Anderson Cancer Center and SWOG and included 125 evaluable patients, 50% of whom achieved a response (17% CR). Subsequent results with this regimen have varied widely, with response rates of 15–57% [42] in different studies. An important observation reported by Yap et al. [43] relates to the importance of achieving a CR with this regimen. In their experience with 331 patients who received CyVADIC, 21% of those who achieved a CR were long-term survivors (>5 years) and were potentially cured.

The major problem with the CyVADIC regimen was the need for hospitalization over the 5 days of DTIC administration. Modifications have thus been made, and three groups have examined an intermittent schedule with the DTIC given on one day [29,44,45] without an apparent reduction in efficacy. An important study by the EORTC randomized patients to the standard CyVADIC, with 5 days of DTIC or a regimen comprising the same doses and agents but given as a split regimen, with doxorubicin and DTIC alternating every 4 weeks with cyclophosphamide and vincristine [5]. An overall response rate of 38% (17% CR) was seen for CyVADIC, but only 14% responses (5% CR) were seen for the other arm ($p = 0.001$), again confirming the importance of maintaining the doxorubicin dose intensity. This study also demonstrated the importance of the Karnofsky performance index (KP) in determining response, with only 14% of those patients presenting with a KP < 80 achieving a remission compared with 41% of those with a KP of 90. Interpretation of data on phase II/III activity of chemotherapy in this disease should obviously be made with the availability of this information.

The M. D. Anderson Hospital modified the CyVADIC regimen further by removing vincristine, which appeared to have only marginal activity as a single agent, and infusing the doxorubicin and DTIC continuously over 4 days (cyclophosphamide was given as a bolus on day 1) in order to reduce toxicity [46]. Fifty patients were treated and a 54% response rate (14% CR) was recorded.

With the demonstration of ifosfamide's activity, several groups investigated its combination with doxorubicin. The first such study involved 24-hour infusions of ifosfamide at doses of 5–8 g/m^2 with doxorubicin 40–60 mg/m^2 repeated every 3 weeks [47]. A 30% response rate (11% CR) was reported and the optimal doses appeared to be doxorubicin 50 mg/m^2 with ifosfamide 5 g/m^2. A subsequent study by the EORTC used this combination in 175 evaluable non-pretreated patients [48]. A response rate of 35% (9% CR) was achieved with a median time to progression for those with a partial remission of 40 weeks and for complete responders of 67 weeks. Although myelosuppression was often severe (grade 3 or 4 in 73% patients), other toxicities were less than had been seen in the EORTC's experience with CyVADIC, and the activity appeared to be at least equivalent.

The Dana Farber combined the three most active single agents — ifosfamide, doxorubicin, and DTIC — in the MAID regimen and carried out an initial phase I study, from which they concluded that the optimal doses were doxorubicin 60 mg/m^2, ifosfamide 7.5 g/m^2, and DTIC 900 mg/m^2 [49]. The chemotherapy was given as a continuous 72-hour infusion every 3 weeks and was generally well tolerated. A subsequent phase II study involving 62 evaluable patients [50] demonstrated a 52% response rate (10% CR) and led to an intergroup randomized study (see later) comparing MAID with the same combination without ifosfamide.

Randomized studies

The majority of randomized studies in advanced soft tissue sarcomas have been performed by the large cooperative groups. The Eastern Cooperative Oncology Group (ECOG) conducted a series of trials and retained single agent doxorubicin as a 'standard' arm. Their initial study attempted to determine whether combination chemotherapy was superior to single agent anthracycline. 210 patients were randomised to single agent doxorubicin 70 mg/m^2 every 3 weeks, doxorubicin 50 mg/m^2 plus cyclophosphamide 750 mg/m^2 and vincristine 1.4 mg/m^2 (ACV) every 21 days or cyclophosphamide 750 mg/m^2 with vincristine 1.4 mg/m^2 and actinomycin D 0.4 mg/m^2 (CVAd) every 3 weeks [4]. The highest response rate (27%) was seen in the single-agent doxorubicin arm, whereas a 19% response rate was seen with ACV and only 11% of patients responded to CVAd. Three important conclusions can be drawn from this trial. The first is that doxorubicin at its maximally tolerated dose intensity of $\geq$70 mg/m^2/21 days provides a greater chance of response than lower doses. Secondly, the addition of cyclophosphamide and vincristine to doxorubicin, by reducing the dose intensity of anthracycline that can be delivered, is inferior to single-agent doxorubicin at the optimal dose. The final conclusion is that actinomycin D is significantly less active in combination than doxorubicin.

In a subsequent three-arm study, the ECOG compared (1) doxorubicin 70 mg/m^2 every 21 days, (2) doxorubicin 20 mg/m^2 days 1–3 every 3 weeks, and (3) doxorubicin 60 mg/m^2 day 1 plus DTIC every 21 days [51]. The combination arm had a significantly higher response rate (30%) than the single-agent arms (arm a, 19%; arm b, 16%; $p = 0.02$), but it was of note that both the doxorubicin arms had lower activity than had ever been seen before.

The combination arm had significantly higher toxicity with greater myelosuppression and vomiting. Survival was identical in all arms, and it was concluded that the 3-weekly bolus therapy with doxorubicin 70 mg/m^2 should be the standard for future comparison.

The SWOG developed their protocols using CyVADIC as the 'standard' arm. They first randomized CyVADIC against the same combination with actinomycin D substituted for DTIC (CyVA-DACT) [52] in 445 patients. Activity was significantly higher in the DTIC arm (52%) than for CyVA-DACT (40%), with a trend for improved median survival for CyVADIC. A subsequent trial drew from the conclusions of the previous studies, which suggested that doxorubicin and DTIC were the most important agents in the treatment of soft tissue sarcomas. Doxorubicin 60 mg/m^2 day 1 and DTIC 250 mg/m^2 daily on days 1–5 were used in each of three arms of the study in 272 patients. In one arm the combination was given alone (AD), in the second cyclophosphamide 500 mg/m^2 was added (ADC), and in the third actinomycin D was added (ADAd). Dose escalation of doxorubicin was mandated in the trial depending on the degree of myelosuppression seen [53]. There was no statistically significant difference in response rates — AD (32%), ADC (35%), and ADAd (24%) — and survival and toxicity were similar with all regimens. Given the lack of benefit from adding agents to doxorubicin and DTIC, the SWOG subsequently attempted to reduce the toxicity of this regimen by comparing bolus administration with continuous infusion (over 96 hours) [54] in 240 evaluable patients. The response rate (17%) was identical in both arms, but toxicity was significantly reduced for the infusion, particularly cardiotoxicity from doxorubicin and nausea and vomiting from DTIC.

Given the activity of ifosfamide and the encouraging results from the MAID combination regimen, an American intergroup study by the SWOG and the Cancer and Acute Leukemia Group B (CALGB) was established to determine the role of ifosfamide in combination chemotherapy [55]. Three hundred and forty eligible patients were randomized to doxorubicin 60 mg/m^2 plus DTIC 1000 mg/m^2 (AD) given by continuous infusion over 4 days or the same combination with ifosfamide (7.5 g/m^2 in the first 154 patients, reduced to 6 g/m^2 subsequently because of myelosuppression) and mesna (MAID). The response rate was significantly ($p < 0.002$) higher for the MAID combination (32%) than for AD (17%), and the time to progression was longer (MAID, 6 months; AD, 4 months; $p < 0.02$). Toxicity (including fatal sepsis) was greater for the ifosfamide-containing regimen, and this resulted in significantly reduced delivered dose intensities of doxorubicin ($p < 0.001$) in the MAID arm. The results from this study suggest that in situations in which the response may be important, such as in a preoperative or adjuvant setting, the addition of ifosfamide may be of value, but the toxicity of the combination would limit it to younger patients. For the palliative management of metastatic disease, the MAID regimen appears to offer no advantages to the two-drug combination.

A large important study by the EORTC was established to determine whether combination chemotherapy was superior to single-agent doxorubicin

[44]. In this study 663 eligible patients were randomized to one of three arms: (1) single-agent doxorubicin (75 mg/m^2 3-weekly), (2) doxorubicin (50 mg/m^2) plus ifosfamide (5 g/m^2) 3-weekly, and (3) CyVADIC (with DTIC given at 750 mg/m^2 on day 1). There was no significant difference in the three arms in any of the important outcome variables. The response rates were 23% in arm 1, 28% in arm 2, and 28% in arm 3. The median remission durations were 46 weeks in arm 1, 48 weeks in arm 2, and 44 weeks in arm 3. The median survival were 52 weeks in arm 1, 51 weeks in arm 2, and 55 weeks in arm 3. Myelosuppression was significantly greater for the ifosfamide arm and cardiotoxicity was more frequent. It was concluded that single-agent doxorubicin remained the standard against which any new therapeutic approaches should be compared and that combination regimens appeared to offer no advantages in the palliative management of this disease. It will, however, be important to perform subset analysis and to obtain longer follow-up information to determine if there is a group of patients who might benefit more from combination therapy.

Role of dose-intensity escalation

Given the dose-response relationship to doxorubicin, it is possible that the reason combination chemotherapy was not found to be superior to single-agent doxorubicin in the EORTC randomized phase III study [44] was that the dose of the anthracycline was only 50 mg/m^2 when used in combination, as compared with 75 mg/m^2 when used alone. The fact that the addition of ifosfamide to the lower dose of doxorubicin resulted in a response rate that was similar to that produced by the most effective dose of doxorubicin suggests that ifosfamide is active in this disease. Unfortunately the myelotoxicity of doxorubicin at a dose of 75 mg/m^2 would preclude its being safely combined with ifosfamide [56]. In order to increase the dose of doxorubicin that can safely be given in combination with ifosfamide, and thereby hopefully to increase the response rate for advanced soft tissue sarcomas, the EORTC conducted a phase II study of the combination of doxorubicin 75 mg/m^2 plus ifosfamide 5 g/m^2 with granulocyte-macrophage–colony-stimulating factor (GM-CSF) support (250 μg/m^2 given subcutaneously for 14 days between each course) [57]. The results of this study, which included 104 eligible patients, indicated such an approach to be feasible with the full protocol dose intensity being administered to the majority of patients and toxicity being comparable, or even less than, previous experience using standard dose therapy. Only 15 of 293 cycles of chemotherapy were complicated by febrile neutropenia, and there were two treatment-related deaths. Encouragingly, the highest response rate (45%) so far seen by the EORTC Sarcoma Group was obtained, with 10% of patients obtaining a complete remission. The median survival of 15 months was also greater than that observed historically by the group. These findings led to the initiation of a randomized phase III trial in which patients receive ifosfamide 5 g/m^2 with doxorubicin 50 mg/m^2 alone or doxorubicin 75 mg/m^2 plus GM-CSF. This large ongoing trial should determine the value of the dose intensity of doxorubicin in adult soft tissue sarcomas.

A phase I/II study at the Mayo Clinic in which 15 patients with soft tissue sarcomas received high-dose combination chemotherapy with ifosfamide, doxorubicin, and cisplatin plus GM-CSF produced encouraging responses [58]. Complete tumor regressions occurred in five patients, and partial responses were seen in another three patients. Of potential importance was the fact that only 3 deaths had occurred during the median follow-up of 17 months (compared with the expected 10 deaths for a risk-matched historical control group). These results have formed the basis for a larger phase II study using the highest feasible dose of chemotherapy with GM-CSF and subsequent attempts at surgical excision of residual disease.

Dose intensification of single-agent doxorubicin using GM-CSF cover was examined in 35 patients by Hoekman et al. [59]. Dose levels of 90 mg/m^2 and 110 mg/m^2 were administered to 9 and 25 patients, respectively. The degree of myelosuppression appeared to have been markedly reduced by GM-CSF, with grade IV neutropenia lasting more than 7 days being seen only after the forth course of chemotherapy. Thrombocytopenia, however, became the dose-limiting toxicity. Response rates at 90 mg/m^2 and 110 mg/m^2 were 33% and 31%, respectively, higher than would be expected with doxorubicin at standard dose.

Early data suggested the potential for a dose-response relationship to ifosfamide, and the potential value of high-dose therapy has therefore been examined in three phase I/II pilot studies. Brain et al. [60] administered ifosfamide 12 g/m^2 as a 72-hour continuous infusion repeated every 4 weeks. Twenty-four pretreated patients were included in this study, 13 of whom had received prior ifosfamide at a standard dose. Of the 23 patients who were evaluable for response, 8 achieved a partial remission (34%) and 5 had stable disease. Of great interest was the observation that 7 of the 8 responders had received prior ifosfamide and 4 had been refractory to this agent at standard dose. Hematological toxicity was severe, with 80% of patients experiencing grade 3–4 neutropenia and seven requiring hospitalization for febrile neutropenia. Hemopoietic growth factors were therefore included in the two other reported studies that employed high-dose therapy. Cerny et al. [61] treated 15 patients (8 with prior standard-dose ifosfamide), with the first 4 receiving 12 g/m^2 ifosfamide over 5 days without growth factor and the subsequent 11 receiving 14 g/m^2 over 5 days with GM-CSF. Despite the higher dose of ifosfamide in the second group, the incidence of infection was reduced from 23% of cycles to 8%. Once again a dose-response effect was seen, with 50% patients who had failed to respond to prior standard dose ifosfamide (<8 g/m^2) achieving a partial remission with the high-dose therapy. Christman et al. [62] used G-CSF between courses of ifosfamide at a starting dose of 10 g/m^2 (given as 96-hour continuous infusions). In this study the intensity of administration was also increased to a 14-day schedule. The regimen appeared feasible, with nine patients receiving at least three cycles every 2 weeks. Dose-limiting thrombocytopenia occurred at a dose of ifosfamide of $12\,g/m^2$. Of seven patients with measurable disease, two achieved partial responses.

There is little information in the literature on the value of high-dose myeloablative therapy with bone marrow or peripheral stem cell support. Two studies have been reported from Lyon. The first involved 22 patients who received a variety of conditioning regimens (some with total-body irradiation), either as intensification following induction therapy (6 patients) or as primary therapy of relapse. The results were encouraging, with a 66% response rate in evaluable patients and median disease-free and overall survivals of 19 and 15 months, respectively. Actuarial survival rates at 2 and 5 years were 40% and 32%, respectively [63]. The second study involved the use of cisplatin, etoposide, and ifosfamide with bone marrow rescue as consolidation after response to first-line therapy [64]. There was a projected 48% 3-year survival rate and 28% 3-year progression-free survival among the 21 patients with metastatic soft tissue sarcomas (excluding those with rhabdomyosarcomas), figures that are superior to those obtained with conventional therapy. The results must obviously be interpreted with caution, given the short follow-up, small numbers, and comparison with historical data. Thirteen patients with metastatic disease were treated with a variety of high-dose conditioning regimens and stem cell rescue at the University of Nebraska [65]. There were two toxic deaths, but three complete and four partial responses were documented (54% response rate). Unfortunately response durations were short and the median overall survival was only 8 months. Clearly, more effective chemotherapy is necessary before this approach will be clinically useful in soft tissue sarcomas, particularly because the active drugs in this disease have severe nonhematological toxicity, which limits the dose escalation that is possible with stem cell support.

Biological response modifiers

Two studies have examined the role of interferon in soft tissue sarcomas. In the first, interferon α-2b was administered at doses of $10–20\,MU/m^2$ 3 times a week for a minimum of 4 weeks to 31 patients [66]. Severe thrombocytopenia, fatigue, and diarrhea resulted in frequent dose reductions, but two partial responses were seen (of 4- and 10-month durations). A subsequent study by the same group treated 28 patients with 5-fluorouracil $750\,mg/m^2$/day given by continuous infusion over 5 days combined with interferon α $5\,MU/m^2$ daily on 6 successive days every 2–3 weeks [67]. The rationale for this study was the in vitro synergistic tumor cell killing seen between these compounds, although 5-fluorouracil has no single-agent activity in sarcomas. The combination was highly toxic, producing severe mucositis, and no activity was seen.

Macrophage colony stimulating factor (M-CSF) was administered by continuous infusion over 7 days every 2 weeks at a dose of 80 μg/kg/day in a study at New York University [68]. Fourteen patients were treated (11 having progressed after prior chemotherapy). The side effects included thrombocytopenia and a flulike syndrome. No activity was demonstrated. Patients with sarcomas have been included in the early trials of interleukin-2 [69], but unfortunately no activity was seen. Similarly, the results of combining interleukin-2 and interferon α-2a in six patients (treated among a larger cohort of other malignancies) revealed no activity despite responses to this combination being seen in renal carcinomas and melanoma in the same study [70].

Preclinical data on a liposomal encapsulated synthetic muramyl tripeptid, MTP/PE, were particularly promising for sarcomas. Stimulation of macrophages occurred and resulted in marked antitumor activity in rodents and dogs. Long-term survival for canine osteosarcoma was a particularly intriguing finding. The EORTC Sarcoma Group [71] treated 19 patients with metastatic disease (who had progressed after prior chemotherapy) with MTP/PE at a dose of 4 mg intravenously every week (the dose that produced biological effects in phase I studies). Treatment was generally well tolerated apart from mild flulike symptoms, but no objective responses occurred.

Conclusions

The treatment of metastatic or locally advanced soft tissue sarcomas remains difficult despite the efforts of well-organized cooperative groups who have carried out a series of phase II and III studies in an attempt to improve the outcome of this disease. It is frustrating to find that 25 years after its introduction to clinical medicine, single-agent doxorubicin remains the standard therapy for this disease, with no benefit being demonstrated for combination regimens [44]. The results for the majority of patients are dismal, and new approaches are clearly needed to improve the outcome. Several approaches are currently under investigation and hold some promise for the future. Dose intensification of doxorubicin with hemopoietic colony-stimulating factors may improve the outcome by allowing optimal dose anthracycline to be given in combination chemotherapy regimens. The availability of the taxoids and topoisomerase 1 inhibitors provides potentially active agents for use in combination regimens. The limited experience with high-dose therapy and stem cell rescue suggests that there may be a subset of patients who can achieve long-term survival, and this should be explored further, although it is probably restricted to patients with proven chemosensitive disease. An approach being increasingly examined is the use of surgery to remove residual disease after a response to chemotherapy. Large studies are necessary to determine the true role of such a strategy. There is an increasing understanding of the biology of soft tissue sarcomas, and novel approaches, such as gene and vaccine therapy, may become available as more information is produced from basic research.

Given the rarity of soft tissue sarcomas, it is essential that patients be treated in trials whenever possible so that new approaches can be explored in the hope that the outcome will be improved. Outside clinical trials, the role of chemotherapy is small and its use must be restricted to patients with rapidly progressive disease that is becoming symptomatic. In this setting, single-agent doxorubicin 70 mg/m^2 is the treatment of choice, with ifosfamide as an alternative in patients for whom anthracyclines are contraindicated. Second-line therapy is of minimal value, and the inclusion of such patients in phase II studies of novel agents should be considered as an alternative. It is only with the continuing concentration on well-organized clinical trials that advances can be made in this disease.

References

1. O'Bryan RM, Luce JK, Talley RW, et al. Phase II evaluation of Adriamycin in human neoplasia. Cancer 32:1–8, 1973.
2. Verweij J, van Oosterom AT, Somers R, et al. Chemotherapy in the multidisciplinary approach to soft tissue sarcomas. Ann Oncol 3:S75–S80, 1992.
3. O'Bryan RM, Baker LH, Gottlieb JE, et al. Dose response evaluation of Adriamycin in human neoplasia. Cancer 39:1940–1948, 1977.
4. Schoenfeld D, Rosenbaum C, Horton J, et al. A comparison of Adriamycin versus vincristine and Adriamycin and cyclophosphamide for advanced sarcoma. Cancer 50:2757–2762, 1982.
5. Pinedo HM, Bramwell VHC, Mouridsen VHC, et al. CyVADIC in advanced soft tissue sarcoma — a randomised study comparing two schedules. Cancer 53:1825–1832, 1984.
6. Bodey GP, Rodriguez V, Murphy WK, Burgess A, Benjamin RS. Protected environment–prophylactic antibiotic program for malignant sarcoma: Randomised trial during remission induction chemotherapy. Cancer 47:2422–2429, 1981.
7. Toma S, Palumbo R, Sogno G, Venturino A, Santi L. Doxorubicin (or epidoxorubicin) combined with ifosfamide in the treatment of adult advanced soft tissue sarcomas. Ann Oncol 3:S119–S123, 1992.
8. Perevodchikova NI, Lichinister MR, Gorbunova VA, et al. Phase II clinical study of carminomycin: Its activity against soft tissue sarcomas. Cancer Treat Rep 61:1705–1707, 1977.
9. Bramwell VHC, Mouridsen HT, Mulder JH, et al. Carminomycin versus Adriamycin in advanced soft tissue sarcoma. An EORTC randomised Phase II study. Eur J Cancer 19:1097–1104, 1983.
10. Mouridsen HT, Bastholt L, Somers R, et al. Adriamycin versus epirubicin in advanced soft tissue sarcomas: A randomised phase II/phase III study of the EORTC Soft Tissue and Bone Sarcoma Group. Eur J Cancer Clin Oncol 23:1477–1483, 1987.
11. Chevalier B, Monteuquet PH, Fachini T, et al. Phase II study of epirubicin in advanced soft tissue sarcomas. Proc Am Soc Clin Oncol 8:323, 1989.
12. Dombernowsky P, Mouridsen H, Nielsen OS, et al. A phase III study comparing Adriamycin versus two schedules of high dose epirubicin in advanced soft tissue sarcoma. Proc Am Soc Clin Oncol 14:515, 1995.
13. Yang JC, Rosenberg SA, Glatstein EJ, Antman KH. Sarcomas of soft tissues. In VT DeVita, Jr., S Hellman, SA Rosenberg, eds. Cancer Principles and Practice of Oncology, 4th ed. Philadelphia: J.B. Lippincott, 199:1436–1488, 1993.
14. Hoefer-Janker H, Scheef W, Gunther U, Huls W. Erfahungen mit der fraktionierten Ifosfamid-Stosstherapie bei generalisierten malignen Tumoren. Med Welt 26:972–979, 1975.
15. Stuart-Harris RC, Harper PG, Parsons CA, et al. High dose alkylating therapy using ifosfamide infusion with mesna in the treatment of adult advanced soft tissue sarcoma. Cancer Chemother Pharmacol 11:69–72, 1983.

16. Bramwell VHC, Mouridsen HT, Santoro A, et al. Cyclophosphamide versus ifosfamide: Final report of a randomised phase II trial in adult soft tissue sarcoma. Eur J Cancer 23:311–321, 1987.
17. Pinedo HM, Bramwell VHC, Mouridsen HT, et al. Chemotherapy of advanced soft tissue sarcoma in adults. Cancer Treat Rev 4:67–86, 1977.
18. Pazdur R, Samson MK, Baker L. Fludarabine phosphate: Phase II evaluation in advanced soft tissue sarcomas. Am J Clin Oncol 10:341–343, 1987.
19. Kurzrock R, Yap BS, Plager C, et al. Phase II evaluation of PALA in patients with refractory metastatic sarcomas. Am J Clin Oncol 7:305–307, 1984.
20. Casper ES, Baselga J, Smart TB, Magill GB, Markman M, Ranhosky A. A phase II trial of PALA plus dipyridamole in patients with advanced soft tissue sarcoma. Cancer Chemother Pharmacol 28:51–54, 1991.
21. Licht JD, Gonin R, Antman K. A phase II trial of trimetrexate in patients with advanced soft tissue sarcoma. Cancer Chemother Pharmacol 28:223–225, 1991.
22. Eisenhauer EA, Wierzbicki R, Knowling M, Bramwell VHC, Quirt IC. Phase II trials of trimetrexate in advanced adult soft tissue sarcomas. Studies of the Canadian Sarcoma Group and National Cancer Institute of Canada Clinical Trials Group. Ann Oncol 2:689–690, 1991.
23. Casper ES, Christman KL, Schwartz GK, Johnson B, Brennan MF, Bertino JR. Edatrexate in patients with soft tissue sarcoma. Activity in malignant fibrous histiocytoma. Cancer 72:766–770, 1993.
24. Borden EC, Amato DA, Edmonson JH, Ritch PS, Shiraki M. Randomised comparison of doxorubicin and vindesine to doxorubicin for patients with metastatic soft tissue sarcomas. Cancer 66:862–867, 1990.
25. van Hoesel QGCM, Verweij J, Catimel G, et al. Phase II study with docetaxel (taxotere) in advanced soft tissue sarcomas of the adult. Ann Oncol 5:539–542, 1994.
26. Blackstein ME, Eisenhauer EA, Bramwell V, Belanger K, Verma S, Beare S. Docetaxel (taxotere) as first line therapy for metastatic or recurrent soft tissue sarcoma: A phase II trial. Eur J Cancer 31A(Suppl 5):S177, 1995.
27. Gian V, Lynch J, McCarley D, Johnson T. Taxol in the treatment of recurrent or metastatic soft tissue or osteosarcomas. Proc Am Soc Clin Oncol 14:516, 1995.
28. Buesa JM, Mouridsen HT, vanOosterom AT, et al. High dose DTIC in advanced soft tissue sarcomas of the adult. A phase II study of the EORTC Soft Tissue and Bone Sarcoma Group. Ann Oncol 2:307–309, 1991.
29. Bernard SA, Capizzi RL, Rudnick SA, Tremont SJ, Raymond RN. A one day combination chemotherapy (CyVADIC) regimen in soft tissue sarcomas. Proc Am Soc Clin Oncol 1:170, 1982.
30. karakousis CP, Holterman OA, Holyoke E. Cisdichlorodiamineplatinum (II) in metastatic soft tissue sarcomas. Cancer Treat Rep 63:2071–2075, 1979.
31. Goldstein D, Cheuvert B, Trump DL, et al. Phase II trial of carboplatin in soft tissue sarcoma. Am J Clin Oncol 13:420–423, 1990.
32. Eisenhauer EA, Wainman N, Boos G, MacDonald D, Bramwell V. Phase II trials of topotecan in patients with malignant gliomas and soft tissue sarcoma. Proc Am Soc Clin Oncol 14:175, 1995.
33. Welt S, Magill GB, Sordillo PP, et al. Phase II trial of VP-16213 in adults with soft tissue sarcomas. Proc Am Soc Clin Oncol 2:234, 1983.
34. Nissen NI, Pajak TF, Leone LA, et al. Clinical trial of VP-16213 (NSC 141540) iv twice weekly in advanced neoplastic disease. Cancer 45:232–235, 1980.
35. EORTC Clinical Screening Group. Epidophyllotoxin VP16213 in treatment of leukemias, haematosarcomas and solid tumours. Br Med J 3:199–202, 1973.
36. Blair SC, Zalupski MM, Baker LH. Ifosfamide and etoposide in the treatment of advanced soft tissue sarcomas. Am J Clin Oncol 17:480–484, 1994.
37. Gottlieb JA. Combination chemotherapy for metastatic sarcoma. Cancer Chemother Rep 58:265–270, 1974.

38. Gottlieb JA, Baker LH, Quagliani JM, et al. Chemotherapy of sarcomas with a combination of Adriamycin and dimethyl triazeno imidazole carboxamide. Cancer 30:1632–1638, 1972.
39. Gottlieb JA, Benjamin RS, Baker LH, et al. Role of DTIC (NDC 45388) in the chemotherapy of sarcomas. Cancer Treat Rep 60:199–203, 1976.
40. Wagner DE, Ramirez G, Weiss AJ. Combination phase I-II study of imidazole carboxamide (NSC-45388). Oncology 26:310–316, 1972.
41. Creagan ET, Hahn RG, Ahmann DL, Edmonson J, Bisel HF, Eagan RT. A comparative clinical trial evaluating the combination of Adriamycin, DTIC and vincristine, the combination of actinomycin D, cyclophosphamide and vincristine, and a single agent methyl CCNU in advanced sarcoma. Cancer Treat Rep 60:1385–1387.
42. Yap B, Baker LH, Sinkovics JG, et al. Cyclophosphamide, vincristine, Adriamycin and DTIC (CYVADIC) combination chemotherapy for the treatment of advanced sarcomas. Cancer Treat Rep 64:93–98, 1980.
43. Yap BS, Sinkovics JG, Benjamin RS, et al. Survival and relapse patterns of complete responders in adults with advanced soft tissue sarcomas. Proc Am Assoc Cancer Res 20:352, 1979.
44. Santoro A, Tursz T, Mouridsen H, et al. Doxorubicin versus CyVADIC versus doxorubicin plus ifosfamide in first-line treatment of advanced soft tissue sarcomas: A randomised study of the EORTC Soft Tissue and Bone Sarcoma Group. J Clin Oncol 13:1537–1545, 1995.
45. Elias A, Ryan L, Sulkes A, et al. Response to mesna, doxorubicin, ifosfamide and dacarbazine in 108 patients with metastatic or unresectable sarcoma and no prior chemotherapy. J Clin Oncol 7:1208–1216, 1989.
46. Benjamin RS, Yap BS. Infusion chemotherapy for soft tissue sarcomas. In LH Baker, ed. Soft Tissue Sarcomas. The Hague, Netherlands: Martinus Nijhoff, 1987.
47. Mansi JL, Fisher C, Wiltshaw E, Macmillan S, King M, Stuart-Harris R. A phase I-II study of ifosfamide in combination with Adriamycin in the treatment of adult soft tissue sarcoma. Eur J Cancer Clin Oncol 24:1439–1443, 1988.
48. Schutte J, Mouridsen HT, Steward WP, et al. Adriamycin plus ifosfamide in previously untreated patients with advanced soft tissue sarcomas. Eur J Cancer 26:558, 1990.
49. Elias A, Antman KH. Doxorubicin, ifosfamide and dacarbazine (AID) with mesna uroprotection for advanced untreated sarcoma: A phase I study. Cancer Treat Rep 70:827–833, 1986.
50. Elias AD, Ryan L, Aisner J, Antman KH. Doxorubicin, ifosfamide and DTIC for advanced untreated sarcoma. Proc Am Soc Clin Oncol 6:134, 1987.
51. Borden EC, Amato D, Enterline HT, et al. Randomised comparison of Adriamycin regimens for treatment of metastatic soft tissue sarcomas. J Clin Oncol 5:840–850, 1987.
52. Benjamin RS, Gottlieb JA, Baker LH. CYVADIC versus CYVADACT — a randomised trial of cyclophosphamide, vincristine and Adriamycin plus either dacarbazine or actinomycin D for advanced soft tissue sarcomas. Proc Am Assoc Cancer Res 17:256, 1976.
53. Baker LH, Frank J, Fine G, et al. Combination chemotherapy using Adriamycin, DTIC, cyclophosphamide and actinomycin D for advanced soft tissue sarcomas. A randomised comparative trial. J Clin Oncol 5:851–861, 1987.
54. Zalupski M, Metch B, Balcerzak S, et al. Phase III comparison of doxorubicin and dacarbazine given by bolus versus infusion in patients with soft tissue sarcomas. A Southwest Oncology Group Study. J Natl Cancer Instit 83:926–932, 1991.
55. Antman K, Crowley J, Balcerzak SP, et al. An Intergroup phase III randomised study of doxorubicin and dacarbazine with or without ifosfamide and mesna in advanced soft tissue and bone sarcomas. J Clin Oncol 11:1276–1285, 1993.
56. Wiltshaw E, Westbury G, Harmer C, McKinna A, Fisher C. Ifosfamide plus mesna with and without Adriamycin in soft tissue sarcoma. Cancer Chemother Pharmacol 18:S10–S12, 1986.
57. Steward WP, Verweij J, Somers R, et al. Granulocyte-macrophage colony-stimulating factor allows safe escalation of dose-intensity of chemotherapy in metastatic adult soft tissue sarcomas: A study of the EORTC Soft Tissue and Bone Sarcoma Group. J Clin Oncol 11:15–21, 1993.

58. Edmonson JH, Long HJ, Kvols LK. Cytotoxic drugs plus subcutanous granulocyte macrophage colony stimulating factor: Can molgramostim enhance antisarcoma therapy? J Natl Cancer Inst 86:312–314
59. Hoekman K, Wagstaff J, van Groeningen CJ, Vermorken JB, Meyer S, Pinedo HM. The treatment of advanced soft tissue sarcoma with high dose doxorubicin plus granulocyte-macrophage colony-stimulating factor. Ann Oncol, in press.
60. Brain E, DeLesne A, LeChevalier T, et al. High dose ifosfamide can circumvent resistance to standard dose ifosfamide in advanced soft tissue sarcomas. Proc Am Soc Clin Oncol 12:470, 1993.
61. Cerny T, Leyvraz S, Daggi H, Varini M, Kroner T, Marti C. Phase II trials of ifosfamide and mesna in advanced sfot tissue sarcoma patients. Proc Am Soc Clin Oncol 11:416, 1992.
62. Christman KL, Crapes ES, Schwartz EK. High intensity scheduling of ifosfamide in adult patients with soft tissue sarcomas. Proc Am Soc Clin Oncol 12:470, 1993.
63. Dumontet C, Biron P, Bouffet E, et al. High dose chemotherapy with ABMT in soft tissue sarcomas: A report of 22 cases. Bone Marrow Transplan 10:405–408, 1992.
64. Blay JY, Bouhour D, Brunat-Mentigny M, et al. High dose chemotherapy (VIC) and bone marrow support in advanced sarcomas. Proc Am Soc Clin Oncol 13:479, 1994.
65. Kessinger A, Petersen K, Bishop M, Schmit-Pokorny K. High dose therapy with autologous hematopoietic stem cell rescue for patients with metastatic soft tissue sarcoma. Proc Am Soc Clin Oncol 13:480, 1994.
66. Salem PA, Benjamin RS, Howard J, Gutterman JU. Phase II trial of recombinant interferon alpha-2b in the treatment of advanced metastatic and refractory sarcomas. Proc Am Assoc Cancer Res 32:200, 1991.
67. Papadopoulos NEJ, Patel SR, Linke K, Benjamin RS. A phase II study of 5-fluorouracil infusion and interferon alpha in metastatic sarcomas. Proc Am Assoc Cancer Res 33:229, 1992.
68. Blum PH, Powers TV, Downey AM, et al. rhGM-CSF for adult soft tissue sarcomas. Proc Am Soc Clin Oncol 12:474, 1993.
69. Rosenberg SA, Lotze MT, Muul LM, et al. A progress report on the treatment of 157 patients with advanced cancer using lymphokine-activated killer cells and IL-2 or high dose IL-2 alone, N Engl J Med 316:889–897, 1987.
70. Rosso R, Sertoli MR, Queirolo P, et al. An outpatient phase I study of a subcutaneous interleukin-2 and intramuscular alpha-2a-interferon combination in advanced malignancies. Ann Oncol 3:559–563, 1992.
71. Verweij J, Judson I, Steward W, et al. Phase II study of liposomal muramyl tripeptide phosphatidylethonolamine (MTP/PE) in advanced soft tissue sarcomas of the adult. An EORTC Soft Tissue and Bone Sarcoma Group Study. Eur J Cancer, 30:842–843, 1994.

12. Adjuvant chemotherapy of soft tissue sarcomas

Jaap Verweij and Herbert M. Pinedo

Introduction

Soft tissue sarcomas tend to metastasize early and hematogenously. Therefore, and despite increasing possibilities of achieving optimal local control by surgery with or without radiotherapy, more than half of patients will die from metastases [1–4]. Clearly, only the elimination of hematogenously borne micrometastases will make a major impact on the survival of these patients. As a result, interest in the use of chemotherapy as an adjunct to local treatment (adjuvant chemotherapy), has developed even though the response rates achieved with single-agent or combination chemotherapy for advanced or metastatic soft tissue sarcomas have been modest.

The underlying rationale is that because the tumor burden is low at the time of initiation of adjuvant therapy, the efficacy of the drugs used might be higher than in the case of a large tumor burden [5]. In addition, chemotherapy may be better tolerated when the tumor burden is low. The primary endpoints of adjuvant therapy, relapse-free survival (RFS) and overall survival (OS), require prolonged follow-up because the therapy must be judged by its ability to reduce the number of tumor recurrences and deaths over time. Therefore, comparison with a randomly assigned control group is essential in these circumstances, because the survival of patients with soft tissue sarcoma has been suggested to improve irrespective of the administration of chemotherapy [1,2,4,6], thus making comparison with historical controls inappropriate. Moreover, with the use of the presently available sophisticated diagnostic tools, such as CT scans and MRI, metastatic disease at first presentation can be detected much more frequently, which makes any comparison with historical controls futile.

Successful adjuvant chemotherapy strategies have been defined for a number of human cancers, including breast cancer, colorectal cancer, and osteosarcoma. However, the role of adjuvant chemotherapy in adult soft tissue sarcoma remains controversial. Only very few clinical trials in soft tissue sarcoma have accrued sufficient numbers of patients, so in most of the studies even random allocation will not avoid imbalances, resulting from the complex interactions of variables, such as the numerous pathologic subtypes, histologic

J. Verweij, H.M. Pinedo, and H.D. Suit (eds). SOFT TISSUE SARCOMAS: PRESENT ACHIEVEMENTS AND FUTURE PROSPECTS.

grades, primary tumor locations, and different local control procedures. In fact, these imbalances are quite likely to occur in small sample-size studies. Imbalances between known prognostic factors may also not be entirely compensated for by prerandomization stratification or postrandomization adjustments.

Clearly large trials are required to draw meaningful conclusions. Unfortunately only two trials of a relatively adequate sample size have been performed until now. In the following we review only randomized studies with emphasis on the two large studies conducted thus far.

Randomized trials of adjuvant chemotherapy

Doxorubicin versus control

The Intergroup Sarcoma Study Group (ISSG) randomized patients to doxorubicin 35 mg/m^2 daily for 2 days, repeated every 3 weeks for a total of six cycles, or to no further treatment. Eighty-six patients were available for analysis, and at a median follow-up of 44 months no differences in disease-free or overall survival were seen [7]. No benefit from doxorubicin therapy was seen for nonextremity sarcomas, but in the preliminary report it was suggested that in patients with extremity tumors there was a trend towards an improved relapse-free survival (RFS) for the doxorubicin-treated group ($p = 0.06$), but OS was not significantly different [8].

Investigators from Boston and from the Eastern Cooperative Oncology Group (ECOG) have jointly reported the results of two separate randomized studies [9]. Both studies accrued patients with American Joint Committee (AJC) stage IIb–IVa tumors stratified for stage, surgical margins, and primary size. Radical surgery or conservative surgery followed by radiotherapy were both permitted as adequate local treatment. Patients with locally recurrent disease were also eligible. Patients in Boston were randomized to five cycles of adjuvant doxorubicin, 90 mg/m^2 every 3 weeks, or two cycles of doxorubicin 90 mg/m^2 preoperatively and three cycles postoperatively, versus no adjuvant treatment postsurgery. Patients treated on the ECOG study received doxorubicin 70 mg/m^2 for seven cycles, with all cycles given after surgery. No significant differences were found with respect to local control, metastasis-free survival, relapse-free survival (RFS), and overall survival (OS). Subgroup analysis did not demonstrate a benefit from doxorubicin therapy for either extremity or nonextremity sarcomas.

Investigators from the Instituto Orthopedica Rizzoli in Bologna evaluated 77 patients with high-grade extremity sarcomas [10,11]. Patients were divided according to three local control procedures:

1. Twenty-eight patients with amputations were randomized to doxorubicin 25 mg/m^2/day for 3 days every 3 weeks for a total of 6 cycles, starting 3 days postoperatively; or to no further treatment.

2. Twenty-nine patients underwent a biopsy, followed by radiotherapy (4500 cGy over 3 weeks) with doxorubicin 75 mg/m^2 repeated once. Conservative surgery was performed, and patients were then randomized to doxorubicin for four cycles (300 mg/m^2) for a total doxorubicin dose of 450 mg/m^2 or to no further treatment.
3. Persistent tumor was suspected in 20 patients who had been treated at another hospital within the previous 3 months. For this reason re-excision of the tumor bed was performed and then these individuals were randomized as in point 1. Patients received postoperative external-beam radiation therapy (4500 cGy) if residual tumor was demonstrated histologically.

Clearly, the patient numbers and this complex design almost preclude any meaningful analysis. The study attempted to utilize a pair-matched stratification for age, site, size of tumor, and stage. The technique of randomization resulted in a large imbalance in patient numbers between the doxorubicin (33 patients) and control (44 patients) groups, and has been extensively criticized [12]. In addition, the control group included an excess number of pelvis/thigh tumors (57% vs. 37.5%), which are generally larger and have a poorer prognosis than distal or upper extremity tumors. At a median follow-up of 68 months, it was suggested that RFS ($p < 0.05$) and OS ($p < 0.05$) were higher in the doxorubicin-treated group. Despite similar durations of follow-up, the RFS for control patients in this study is worse (47%) than that for comparable control groups of other studies. In view of this criticism, the reader is advised to interpret these data with extreme caution.

At the University of California at Los Angeles (UCLA) 119 patients with grade III extremity soft tissue sarcomas were treated with preoperative intraarterial doxorubicin (20–30 mg/24 hours for 3 days), followed by external-beam radiation therapy to the primary tumor, and surgical excision of the tumor 1 week after the completion of radiation. Patients were subsequently randomized within 6 weeks of surgery to receive doxorubicin 45 mg/m^2/day for 2 days each month for 5 courses or to no further therapy. With a median follow-up of 28 months, there were no significant differences in terms of RFS or OS. A slightly lower local recurrence rate in those patients who received adjuvant systemic doxorubicin did not reach statistical significance. The infusion of doxorubicin intraarterially to all patients may have obscured any differences between the treatment groups [6].

The most relevant study, and by far the largest evaluating adjuvant single-agent doxorubicin, was performed by the Scandinavian Sarcoma Group (SSG) [13]. They randomized 240 patients with high-grade (Broder grade III or IV) sarcomas to receive either doxorubicin 60 mg/m^2 monthly for nine courses or no systemic treatment. Sixty-nine patients (29%) were not evaluable, with the most common reasons for exclusion being ineligible histologies (22 patients) or marginal excisions not followed by radiotherapy (25 patients). It should be noted that exclusion of the latter patients, who might have a higher rate of local recurrence and possibly distant metastasis, might be expected to improve the results for the study as a whole. This high rate of ineligibility is similar to that reported for the European Organization for Research and Treatment of Cancer (EORTC) trial, to be discussed later. This emphasizes the difficulty of such multicenter multinational studies, which lack effective quality control mechanisms [14]. Thirty-four patients who underwent marginal resection received radiotherapy postoperatively before being randomized and were analyzed separately. Chemotherapy was started within 6 weeks after surgery, except for patients receiving postoperative radiotherapy, who started chemotherapy within 10 weeks of surgery. No patients were lost to follow-up, and the median duration of follow-up was 40 months. No significant differences between the treatment and the control groups were seen with respect to local recurrence, RFS (Fig. 1), or OS (Fig. 2), either for the 181 evaluable or the 240 total randomized patients. Amputation was performed in 26 of 155 (17%) patients with extremity sarcomas. Radical surgery was performed wherever feasible, and radiotherapy was only given to patients undergoing regional excision (27 patients, 17%). The local recurrence rates were low for radically excised patients (8% in both the doxorubicin and control groups) but slightly higher in patients treated by marginal excision and radiotherapy (14% in the doxorubicin group and 10% in the control group; $p = 0.72$). The authors concluded that adjuvant chemotherapy with single-agent doxorubicin given at these doses does not have an impact on the survival of patients with high-grade sarcomas.

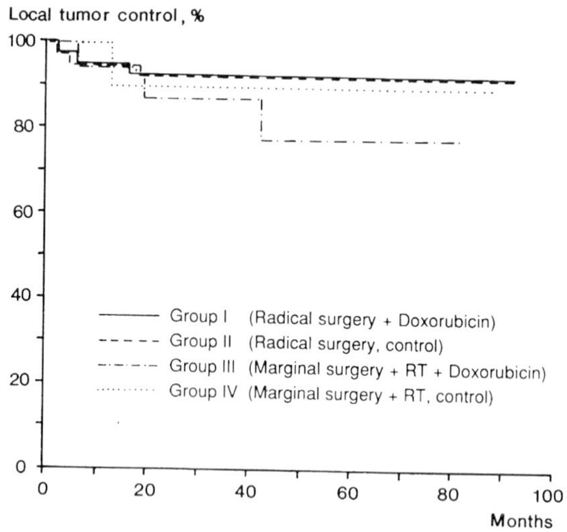

Figure 1. Relapse-free survival in patients randomized to adjuvant single-agent doxorubicin or no chemotherapy). (From Alvegard et al. [13], with permission.)

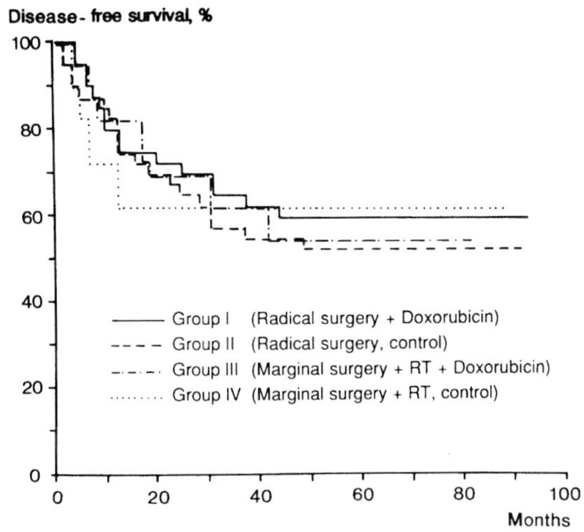

Figure 2. Overall survival in patients randomized to adjuvant single-agent doxorubicin or no chemotherapy. (From Alvegard et al. [13], with permission.)

Combination chemotherapy versus control

At the National Cancer Institute (NCI) a trial was performed in which patients with stage IIA–IIIB (AJC) extremity soft tissue sarcoma underwent either amputation or limb-sparing surgery followed by radiotherapy. Patients were then randomized to receive a chemotherapy regimen of doxorubicin 50 mg/m^2 day 1 (escalated each cycle, as tolerated, by 10 mg/m^2 to a maximum of 70 mg/m^2/cycle and a maximum cumulative dose of 500–550 mg/m^2) and cyclophosphamide 500 mg/m^2 IV (escalated by 100 mg/m^2 per course, if tolerated, to a maximum of 700 mg/m^2). Cycles were repeated every 4 weeks. After achieving the maximum cumulative dose of doxorubicin, chemotherapy was switched to six additional cycles of 4-weekly high-dose methotrexate (50–250 mg/kg) and leucovorin rescue after a maximum cumulative dose of doxorubicin (500–550 mg/m^2) was administered. Patients randomized to chemotherapy who required radiation therapy received their first chemotherapy course 3 days prior to the initiation of radiation, with the second course administered during radiation therapy. Other patients received their chemotherapy within 3–4 weeks following surgery. At a median follow-up of 7.1 years [15], the 5-year RFS was better for patients who received chemotherapy (two-sided $p = 0.04$). The difference in OS was not statistically significant. The local recurrence rate was favorably influenced by chemotherapy (two-sided $p < 0.05$). Criticisms of this study include its relatively small size, as well as an unusual randomization procedure, leading to an imbalance in the total numbers of patients entered into each treatment arm. In addition, a higher proportion of chemotherapy-treated patients had distal extremity lesions (41% vs. 25% for the no-treatment arm).

A similar trial included soft tissue sarcomas of head and neck, breast, and trunk [16]. Only 31 patients were entered into this study after complete resection of gross tumor and postoperative radiotherapy. The chemotherapy regimen was similar to that used for patients with extremity sarcoma. Six patients also received immunotherapy with *Corynebacterium parvum*, and analysis of the data with and without these subjects did not influence the results. The 3-year OS was not different (68% for the chemotherapy arm vs. 58% of controls; $p = 0.38$). In a further study, 37 patients with resectable retroperitoneal sarcomas were randomized to receive the same adjuvant chemotherapy or no further treatment after definitive surgical resection followed by adjuvant radiation therapy, and there was no difference in RFS ($p = 0.54$) [17].

Subsequently the NCI team randomized 88 patients to the same chemotherapy regimen or a lower dose regimen that eliminated methotrexate and administered only 5 courses of doxorubicin and cyclophosphamide to a maximum cumulative dose of doxorubicin of 350 mg/m^2 in order to reduce the risk of occurrence of doxorubicin cardiotoxicity. A third (control) arm was unfortunately not included in this study. RFS and OS were similar between the two arms, but the statistical power to detect an important difference was limited [15]. None of the patients in both arms developed congestive heart failure.

At the Mayo Clinic 61 patients, stratified according to primary or recurrent disease, site of origin (somatic or visceral), and Broder grade I–II or III–IV, were randomized to therapy with vincristine 1.2 mg/m^2 on days 1 and 5; cyclophosphamide 250 mg/m^2 IV on days 1, 3, and 5; and dactinomycin 0.325 mg/m^2. This regimen was alternated every 6 weeks with vincristine 1.2 mg/m^2 on days 1 and 5, doxorubicin 50 mg/m^2 on day 3, and dacarbazine 250 mg/m^2/day on days 1–5. Chemotherapy was administered for a total of eight courses. Six control and seven doxorubicin-treated patients were also given methanol extraction residue (MER) of bacillus Calmette-Guérin (BCG) intracutaneously. Local excision or amputation was permitted, but adjuvant radiation therapy was not given. Patients relapsing after therapy were given surgical resection of metastases and local recurrence. There was no statistically significant survival benefit for chemotherapy, but this chemotherapy regimen made largely use of drugs presently known to be ineffective in soft tissue sarcoma treatment, while the active drugs doxorubicin and dacarbazine were only given at 6-weekly intervals. This drawback may well explain the disappointing results. Adjuvant chemotherapy was associated with a reduced requirement for salvage surgical excision of pulmonary metastases (30% of chemotherapy-treated patients vs. 55% of the untreated group) and metastases at other sites. However, the rate of salvage surgery for local recurrences was not reduced by adjuvant chemotherapy. It is likely that the high local recurrence rate (28%) reflects the omission of adjuvant radiotherapy after local excision [18]. Clearly, and as already mentioned, the study design would not meet modern standards.

At the M. D. Anderson Hospital in Houston, a randomized clinical trial of combination chemotherapy versus observation was performed in the early 1970s. The chemotherapy consisted of doxorubicin 60 mg/m^2, vincristine 2 mg every week for 9 weeks, and cyclophosphamide 200 mg/m^2/day days 3–5 orally, administered for seven 4-weekly cycles. Doxorubicin was then replaced by dactinomycin 0.3 mg/m^2/day on days 1–5, and the cycle interval was extended to 8 weeks. Treatment was given for a total of 2 years. Patients with stage IIB and IIIB (AJC) lesions were entered, and patients were stratified for histology but not for grade or size of tumor. All patients underwent local resection and radiotherapy. After accrual of a small number of patients and at 18 months median follow-up, the study was terminated early because of unacceptable toxicity and a poor RFS for the chemotherapy group (76% vs. 83% for controls). In view of the initial results obtained by the National Cancer Institute Surgery Branch in extremity soft tissue sarcoma, this trial was reanalyzed after 10 years of follow-up. The 20 patients with extremity lesions treated with chemotherapy had significantly better RFS ($p = 0.04$) compared with the 23 patients who received no further therapy. This could almost entirely be accounted for by a difference in the rate of local recurrence, whereas the incidence of metastasis and OS were not significantly different [19].

Over a period of 8 years, investigators from the Fondation Bergonie in Bordeaux, France randomized 65 patients to chemotherapy with cyclophosphamide/vincristine/doxorubicin/DTIC (CyVADIC) or no further therapy [20]. Stratification according to known prognostic variables was not performed, and most patients underwent conservative surgery and radiotherapy. The chemotherapy regimen was almost similar to the one used in the EORTC study, discussed later, and consisted of cyclophosphamide 500 mg/m^2 IV on day 3, vincristine 1.5 mg/m^2 on day 1, doxorubicin 50 mg/m^2 on day 2, and DTIC (dacarbazine) 400 mg/m^2/day on days 1–3. The main differences were that in this study chemotherapy courses were repeated with 21-day intervals and chemotherapy was commenced no later than 30 days after surgery, while most patients received their first course of chemotherapy during the first 3 days of therapy with radiation (which started on the 14th postoperative day). Despite the difference in cycle intervals, the dose intensity received may not have differed between the two studies. With a median follow-up of 4.4 years, statistically significant differences were found in terms of RFS (84% vs. 43%, $p = 0.0003$) and OS (87% vs. 54%, $p = 0.002$), both favoring the chemotherapy arm. Although there was a delay in the development of local recurrences in the chemotherapy arm and the actual number of local recurrences was lower (3% in the chemotherapy arm vs. 18% for controls), this difference was not significant ($p = 0.17$), perhaps because of the overall small size of the study.

The most important defects of this study are its small sample size as well as the imbalance in histologic subtypes between the two treatment arms. In addition, a higher proportion of patients on the chemotherapy arm had extremity primaries, which usually have a better prognosis. The most recent report restricts OS to disease-related deaths, leaving four deaths initially reported unaccounted for. As in the Bologna trial, the OS of the control group appears to be lower than that found in other trials.

With 468 patients accrued the study of the EORTC is the largest randomized trial of adjuvant chemotherapy in soft tissue sarcoma [21]. Patients with a primary or locally recurrent tumor were eligible provided surgery comprised complete macroscopic removal. If microscopic residual disease was present at the resection margins or the healthy tissue margin surrounding the tumor was <1 cm, postoperative radiotherapy up to a dose of 50 Gy had to be given. Chemotherapy consisted of 8 cycles of cyclophosphamide 500 mg/m^2 IV on day 1, vincristine 1.4 mg/m^2 on day 1, doxorubicin 50 mg/m^2 on day 1, and DTIC 400 mg/m^2/day on days 1–3, with cycles to be repeated every 4 weeks. Chemotherapy had to start within 13 weeks of initial surgery. Patients were stratified to primary or recurrent disease, site of disease, and whether or not radiotherapy was to be given. The 468 patients were equally distributed over both arms. As in the SSG study [13], this study suffered from a relatively high ineligibility rate (32%), mainly related to inappropriate application of radiotherapy (indications). Compliance with chemotherapy was not optimal, and only 52% of patients completed the full chemotherapy. Seventy percent of patients received at least four courses. At a median follow-up of 80 months actuarial percentage survival figures at 7 years were compared. The RFS was significantly better after CyVADIC (56% vs. 43% for controls; $p = 0.007$), and local recurrence was significantly reduced by CyVADIC (17% vs. 31%; $p = 0.01$). This result appeared to be confined to head, neck, and trunk tumors. In contrast, distant metastases rates were similar in both arms, as were overall survival rates (63% vs. 56%; $p = 0.64$; Fig. 3). Inclusion of the ineligible patients into the analysis did not change the conclusions (Fig. 4). In addition, the design was criticized for the delay between definitive surgery and the start of chemotherapy. In effect, there was a median delay of 6 weeks and the maximum time was 13 weeks. Analysis of the outcome by groups with delays less than 6 weeks, 6–13 weeks, or more than 13 weeks did not show any differences in any of the results.

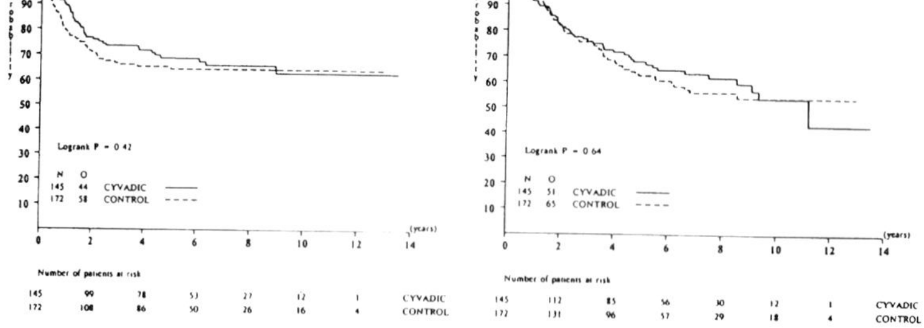

Figure 3. Relapse-free (left) and overall (right) survival for the CyVADIC versus control groups in eligible patients. (From Bramwell et al. [21], with permission.)

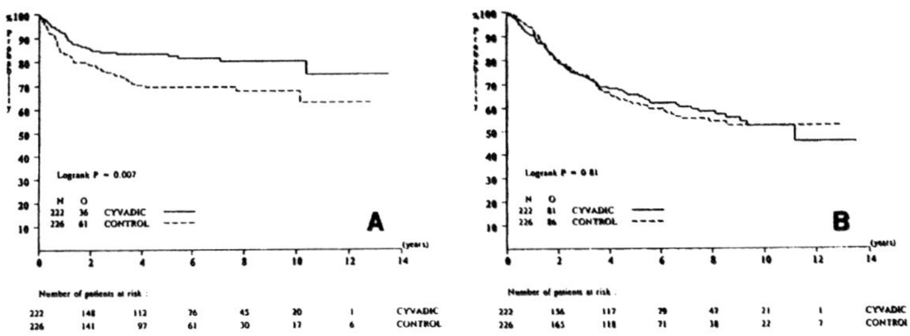

Figure 4. Relapse-free (**A**) and overall (**B**) survival for the CyVADIC versus control groups in all randomized patients. (From Bramwell et al. [21], with permission.)

Meta-analysis

A meta-analysis was performed on 13 randomized trials of adjuvant chemotherapy versus control in soft tissue sarcoma, including >1400 patients [22]. The analysis separates the three sites (extremity; head, neck, and trunk; and retroperitoneal) identified in the various reports and includes a study of uterine sarcomas [23]. Although this analysis suggests that overall survival is increased by 9% (odds ratio 0.71, $p = 0.01$), and both distant (odds ratio 0.62, $p = 0.001$) and local recurrences (odds ratio 0.42, $p = 0.0003$) were reduced, with a trend favoring combination chemotherapy over single-agent doxorubicin, these results should also be viewed with caution. The reason for this is that trials not only largely vary in their design but also in terms of the types of outcome data reported. In addition, the number of trials evaluated for outcome in terms of survival, distant failure, and local failure were 10, 8, and 6, respectively. Therefore, definitive recommendations can not be made. Even once the full analysis is published, this will not provide proper guidance as to the most appropriate approach.

Late toxicities

The chemotherapy used in these trials coincided with the usual side effects, such as alopecia, nausea and vomiting, myelosuppression, and the possibility of granulocytopenia-associated sepsis and mucositis. However, in some studies the frequency of doxorubicin-associated cardiomyopathy has caused concern because this is difficult to treat, often irreversible, and frequently lethal. The incidences of clinical doxorubicin-associated congestive heart failure were 4–10% [7,13]. However, in the EORTC and Bologna studies, no patient developed congestive heart failure (CHF) [11,21], and it is quite likely that the incidence of CHF will remain low as long as cumulative doses of doxorubucin can be restricted. The other possibility for reducing the risk of cardiotoxicity is to administer doxorubicin at longer infusion times [24].

Another concern related to adjuvant chemotherapy is the occurrence of secondary leukemias. This was specifically mentioned not to occur only in the EORTC study. Apparently, with the chemotherapy used in soft tissue sarcomas this risk is negligible. However, once more effective regimens lead to an improvement in survival, the risk of secondary leukemia may again become a concern. Finally, in view of the use of anttracycline-based chemotherapy, the synergistic toxicity of radiotherapy plus chemotherapy might be a concern. Such an increased toxicity was not observed in any of the studies in which radiotherapy was not given at the same time as chemotherapy. The only study that applied radiotherapy and anthracyclines at the same time was the study performed at the Fondation Bergonie [20]. Indeed, this study resulted in great local toxicity, necessitating amputations in several instances. In view of this, simultaneous application of chemotherapy and radiotherapy appears not to be recommended.

Discussion

Clearly the only two studies with relative large sample sizes (SSG and EORTC) [13,21] do not support the use of adjuvant chemotherapy as standard treatment for soft tissue sarcomas. The only studies that have shown significant differences in RFS and OS (Bologna, Bordeaux, and NCI) have been extensively criticized on various grounds, and also the reported meta-analysis does not come to solid conclusions.

Reductions in local recurrence rates have been noted in several studies, particularly those using combination chemotherapy, although in most cases this has not been accompanied by significant reductions in metastases or improvements in overall survival. The only study of combination chemotherapy that does not show this effect [17] differed from the others in omitting local radiotherapy, leading to a high overall rate of local recurrence, and based on current information it is likely that the chemotherapy administered was inadequate. The variable patterns of improvement in local control also complicate interpretation. The EORTC study found reduced local recurrence rates in head, neck, and trunk sarcomas. In contrast, a significant reduction in the local recurrence rates in patients with extremity sarcoma was noted in the study from the NCI. A reduction in local recurrence rates in extremity sarcomas was reported in the Fondation Bergonie trial, although these data must be interpreted cautiously in view of its small size and the possible imbalance in prognostic factors between treatment arms.

In considering the use of adjuvant chemotherapy outside of a clinical trial setting, the modest clinical gain in local control and the equivocal results in terms of survival must be counterbalanced by the often substantial toxicity of these regimens. Although adjuvant chemotherapy is often given to young patients with high-grade extremity sarcomas, the data to support this type of treatment are scanty, and the largest study of adjuvant chemotherapy

(EORTC) supports its use in an entirely different group of patients. Even so, such treatment may only reduce the unpleasant consequences of local recurrence in difficult sites in the head, neck, and trunk, without influencing survival.

Future prospects

Early nonrandomized studies had suggested benefits from adjuvant chemotherapy when compared with historical controls. Such a design would now be unacceptable, and recent trials have been mostly randomized. Nevertheless, they have produced conflicting results, and it is difficult to make firm recommendations on the use of adjuvant chemotherapy outside the setting of well-constructed research protocols. However, the introduction of new concepts and even the inconclusive results from published studies provide the stimulus for further research in this area. Investigators at the NCI Surgery Branch are currently randomizing patients with resected extremity soft tissue sarcoma who have also received 5 monthly cycles of adjuvant chemotherapy with cyclophosphamide (700 mg/m^2) and doxorubicin (70 mg/m^2) to postoperative radiotherapy or no further treatment. This is the first study assessing the value of postoperative radiotherapy in a randomized manner. The radiotherapy in the treatment arm will start within 2–3 days of the start of chemotherapy. The primary aims of the study are to evaluate the combined toxicities and to document any differences in the rates of local control. Patients with soft tissue sarcomas arising in the head and neck regions, breast, or trunk will all be treated by surgery and radiation therapy, and then randomized to a combination of cyclophosphamide and doxorubicin, or to no chemotherapy.

Despite the seemingly positive results of their previous randomized study [10,11], in Italy the presently ongoing study still includes an arm without chemotherapy. Patients are stratified into three groups for local treatment: radical surgery, conservative surgery + radiotherapy, and preoperative radiotherapy followed by surgery. In the first group chemotherapy is to start within 4 weeks from surgery, in the second 12–13 weeks from surgery, and in the third 9–10 weeks from radiotherapy start. Patients are randomized to chemotherapy or control, and chemotherapy consists of epirubicin 60 mg/m^2/day on days 1 + 2 and ifosfamide 1.8 g/m^2/day on days 1–5, with cycles to be repeated every 3 weeks for 5 times and supported with granulocyte–colony-stimulating factor (G-CSF) 300 μg/day on days 8–15. Although previous studies have shown that epidoxorubicin may have disadvantages rather than advantages, at least for the treatment of metastatic soft tissue sarcomas [26,27], the inclusion of high doses of ifosfamide still makes this study an interesting one. However, the initially planned 200-patient population appears to be too low a number.

In a study aiming for the accrual of over 500 patients, the EORTC has recently started randomizing five 3-weekly cycles of combination of doxorubicin 75 mg/m^2 on day 1 and ifosfamide 5 g/m^2 on day 1, with G-CSF support, versus no chemotherapy. Patients with high-grade soft tissue sarcomas are eligible. Chemotherapy will start within 4 weeks of definitive surgery, and radiotherapy, if indicated, will commence after the completion of chemotherapy.

Neoadjuvant chemotherapy (chemotherapy delivered before primary or local therapy) has some advantages over postoperative treatment, because the presence of evaluable tumor allows the determination of chemotherapy sensitivity clinically as well as pathologically, and valuable prognostic information may be obtained. The primary tumor may also be downstaged, and some lesions that were technically unresectable may be more amenable to surgical intervention. In addition, drug delivery to the primary tumor may be improved because surgery and radiation therapy have not yet been delivered and the tumor's vascular supply remains undisturbed. The EORTC is currently analyzing a completed randomized trial on neoadjuvant chemotherapy in patients with soft tissue sarcomas of the extremities, head, neck, and trunk. Only poor-risk patients were eligible, based on tumor size (>8 cm) or intermediate/high histological grade (mitotic count ≥3/10 high-power fields). Three courses of chemotherapy with doxorubicin, ifosfamide, and mesna were administered before definitive surgery and radiotherapy. Chemotherapy had to start within 6 weeks of biopsy or of an attempt at definitive surgery. Patients in the control group proceded to immediate surgery and postoperative radiotherapy. This trial again suffered from low accrual, related to complex referral patterns in several countries. However, it is unique in its design, and the results in the 150 patients entered are awaited with interest.

Fortunately, the concept of neoadjuvant chemotherapy is now also being studied by other groups. At the M. D. Anderson Hospital a study is being initiated in patients with poor-prognosis extremity primaries ≥5 cm in diameter. All patients will receive six cycles of neoadjuvant chemotherapy with DX 75 mg/m^2 and ifosfamide 10 g/m^2 with growth factor support. Responding patients will than be randomized to surgery or to surgery + radiotherapy, and subsequently all will receive three additional cycles of chemotherapy. Nonresponding patients will then undergo surgery. A somewhat different approach is being studied by the Radiation Therapy Oncology Group, based on a pilot study performed at the Massachusetts General Hospital. Patients with grade II–III, ≥8 cm in diameter, soft tissue sarcomas of the extremities, head/neck, or trunk will be randomized to undergo, within 6 weeks of biopsy, either preoperative radiotherapy (total dose 50 Gy) followed by surgery, or neoadjuvant chemotherapy + radiotherapy followed by surgery and four cycles of adjuvant chemotherapy. The chemotherapy will consist of a modified mesna/doxorubicin/ifosfamide/DTIC (MAID) regimen, as well as mesna, including ifosfamide 2500 mg/m^2/day on days 1–3, doxorubicin 20 mg/m^2/day on days 1–3, and DTIC 225 mg/m^2/day on days 1–3, with all drugs given by continuous infusion approximately every 3 weeks. In the preoperative treatment using both modalities (chemotherapy and radiotherapy), MAID will be given days 1–3, the first total 22 Gy of radiotherapy between days 7 and 22, the second cycle of MAID on days 23–26, and the second 22 Gy of radiotherapy on days 30–45. Surgery will follow on day 66. Obviously this aggressive preoperative regimen will be supported by G-CSF.

Finally, a subgroup of patients has been identified that clearly benefits from resection of lung metastases [25]. Even though the results are interesting, a further improvement in the survival of these patients should also be pursued. Therefore, EORTC will start a study randomizing patients eligible for radical lung metastasectomy to two cycles of preoperative neoadjuvant chemotherapy followed by surgery or to surgery alone. Patients with an objective clinical response to the preoperative chemotherapy with doxorubicin and ifosfamide, or >50% at histological examination, will receive another three cycles of the same chemotherapy postoperatively. This study will be performed as an Intergroup study with the SSG and ECOG. This Intergroup approach deserves further support because the major drawback in clinical research on adjuvant chemotherapy for soft tissue sarcomas is clearly the limited numbers of patients accruable by each separate group, and meaningful conclusions can only be based on studies of a large sample size.

References

1. Enneking WF, Spanier SS, Malawer MM. The effect of the anatomic setting on the results of surgical procedures for soft part sarcoma of the thigh. Cancer 47:1005–1023, 1981.
2. Russell WO, Kohen J, Enzinger F, Hajdu SI, Heise H, Martin RG, Meissner W, Miller WT, Schmitz RL, Suit HD. A clinical and pathological staging system for soft tissue sarcomas. Cancer 40:1562–1570, 1977.
3. Romsdahl MM, Lindberg RD, Martin RG. Patterns of failure after treatment of soft tissue sarcoma. Cancer Treat Symp 2:251–258, 1983.
4. Suit HD. Patterns of failure after treatment of sarcoma of soft tissue by radical surgery or by conservative surgery and radiation. Cancer Treat Symp 2:241–246, 1983.
5. Schable FM. Rationale for adjuvant chemotherapy. Cancer 39:2875–2882, 1977.
6. Eilber FR, Giuliano AE, Huth JF, Morton DL. A randomized prospective trial using postoperative chemotherapy (Adriamycin) in high grade extremity soft-tissue sarcoma. Am J Clin Oncol (CCT) 11:39–45, 1988.
7. Antman K, Ryan L, Borden E, Wood WC, Lerner HL, Corson JM, Carey R, Suit H, Balcerak S, Elias A, Baker L. Pooled results from three randomized adjuvant studies of doxorubicin versus observation in soft tissue sarcoma: 10 year results and review of literature. In SE Salmon, ed. Adjuvant Therapy of Cancer VI. Philadelphia: WB Saunders, 1990:529–543.
8. Baker LH. Adjuvant therapy for soft tissue sarcomas. In JR Ryan, LO Baker, eds. Recent Concepts in Sarcoma Treatment. Dordecht, the Netherlands: Kluwer Academic, 1988:131–136.
9. Wilson RE, Wood WC, Lerner HL, Antman K, Amato D, Corson JM, Proppe K, Harmon D, Carey R, Greenberger J, Suit H. Doxorubicin chemotherapy in the treatment of soft tissue sarcoma: Combined results of two randomized trials. Arch Surg 121:1354–1359, 1986.
10. Gherlinzoni F, Bacci G, Picci P, Capanna R, Calderoni P, Lorenzi EG, Bernini M, Emiliani E, Barbieri E, Normand A, Campanacci M. A randomized trial for the treatment of high grade soft tissue sarcomas of the extremities: Preliminary observations. J Clin Oncol 4:552–558, 1986.
11. Gherlinzoni F, Pignatti G, Fontana M, Giunti A. Soft tissue sarcomas: The experience at the Istituto Ortopedico Rizzoli. Chir Organi Mov 75:150–154, 1987.

12. Sylvester R. Soft-tissue sarcomas of the extremities [letter]. J Clin Oncol 5:321–322, 1987.
13. Alvegard TA, Sigurdsson H, Mouridsen H, Solheim O, Unsgaard B, Ringborg U, Dahl O, Nordentoft AM, Blomqvist C, Rydholm A, Stener B, Ranstam J. Adjuvant chemotherapy with doxorubicin in high grade soft tissue sarcoma: A randomized trial of the Scandinavian Sarcoma Group. J Clin Oncol 7:1504–1513, 1989.
14. Steward WP, Vantongelen K, Verweij J, Thomas D, Van Oosterom AT. Chemotherapy administration and data collection in an EORTC Collaborative group—can we trust the results? A study of the EORTC Soft Tissue and Bone Sarcoma Group. Eur J Cancer 29A:943–947, 1993.
15. Chang AE, Kinsella T, Glatstein E, Baker AR, Sindelar WF, Lotze MT, Danforth DN, Sugarbaker PH, Lack EE, Steinberg SM, White DE, Rosenberg SA. Adjuvant chemotherapy for patients with high grade soft tissue sarcomas of the extremity. J Clin Oncol 6:1491–1500, 1988.
16. Glenn J, Kinsella T, Glatstein E, Tepper J, Baker A, Sugarbaker P, Sindelar W, Roth J, Brennan M, Costa J, Seipp C, Wesley R, Young RC, Rosenberg SA. A randomized, perspective trial of adjuvant chemotherapy in adults with soft tissue sarcomas of the head and neck, breast and trunk. Cancer 55:1206–1214, 1985.
17. Rosenberg SA. Adjuvant chemotherapy of adult patients with soft tissue sarcoma. In V DeVita, S Hellman, S Rosenberg, eds. Important Advances in Oncology. Philadelphia: JB Lippincott, 1985:273–294.
18. Edmonson JH, Fleming TR, Ivans JC, Burgert O, Soule EH, O'Connell MJ, Sim FH, Ahmann DL. A randomized study of systemic chemotherapy following complete excision of nonosseous sarcomas. J Clin Oncol 2:1390–1396, 1984.
19. Benjamin RS, Terjanian TO, Genoglio CJ, Barkley HT, Evans HC, Murphy WK, Martin RG. The importance of combination chemotherapy for adjuvant treatment of high risk patients with soft tissue sarcomas of the extremities. In SE Salmon, ed. Adjuvant Therapy of Cancer V. New York: Grune & Stratton, 1987:735–744.
20. Ravaud A, Bui NB, Coindre JM, Kantor G, Stockle E, Lagarde P, Becouarn Y, Chauvergne J, Bonichon F, Maree D. Adjuvant chemotherapy with CyVADIC in high risk soft tissue sarcoma: A randomized prospective trial. In SE Salmon, ed. Adjuvant Therapy of Cancer VI. Philadelphia: WB Saunders, 1990:556–566.
21. Bramwell V, Rouésse J, Steward W, Santoro A, Schraffordt-Koops H, Buesa J, Rinka W, Priario J, Wagener Th, Burgers M, van Unnik J, Contesso G, Thomas D, Van Glabbeke M, Markham D, Pinedo H. Adjuvant CYVADIC chemotherapy for adult soft tissue sarcoma—Reduced local recurrence but no improvement in survival: A study of the European Organization for Research and Treatment of Cancer Soft Tissue and Bone Sarcoma Group. J Clin Oncol 12:1137–1149, 1994.
22. Jones GW, Chouinard E, Patel M. Adjuvant Adriamycin (doxorubicin) in adult patients with soft-tissue sarcomas: A systematic overview and quantitative meta-analysis (abstr). Clin Invest Med 14(Suppl 19):A772, 1991.
23. Omura GA, Blessing JA, Major F, Lifshitz S, Ehrlich CE, Mangan C, Beecham J, Patk R, Silverberg S. A randomized clinical trial of adjuvant Adriamycin in uterine sarcomas: A Gynecologic Oncology Group Study. J Clin Oncol 3:1240–1245, 1985.
24. Casper ES, Gaynor JJ, Hajdu SI, Magill GB, Tan C, Friedrich C, Brennan MF. A prospective randomized trial of adjuvant chemotherapy with bolus versus continuous infusion of doxorubicin in patients with high-grade extremity soft tissue sarcoma and an analysis of prognostic factors. Cancer 68:1221–1229, 1991.
25. Van Geel AN, Pastorino U, Jauch KW, Judson R, Coevorden F, Pietraszak A, Buesa JM, Nielsen OS, Boudinet A, Steward WP, Woll PJ, Vaneerdeweg W, Hoekstra HJ, Tursz T, Schmitz PIM. Surgical treatment of lung metastases: The EORTC Soft Tissue and Bone Sarcoma Group study of 255 patient. Cancer 77:675–682, 1996.
26. Mouridsen HT, Bastholt L, Somers R, Santoro A, Bramwell V, Mulder JH, Van Oosterom AT, Buesa J, Pinedo HM, Thomas D, Sylvester R. Adriamycin versus epirubicin in advanced

soft tissue sarcomas. A randomized phase II/phase III study of the EORTC Soft Tissue and Bone Sarcoma Group. Eur J Cancer Clin Oncol 23:1477–1483, 1987.

27. Dombernowsky P, Mouridsen H, Nielsen OS, Crowther D, Verweij J, Buesa J, Steward W, Tursz T for the EORTC Soft Tissue and Bone Sarcoma Cooperative Group. A phase III study comparing Adriamycin vs. two schedules of high dose epirubicin in advanced soft tissue sarcoma. Proc Am Soc Clin Oncol 14:1688, 1995.

13. Isolated limb perfusion with high-dose tumor necrosis factor-α for locally advanced extremity soft tissue sarcomas

A.M.M. Eggermont, H. Schraffordt Koops, J.M. Klausner, P.M. Schlag, B.B.R. Kroon, G. Ben-Ari, and F.J. Lejeune

Introduction

Extremity soft tissue sarcoma

Sixty percent of the 6000 new cases of soft tissue sarcomas diagnosed in the United States each year occur in the extremities and are often large at the time of initial diagnosis [1]. Surgery for locally advanced extremity soft tissue sarcomas may consist of an amputation or exarticulation. Limb-sparing surgical procedures in these advanced cases, if at all possible, usually consist of extensive but still marginal resections requiring adjuvant radiation therapy to a large area. In those cases where location of the tumor dictate the sacrifice of functionally crucial muscles and or joint-spanning radiation therapy treatment may mutilate and compromise limb function considerably, some form of induction therapy prior to surgery should be considered. Preservation of the limb and limb function has become all the more important in light of evidence that amputations do not improve survival rates because the prognosis in patients with large (>5 cm) deep-seated, high-grade soft tissue sarcomas is not, or is only marginally, influenced by the extent of the procedure dealing with the primary tumor [2]. Although local recurrence rates vary according to the initial surgical procedure and improved local control has been reported to correlate with better survival [3], several recent studies have not been able to show that 'inadequate treatment,' that is, marginal excisions with a high risk for local recurrence, influences survival significantly [2,4–7].

Strategies to improve local tumor control

Preoperative therapies to improve local tumor control rates have been used. Suit and coworkers reported on a favorable outcome using preoperative radiation therapy followed by limb-sparing surgery [8]. Neoadjuvant chemotherapy in a series publicized by Rouësse and collegues was reported to yield a 38% overall response rate (6% complete response [CR] and 32% partial response [PR]), which was considered in some cases to have facilitated limb-sparing surgery [9]. Eilber and collegues developed a multimodality approach combin-

J. Verweij, H.M. Pinedo, and H.D. Suit (eds). SOFT TISSUE SARCOMAS: PRESENT ACHIEVEMENTS AND FUTURE PROSPECTS.

ing preoperative (intraarterial or systemic) chemotherapy and radiotherapy [10,11]. When applied in the general patient population with extremity soft tissue sarcomas, limb salvage and local tumor control rates of over 90% were achieved. This has been confirmed by other centers in a series of patients with tumors of a rather modest median size of 7 cm [12].

Amputation may be avoided and local control improved by applying brachytherapy techniques to the tumor bed in the context of marginal resections. Shiu and coworkers reported a 70% limb salvage rate in patients with truly locally advanced soft tissue sarcoma abutting the neurovasular bundle [13]. Yet another strategy, and one we consider reserved only for truly locally advanced cases, is to perform an isolated limb perfusion (ILP).

Isolated limb perfusion with only cytostatic drugs

Isolated limb perfusion was first described by Creech et al. [14] and is most commonly used to treat melanoma in-transit metastases in the extemity. Regional cytostatic concentrations during ILP are 15–20 times higher than those reached after systemic administration, with minimal systemic toxicity [15]. Isolated limb perfusion may render an irresectable tumor resectable and may reduce the local recurrence rate. In cases with widespread metastases, it can be used palliatively for alleviation of pain and to avoid ablative surgery [16,17]. Melphalan is the standard drug for ILP in the treatment of melanoma [16]. Because of its excellent perfusion properties, it has also been used alone or in combination with other drugs in the treatment of extremity soft tissue sarcoma.

The results of ILP with melphalan, as well as with other drugs, have been rather disappointing, however [17–25]. Krementz et al. reported only 4 CRs (10%) and 8 PRs (21%) in 39 patients with extremity soft tissue sarcoma (resectable, various sizes) after ILP with melphalan ± nitrogen mustard ± actinomycin D. In 17 patients with truly locally advanced disease, 0 CRs (0%) and only 6 PRs (35%) were observed [17].

Doxorubicin has also been investigated in the ILP setting. In a series of 26 patients from the Netherlands, a 0% reponse rate was seen in 22 grade II–III sarcomas with 3 amputations because of toxicity, while 4 CRs were observed only in patients with low-grade sarcomas, and only when doxorubicin was combined with melphalan [18]. In a recent study >50% necrosis in soft tissue sarcoma tumors after ILP with doxorubicin was observed in 16 of 23 patients, but no clinical response data were provided and, most importantly, no complete remissions were observed [19]. Others reported high local recurrence rates and amputation rates of up to 41% after ILP with melphalan in combination with other cytostatic agents [20].

Most other reports on the use of ILP in soft tissue sarcoma patients concern adjuvant ILPs in situations where the sarcomas had already been (nonradically) resected or were resected immediately after the limb perfusion [21–26]. These reports, therefore, do not provide information on response rate nor on the role of ILP in limb salvage. Because of the modest results achieved by ILP with cytostatic drugs alone, this procedure was abandoned in most centers for the management of locally advanced extremity STS.

Introduction of tumor necrosis factor-α in isolated limb perfusion

This lack of efficacy prompted Lejeune and coworkers to investigate the addition of high doses of tumor necrosis factor (TNF). The initial experience with high CR rates after treatment of 19 stage III melanoma patients and 4 soft tissue sarcoma patients was published in 1992 [26]. In a multicenter study protocol, rules for the perfusion, resection of residual tumor, and preoperative and postoperative evaluation were defined. Results of the initial experience with the triple regimen, for example, TNF + melphalan + IFN, have been reported recently [27,28]. Here we present an overview of the experience with the application of high-dose TNF-α in the setting of ILP as an induction biochemotherapy procedure in 125 patients. In this study 55 consecutive patients were treated with the combination of TNF with interferon-γ (IFN) and melphalan at the four centers that were initially involved in a multicenter trial. Over time the number of centers involved in the TNF perfusion program has expanded to seven centers. Interferon was left out of the treatment schedule in the expanded program. Seventy patients were treated in the seven centers not using IFN.

Patient and methods

Patients. One hundred and twenty-five patients with unresectable soft tissue sarcomas of the leg (105) or arm (20) underwent 137 ILPs in the period May 1991 through August 1994; 6 patients received a second perfusion prior to resection, and another 6 patients received a second or even third perfusion because of local tumor recurrence. There were 70 males and 55 females, with a median age of 49 years (range 13–84). There were primary sarcomas and local recurrences in about 50% of patients. The fact that most patients considered eligible only for amputations were referred for ILP is illustrated by the unusual composition of this series: 28 patients had multiple tumors (22%), either multifocal primary tumors or multiple recurrences, often after inadequate previous surgical procedures with tumor spill, and 20 patients (16%) had systemic metastases evident at the time the ILP was being performed only to control rapid local tumor growth.

Criteria for unresectablility. All patients were referred to the seven participating cancer centers because their sarcomas were considered unresectable by the referring specialists, who would have otherwise performed an amputation. All tumors were considered unresectable or resectable at the cost of unacceptable (functional) mutilation by several surgeons from a team of specialists at the referral centers because of either multifocal disease or single tumors with fixation/invasion to the neurovascular bundle and/or bone. Radical resections, for example, resections with a margin of healthy tissue, were not possible in these 125 patients. Tumors were very large, with a median size of 18 cm (range 2–35 cm) in the first 55 patients treated with TNF + IFN + melphalan, and a median size of 16 cm (range 2–38 cm) in the next 70 patients treated with TNF + melphalan.

Histological types and grades. Most tumors (110 in 125) were high-grade tumors (grade II–III) of a great variety of histological types (at least 16 different histological types). Grading was according to the method of Trojani et al. [29].

Drugs and treatment schedule. Recombinant human TNF-α (0.2 mg/ampule, 4.9–5.8 $\times$ 10^7 U/mg) and recombinant human IFN-α (0.2 mg or 1.5 $\times$ 10^6 U/ampule) were gifts from Boehringer Ingelheim GmbH, Ingelheim/Rhein, Germany. The cytostatic drug melphalan (Alkeran) was obtained as a sterile powder (100 mg) and was dissolved aseptically using solvent and diluent provided by Burroughs Wellcome (London, England). Fifty-five patients received 0.2 mg IFN subcutaneously on the 2 days prior to the ILP as well as 0.2 mg IFN in the perfusate during ILP. Seventy patients did not receive IFN at all. Isolated limb perfusions were carried out under general anesthesia, and the procedure usually took 3–5 hours. ILP consisted of a 90-minute long perfusion with 0.2 mg IFN, 3 mg (arm) to 4 mg (leg) TNF, and 10 mg/l (leg) or 13 mg/l (arm) melphalan under mild hyperthermia (39–40°C). The composition of the perfusate was as follows: the priming volume of 700–850 ml consisted of 400–500 ml blood (50% red blood cells, 50 plasma), 200–400 ml 5% dextran 40 in glucose 5% (Isodex, Pharmacia, Uppsala, Sweden) of Haemaccel, 10–30 ml of 8.4% sodium bicarbonate, and 0.5 ml of 2500–5000 IU heparin. IFN and TNF were injected as successive boluses into the arterial line, provided the limb tissue temperature was >38°C. Melphalan was administered 30 minutes later at limb temperatures between 39 and 40°C. Flow rates were kept at 40–60 ml/min per liter limb volume. At the end of the ILP, the limb was washed with at least 1 l of Haemaccel and 1 l of 6% dextran 70 (Macrodex, Pharmacia, Uppsala, Sweden).

Leakage monitoring. Throughout the perfusion period any potential drug leakage was monitored using a radioactive tracer. A small calibration dose of human serum albumin radiolabeled with ^{131}I or ^{99m}Tc was injected into the systemic circulation, and a (10-fold) higher dose of the same isotope was injected into the isolated extremity. Continuous monitoring was performed with a precordial scintillation probe. Systemic leakage was expressed quantitatively as a percentage such that 100% leakage represented a homogeneous distribution of the isotope in the body [30,31].

Cardiopulmonary and hemodynamic monitoring. Perioperative cardiopulmonary and hemodynamic monitoring consisted of ECG, urine output, blood pressure, venous and pulmonary pressures, and arterial wedge pressures in most patients until the second postoperative day. Preoperative and postoperatively dopamine was routinely given in two centers (23 patients) at 2–4 μg/kg/min for up to 48 hours; in the other centers it was given only when indicationed, that is, only occasionally (to <10% of the patients). Fluid loading was used during the operation before releasing the tourniquet after completion of the limb washout.

Assessment of tumor response. Complete remissions (CR), partial remissions (PR), no change (NC), and progressive disease (PD) were assessed using the standard WHO criteria [32]. Extensive histopathological examination of the resected specimens was performed, and the percentage of necrosis was estimated on the basis of macroscopic evaluation of necrotized tissue and histologic examination of tissue surrounding the necrotic area, with tissue without identifiable nuclei being considered necrotic. If no clinically detectable tumor was seen (clinical CR) but resection of the tumor bed revealed vital tumor cells, the final outcome was *downgraded* to a PR. If the clinical response was a PR, the final outcome response could only be *upgraded* to a CR if histological examination showed 100% necrosis of the tumor remnant. Likewise, a clinical minimal regression of <50%, but still rendering the tumor resectable, could be upgraded to a PR if histological examination showed the tumor remnant to be necrotic for 50% or more.

Marginal resection of the tumor remnant. Resections of the tumor remnants were usually performed between 4 and 24 weeks after ILP. The average period was 10 weeks. Usually this period allowed for enough shrinkage of the tumor to become mobile or to shrink for more than 50%. Margins were usually not more than 1 mm, and all resections were marginal resections and often could be described as 'shell-out' procedures. No grossly evident residual disease was left in the surgical bed. The presence of tumor cells close by or clearly in the margin (microscopic irradicality) prompted adjuvant radiation therapy in 28 patients.

Assessment of toxicity. Systemic toxicity was graded by the Eastern Cooperative Oncology Group (ECOG) — World Health Organization (WHO) grading system [32]. Regional toxicity was graded according to Wieberdinks classification: 1 = no toxicity; 2 = redness and slight edema; 3 = considerable erythema or edema with some blistering, slightly disturbed mobility possible; 4 = extensive epidermiolysis or obvious damage to the deep tissues, causing definite functional disturbances, threatening or manifest compartmental syndrome; and 5 = reaction requiring amputation [33].

Ethical committe approval and informed consent. The protocol was approved by the ethical committees of all institutions involved in the study. Informed consent was obtained from all patients prior to treatment.

Results

Treatment outcome

Table 1 summarizes the clinical and histopathological response rates as well as the final outcome and limb salvage rates in all 125 patients. In the 55 patients treated with the triple regimen, including IFN, the following clinical response rates were observed after one ILP: 10 CR (18%), 35 PR (64%), and 10 no change (NC; 18%). After resection of the tumor remnant; histopathological exams determined whether a clinical CR would be downgraded to a PR (vital tumor cells in a scar area) or whether a clinical PR or NC was upgraded on the basis of the percentage of necrosis to a CR (100% necrosis) or PR (50–99% necrosis) in the resected tumor remnant. Resections or biopsies were performed in 43 patients. Thus two clinical CRs were *downgraded* to a PR, whereas 10 clinical PRs were *upgraded* to a CR; 3 patients with no change clinically (up to 45% regression) were *upgraded* to PRs because of >50% necrosis in the resection specimen. Thus the final outcome in 55 patients was 20 CR (36%), 27 PR (51%), and 7 NC (13%); the overall response rate was 87%. Limb salvage at a median follow-up of 2.5 years (range 20–50 months) was observed in 45 patients (82%). Amputations were done for lack of tumor response or local tumor recurrence in seven patients and in three patients due to acute local problems after ILP (one patient) or chronic local problems after ILP (two patients: osteomyelitis, chronic erysipelas) in spite of a histopathological CR in these three patients.

Table 1. Treatment outcome after one TNF-based isolated limb perfusion

TNF + IFN + melphalan			TNF + melphalan		
Clinical (55 pts)	Histology (43 pts)	Final outcome (55 pts)	Clinical (70 pts)	Histology (58 pts)	Final outcome (70 pts)
10 CR 18%	15 CR	20 CR 36%	15 CR 21%	14 CR	19 CR 27%
35 PR 64%	21 CR	28 PR 51%	32 PR 46%	33 PR	39 PR 56%
10 NC 18%	7 NC	7 NC 13%	22 NC 32%	11 NC	11 NC 16%
0 PD 0%	12 ND		1 PD 1%	12 ND	1 PD 1%
	Limb salvage[a] 45/55 = 82%			Limb salvage[b] 57/70 = 81%	

[a] Limb salvage at median follow-up of 2.5 years.
[b] Limb salvage at median follow-up of 1.5 years.
CR = complete remission; PR = partial remission; NC = change; PD = progressive disease; ND = not done.

In the 70 patients treated with TNF + melphalan, without IFN, the following clinical response rates were observed: 15 CR (21%), 32 PR (46%), 22 NC (32%), and 1 PR (1%). Histopathological exams in 59 patients revealed 14 CR (100% necrosis), 33 PR (>50% necrosis), and 11 NC (0–50% necrosis). The final outcome after one ILP in 70 patients was 19 CR (27%) 39 PR (56%), 11 NC (16%), and 1 progressive disease (PD; 1%). The overall response rate was 83%. Four patients who achieved a clinical PR after their first ILP received a second ILP 6–8 weeks later and a CR was acheived. Therefore in the 70 patients treated with TNF + melphalan, eventually 23 CR (31%), 35 PR (52%), 11 NC (16%), and 1 PD (1%) were seen. Limb salvage at a median follow-up of 1.5 years (range 9–38) was observed in 57 patients (81%). Amputations were done in spite of a CR but without further soft tissue coverage of the lower limb in one patient, and in spite of a lack of tumor response or local recurrence in 12 other patients.

Local tumor control

Patients treated by a resection of the tumor remnant after ILP had excellent local tumor control. Seven local recurrences were observed in 85 patients (8%). The 20 patients with metastases at the time of ILP did not undergo a resection of their tumor, nor did 20 of the 28 patients with multiple tumors. In these 40 patients local recurrence or a re-outgrowth of their completely or partially regressed tumors occurred in 14 patients (35%). Limb salvage was achieved in most patients because they were dying of systemic disease.

Systemic metastases and survival

At a median follow-up of 2.5 years in the 55 patients treated with IFN + TNF + melphalan, 15 of the 46 patients who underwent ILP without evidence of systemic metastases have been diagnosed with systemic disease (33%). Of these 15 patients, 13 (87%) have died thus far. Nine patients (16%) underwent an ILP for local tumor control with known widespread metastatic disease. Seven of these nine (78%) have died thus far. At a median follow-up of 1.5 years in the 70 patients treated with TNF + melphalan, 19 of the 59 patients who were treated with an ILP without known systemic metastases have been diagnosed with systemic disease (32%). Thirteen of these 19 patients (70%) have died thus far. Eleven patients (16%) already had distant metastases at the time of ILP, and they have all died.

Regional toxicity

Regional toxicity, scored according to Wieberdink et al. [33], was moderate. Almost all patients had a perfusion reaction of grade II–III. This is similar to the toxicity observed after ILP with melphalan alone. In seven patients grade IV toxicity and in one patient grade V toxicity immediately followed ILP.

When radiation therapy followed resection of the tumor remnant, no enhanced toxicity was observed in patients with grade I–II toxicity after ILP. However, in some patients with grade III–IV toxicity radiation therapy was tolerated less well. In one patient with grade IV toxicity, recurrent bouts of erysipelas led to skin ulcerations and eventually prompted a late amputation. Short-lived (<6 months) post-ILP neurapraxia, consisting of hypesthesia and paresthesias in the fingertips and soles of the foot, was relatively frequently observed (15–20%), but longlasting and then often permanent neurapraxia was observed in only 5% of patients. In four of the latter cases, the peroneal nerve was involved and loss of its function was compensated for by a peroneal brace.

Systemic toxicity

Systemic toxicity was moderate and easily managable. All patients developed fever and chills within 4 hours of the ILP, which was treated effectively with paracetamol or indomethacin.

Cardiovascular. All patients developed a hyperdynamic state, with an increased pulse rate and cardiac output in spite of a sometimes transient lowering of the blood pressure, which was easily managed by administering fluid. Low-dose dopamine was standardly given for 48 hours in two centers in the early years of the TNF program; in the other centers it was only given on indication, and only for a short period (<8 hours). At present dopamine is no longer routinely administered.

Pulmonary. Adult respiratory distress syndrome was seen in one patient. This patient developed a multiple organ failure (MOF) during the first 3 weeks after ILP.

Renal. Creatinine levels remained normal in most patients, but one patient experienced grade IV renal toxicity (the patient with MOF).

Hepatic. Hepatic toxicity was very modest and was mainly reflected in an isolated transient rise in transaminases. Grade III–IV peak levels of the transaminases ASAT and ALAT were seen in 10% of the patients. This was of no clinical significance as levels normalize within a few days. Other parameters, notably bilirubin, usually did not rise at all, except in the one patient with MOF (grade IV).

Hematological. Transient grade III–IV leukopenia and grade III–IV thrombocytopenia (usually around day 3) occurred in less than 10% of patients. It was without clinical consequences because these low numbers only lasted for 1 or 2 days, and did not require intervention.

Evaluation of the effect of TNF-α perfusion on tumor vascularity

To document the effects of an ILP with TNF, IFN, and melphalan on the vascular bed of these often very large sarcomas, angiograms were performed before and 1–2 weeks after the ILP. Pre-ILP angiographies demonstrated a very large, well-developed tumor vascular bed in many patients. Angiography 1–2 weeks after the ILP with TNF showed that all tumor-associated vessels had disappeared. One typical case is shown in Figure 1, which illustrates the hypervascular sarcoma of a patient depicted on a preoperative angiogram and the disappearance of all tumor-associated vessels 3–4 weeks after ILP, without damage being inflicted on the normal vessels. This patient was a 63-year-old woman with a rapidly growing grade III malignant fibrous histiocytoma (MFH) in the popliteal fossa of her right leg, which progressed during two courses of systemic induction chemotherapy with doxorubocin and ifosfamide. The tumor was fixed to the vessels and bones, and had caused a popliteal nerve palsy by invading the peroneal nerve. The patient had an excellent response to the ILP

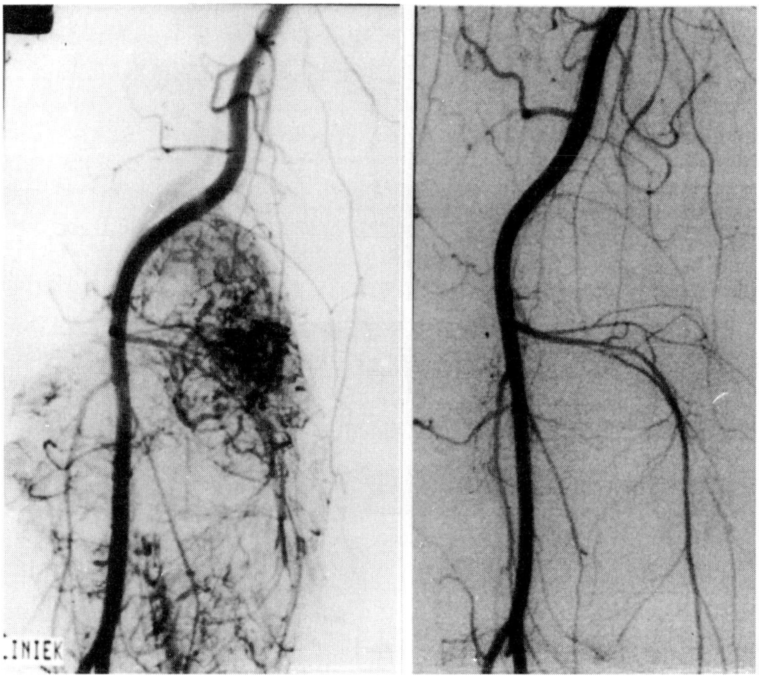

Figure 1. A pre-ILP angiogram of a hypervascular grade III malignant fibrous histiocytoma in the right popliteal fossa of a 63-year-old woman is shown on the left. The tumor was fixed to the vessels and bone, and had invaded the popliteal nerve, causing popliteal nerve palsy (drop foot). On the post-ILP angiogram, the disappearance of all tumor-associated vessels 3–4 weeks after ILP is seen, but no damage seems to have been inflicted on the normal vessels. The patient had a rapid clinical response with softening of the tumor and >50% regression, rendering the tumor mobile again. Resection of the tumor remnant, 6 weeks after ILP, revealed 100% necrosis.

with IFN + TNF + melphalan. A rapid clinical PR allowed for the tumor remnant to be resected by a shell-out procedure. Histopathological examination revealed 100% necrosis. No radiation therapy was given to the tumor bed. The patient remains disease-free more than 4 years after the resection.

Discussion

The results of our experience in these 125 patients show that longlasting complete remissions and valuable partial remissions, which render unresectable extremity sarcomas resectable, can be obtained by ILP with TNF and melphalan. The 87% objective response rate and the 82% limb salvage rate in 55 patients treated with IFN + TNF + melphalan, and the 83% overall response rate and 81% limb salvage rate in 70 patients treated without IFN, demonstrate the efficacy of this two-step approach in achieving limb salvage in patients with locally very advanced disease in an unusual series of patients, given the fact that 23% had multiple tumors in the extremity and 16% already had systemic metastases at the time of ILP. It is hard to find a comparable series of patients with comparably advanced tumors. Krementz et al. [17] described, in a noncomparable series of 39 patients with resectable extremity soft tissue sarcomas, only 4 CRs (10%) and 8 PRs (21%) after ILP with melphalan ± nitrogen mustard ± actinomycin D. In another 17 patients, comparable with our series of patients with irresectable sarcomas and a delayed resection after ILP, 0 CRs (0%) and only 6 PRs (35%) were observed [17]. These results are quite inferior to ours, including TNF-α. Whether melphalan, the best perfusion drug for melanoma in-transit metastases, is also the ideal drug for the perfusion of soft tissue sarcomas in unclear. ILP with doxorubicin may seem attractive for sarcomas, but was reported to cause considerable regional toxicity and to be ineffective when used alone. In a Dutch report on 26 patients, a 0% reponse rate was seen in 22 grade II–III sarcomas with three amputations because of toxicity, while 4 CRs were observed only in patients with low-grade sarcomas and only when doxorubicin was combined with melphalan [18]. The study by Rossi et al., in contrast, reported a >50% necrosis in soft tissue sarcoma tumors after ILP with doxorubicin in 16 of 23 patients. Because no clinical response data were provided and, most importantly, no complete remissions were observed, the value of ILP with doxorubicin alone remains unclear [19]. Others reported high local recurrence rates and amputation rates up to 41% after ILP with melphalan in combination with other cytostatic agents [20]. Overall it seems fair to conclude that the addition of TNF markedly improves results.

Other multimodality approaches, such as the combination of preoperative intraarterial infusions with doxorubicin and radiation therapy followed by resection of the soft tissue sarcoma, may also result in excellent local control rates, but these are acheived in rather unselected and thus differently composed patient populations [10–12]. Again, reports on patients with disease as advanced as seen in this series are very hard to find, as illustrated by the study of Wanebo et al. [12]. In their series of 66 patients, the median tumor size was only 7 cm (vs. an 18-cm median size in our first series of 55 patients) and local wide resections (margins of 2–4 cm of normal tissue) were possible in 58%, whereas these wide resections were not possible in our patients.

ILP with TNF + IFN + melphalan seems of particular palliative value in patients with widespread metastatic disease and an uncontrollable rapidly growing tumor that threatens the limb. In all but 2 of these 20 patients, a single ILP with TNF + IFN + melphalan provided rapid and long-lasting (up to >2 years; median 9 months) local control.

Assessment of necrosis of soft tissue sarcomas after ILP is difficult. The disappearance of the vascular bed, as demonstated by postoperative angiograms, is usually a good indicator of the induction of massive necrosis, and it may be valuable to be patient and wait for a slowly regressing tumor to shrink to such a degree that a resection can be done with as little mutilation as possible. New techniques, such as MRI and PET scanning, may be quite useful to assess the extent of necrosis and to predict the quality of the response and thus influence clinical decision making regarding the type and timing of the resection of the tumor as well as the decision to add radiation therapy [34,35].

It is clear that ILP with TNF is safe and is associated with little to moderate regional and systemic toxicity. Systemic toxicity is related to the leakage rate during perfusion. As soon as all centers began using a physiological (low) perfusion flow rate of 40–50 ml/min/l limb volume in combination with continuous leakage monitoring, toxicity became minor and easily manageable, obviating the routine application of Swan Ganz catheters and/or dopamine. The importance of continuous leakage monitoring is further underscored by the observation that two other reports on TNF-ILPs mentioned cases with considerable to severe toxicity in a setting where continuous leakage monitoring was not carried out [36,37], whereas Thom et al. [38] and Swaak et al. [39] have demonstrated in their reports on ILPs with TNF + IFN + melphalan that very little toxicity was seen in the absence of leakage during ILP. Furthermore, especially after iliac and femoral perfusions, we have intensified the washout procedure at the end of the ILP, using up to 6 of Marcodex or Haemaccel, and signs of TNF-related toxicity and postoperative peak levels of TNF have been further reduced [40].

Regarding the role of IFN-α, our data do not indicate that IFN plays a crucial role, but it is clear that melphalan is crucial because ILPs with TNF-α alone induce no or only very short-lived responses in patients with melanoma [41], in those with soft tissue sarcoma (DL Fraker, NCI Surgery Branch, Bethesda, MD, personal communication), and in an isolated limb perfusion model using a nonimmunogenic soft tissue sarcoma in rats [42]. In the ILP setting human tumors are exposed to extremely high levels of TNF (perfusate TNF-α levels are usually in the range of 3–5 μg/ml). The disappointing results of the systemic administration of TNF in humans in phase I–II trials [43–46] may well be due to the fact that TNF toxicity in humans allowed only 1th/20th to 1/50th of the dose required for antitumor effects in murine experimental tumor models [47]. A gap of this magnitude can only be overcome in an ILP setting and in humans also produces the typical acute antitumor effects of TNF. This supports the hypothesis that, apart from direct antitumor effects [48,49], TNF has mainly important indirect (vascular) antitumor effects in humans. These intravascular effects, such as thrombocyte aggegation, erythrostasis, and endothelial and vascular destruction, have already been described [50,51] and resemble many of the phenomena reported in experimental tumor systems [52–55]. Moreover, the selective destructive effects of TNF-ILP on tumor-associated vessels are illustrated in Figure 1.

Neutrophils may also play an important role in the antitumor effects because extravasation and invasion of the tumor by neutrophils can be observed after ILP with TNF-α [50]. Observations in the sarcoma perfusion model in rats in our laboratory suggest strongly that neutrophils play a crucial role because much of the TNF antitumor effect is lost in rats with severe radiation-induced neutropenia [56]. The evidence that the greatest common denominator, that is, the tumor vascular bed, is the 'aselective' target for TNF would predict that any histological type of solid tumor is likely to be sensitive to the effects of TNF. The observation that 16 types of sarcomas, melanomas, and a range of other extremity tumors (unpublished observations) have all been affected is attractive and may indicate a widening field of indications for the use of TNF.

Conclusions

The results in the 125 patients described in this chapter demonstrate that typical TNF-mediated antitumor effects can be obtained in humans, provided sufficiently high TNF levels can be delivered to the tumor site. Therefore, clinically effective applications of TNF may well be restricted to locoregional administration of this cytokine. High-dose TNF can be administered safely via isolation perfusion, provided that leakage during ILP is well controlled and monitored and that adequate cardiovascular monitoring is performed. rTNF-α may establish itself as an important drug in isolation perfusion for a number of tumors and in a number of settings, such as the isolated lung [57], liver [58,59], and kidney [60]. Isolated limb perfusion with TNF is a new option in the management of locally advanced and unresectable soft tissue sarcomas of the extremities. The procedure merits further evaluation in an increasing number of centers that deal with the treatment of soft tissue sarcomas to further define its value and place in the management of extremity tumors.

References

1. Boring CC, Squires TS, Tong T, Montgomery S. Cancer Statistics, 1994. CA Cancer J Clin 44:7–26, 1994.

2. Gaynor JJ, Tan CC, Casper ES, et al. Refinement of clincopathologic staging for localized soft tissue sarcoma of the extremity: A study of 423 adults. J Clin Oncol 10:1317–1327, 1992.
3. Suit HD, Tepper JE. Impact of improved local control on survival in patients with soft tissue sarcoma. Int J Radiat Oncol Biol Phys 12:699–700, 1986.
4. Brennan MF, Shiu MH, Collin C, et al. Extremity soft tissue sarcomas. Cancer Treat Symp 3:71–81, 1985.
5. Potter DA, Kinsella D, Gladstein E, et al. High grade soft tissue sarcomas of the extremities. Cancer 59:190–205, 1986.
6. Stotter AT, A'Hearn RP, Fisher C, Mott AF, Fallowfield ME, Westbury G. The influence of local recurrence of extremity soft tissue sarcoma on metastasis and survival. Cancer 65:1119–1129, 1990.
7. Gustafson P, Rööser B, Rydholm A. Is local recurrence of minor importance for metastases in soft tissue sarcoma? Cancer 67:2083–2086, 1991.
8. Suit HD, Proppe KH, Mankin HJ, Wood WC. Preoperative radiation therapy for sarcoma of soft tissue. Cancer 47:2269–2274, 1981.
9. Rouësse JG, Friedman S, Sevin DM, et al. Preoperative induction chemotherapy in the treatment of locally advanced soft tissue sarcomas. Cancer 60:296–300, 1987.
10. Eilber FR, Mirra JJ, Grant T, Weisenburger T, Morton DL. Is amputation necessary for sarcoma: A 7-year experiment with limb salvage. Ann Surg 192:431–437, 1980.
11. Eilber FR, Morton DL, Eckhardt J, Grant T, Weisenburger T. Limb salvage for skeletal and soft-tissue sarcomas: Multidisciplinary preoperative therapy. Cancer 53:2579–2584, 1984.
12. Wanebo HJ, Temple WJ, Popp MB, Constable W, Aron B, Cunningham SL. Preoperative regional therapy for extremity sarcoma: A tricenter update. Cancer 75:2299–2306, 1995.
13. Shiu MH, Hilaris BS, Harrison LB, Brennan MF. Brachytherapy and function-saving resection of soft tissue sarcoma arising in the limb. Int J Radiat Oncol Biol Phys 21:1485–1492, 1991.
14. Creech OJ, Krementz ET, Ryan RF, Winblad JN. Chemotherapy of cancer: Regional perfusion utilizing an extracorporeal circuit. Ann Surg 148:616–632, 1958.
15. Benckhuijsen C, Kroon BBR, Van Geel AN, Wieberdink J. Regional perfusion treatment with melphalan for melanoma in a limb: Evaluation of drug kinetics. Eur J Surg Oncol 14:157–163, 1988.
16. Thompson JF, Gianoutsos MP. Isolated limb perfusion for melanoma: Effectiveness and toxicity of cisplatin compared with that of melphalan and other drugs. World J Surg 61:227–233, 1992.
17. Krementz ET, Carter RD, Sutherland CM, Hutton I. Chemotherapy of sarcomas of the limbs by regional perfusion. Ann Surg 185:555–564, 1977.
18. Klaase JM, Kroon BBR, Benckhuysen C, Van Geel AN, Albus-Lutter ChE, Wieberdink J. Results of regional isolation perfusion with cytostatics in patients with soft tissue tumors of the extremities. Cancer 64:616–621, 1989.
19. Rossi CR, Vecchiato A, Foletto M, et al. Phase II study on neoadjuvant hyperthermic-antiblastic perfusion with doxorubicin in patients with intermediate of high grade limb sarcomas. Cancer 73:2140–2146, 1994.
20. Filippo FD, Calabro AM, Cavallari A, et al. The role of hyperthermic perfusion as a first step in the treatment of soft tissue sarcomas of the extremities. World J Surg 12:332–339, 1988.
21. McBride CM. Sarcomas of the limbs: Result of adjuvant chemotherapy using isolation perfusion. Arch Surg 109:304–308, 1974.
22. Stehlin JS, de Ipolyi PD, Giovanella BC, Gutierrez AE, Anderson RF. Soft tissue sarcomas of the extremity: Multidisciplinary therapy employing hyperthermic perfusion. Am J Surg 130:643–646, 1975.
23. Lethi PM, Stephens MH, Janoff K, Stevens K, Fletcher WS. Improved survival for soft tissue sarcoma of the extremities by regional hyperthermic perfusion, local excision and radiation therapy. Surg Gynecol Obstet 162:149–152, 1986.
24. Hoekstra HJ, Schraffordt Koops H, Molenaar WM, Oldhoff J, Results of isolated regional

perfusion in the treatment of malignant soft tissue tumors of the extremities. Cancer 60:1703–1707, 1987.
25. Braat RP, Wieberdink J, van Slooten EA, Olthuis G. Regional perfusion with Adriamycin in soft tissue sarcomas. In K Schwemmle, K Aigner, eds. Vascular Perfusion in Cancer Therapy. Recent Results in Cancer Research, Vol. 86. Berlin: Springer-Verlag, 1983:260–263.
26. Liénard D, Delmotte JJ, Renard N, Ewalenko P, Lejeune FJ. High doses of rTNF-α in combination with IFN-gamma and melphalan in isolation perfusion of the limbs for melanoma and sarcoma. J Clin Oncol 10:52–60, 1992.
27. Eggermont AMM, Liénard D, Schraffordt Koops H, Van Geel AN, Hoekstra HJ, Lejeune FJ. Limb salvage by high dose tumor necrosis factor-alpha (TNF), gamma-interferon (IFN) and melphalan isolated limb perfusion (ILP) in patients with irresectable soft tissue sarcomas (abstr). Proc Am Soc Cin Oncol 11:412, 1992.
28. Eggermont AMM, Schraffordt Koops H, Liénard D, Kroon BBR, Van Geel AN, Hoekstra HJ, Lejeune FJ. Isolated limb perfuson with high-dose tumot necrosis factor-α in combination with inteferon-γ and melphalan for irresectable extremity soft tissue sarcomas: A multicenter trial. J Clin Oncol 14:2556–2565, 1996.
29. Trojani M, Contesso G, Coindre JM, et al. Soft-tissue sarcomas of adults; study of pathologic prognostic variables and definition of a histopathological grading system. Int J Cancer 33:37–42, 1984.
30. Hoekstra HJ, Naujocks T, Schraffordt Koops H, et al. Continuous leakage monitoring during hyperthermic isolated regional perfusion of the lower limb: Techniques and results. Reg Cancer Treat 4:301–304, 1992.
31. Klaase JM, Kroon BBR, Van Geel AN, Eggermont AMM, Franklin HR. Systemic leakage during isolated limb perfusion for melanoma. Br J Surg 80:1124–1126, 1993.
32. WHO Handbook for Reporting Results of Cancer Treatment. WHO Offset Publication No. 48. Geneva: WHO, 1979.
33. Wieberdink J, Benckhuijsen C, Braat RP, Van Slooten EA, Olthuis GAA. Dosimetry in isolation perfusion of the limbs by assessment of perfused tissue volume and grading of toxic tissue reactions. Eur J Cancer Clin Oncol 18:905–910, 1982.
34. Sijens PE, Eggermont AMM, Van Dijk P, Oudkerk M. ^{31}P magnetic resonance spectroscopy as predictor for clinical response in human extremity sarcomas treated by single dose TNFα + melphalan isolated limb perfusion. NMR Biomed 8:215–224, 1995.
35. Nieweg OE, Pruim J, Hoekstra HJ, et al. Positron emission tomography with fluorine-18-fluorodeoxyglucose for the evaluation of therapeutic isolated regional limb perfusion in a patient with soft-tissue sarcoma. J Nucl Med 35:90–92, 1994.
36. Hill S, Fawcett WJ, Sheldon J, Soni N, Williams T, Thomas JM, Low-dose tumour necrosis factor α and melphalan in hyperthermic isolated limb perfusion. Br J Surg 80:995–997, 1993.
37. Vaglini M, Belli F, Ammatuna M, et al. Treatment of primary or relapsing limb cancer by isolation perfusion with high-dose alpha-tumor necrosis factor, gamma-interferon and melphalan. Cancer 73:483–492, 1994.
38. Thom AK, Alexander HR, Andrich MP, Barker WC, Rosenberg SA, Fraker DL. Cytokine levels and systemic toxicity in patients undergoing isolated limb perfusion with high-dose tumor necrosis factor, interferon gamma, and melphalan. J Clin Oncol 13:264–273, 1995.
39. Swaak AJG, Liénard D, Schraffordt Koops H, Lejeune FJ, Eggermont AMM. Effects of recombinant tumour necrosis factor (rTNF-α) in cancer. Observations on the acute phase protein reaction and immunoglobulin synthesis after high dose recombinant TNF-α administration in isolated limb perfusions in cancer patients. Eur J Clin Invest 23:812–818, 1993.
40. Lejeune FJ, Liénard D, Eggermont AMM, et al. Clinical experience with high-dose tumor necrosis factor alpha in regional therapy of advanced melanoma. Circ Shock 43:191–197, 1994.
41. Posner M, Liénard D, Lejeune FJ, Rosenfelder D, Kirkwood JM. Hyperthermic isolated limb perfusion (HILP) with tumor necrosis factor (TNF) alone for metastatic intransit melanoma (abstr). Proc Am Soc Clin Oncol 13:1351, 1994.
42. Manusama ER, Nooijen PTGA, Stavast J, Durante NMC, Marquet RL, Eggermont AMM.

Synergistic antitumour effect of recombinant human tumour necrosis factor α with melphalan in isolated limb perfusion in the rat. Br J Surg 83:551–555, 1996.
43. Spriggs DR, Sherman ML, Michie H, et al. Recombinant human tumor necrosis factor administered as a 24 h intravenous infusion. A phase I and pharmacologic study. J Natl Cancer Inst 80:1039–1044, 1988.
44. Blick MB, Sherwin SA, Rosenblum M, et al. A phase I trial of recombinant human tumor necrosis factor in cancer patients. Cancer Res 47:2986–2989, 1987.
45. Chapman PB, Lester TJ, Casper ES, et al. Clinical pharmacology of recombinant human tumor necrosis factor in patients with advanced cancer. J Clin Oncol 5:1942–1951, 1987.
46. Feinberg B, Kurzrock R, Talpaz M, et al. A phase I trial of intravenously administered recombinant tumor necrosis factor alpha in cancer patients. J Clin Oncol 6:1328–1334, 1988.
47. Asher AL, Mule JJ, Reichert CM, Shilone E, Rosenberg SA. Studies of the antitumor efficacy of systemically administered recombinant tumor necrosis factor against several murine tumors in vivo. J Immunol 138:963–974, 1987.
48. Carswell EA, Old LJ, Kassel RL, et al. An endotoxin induced serum factor that causes necrosis of tumors. Proc Natl Acad Sci USA 72:3666–3370, 1975.
49. Sugarman BJ, Aggarwal BB, Hass PE, et al. Recombinant tumor necrosis factor-alpha: Effects on proliferation of normal and transformed cells in vitro. Science 230:943–945, 1985.
50. Renard N, Liénard D, Lespagnard L, Eggermont AMM, Heimann R, Lejeune FJ. Early endothelium activation and polymorphonuclear cell invasion precede specific necrosis of human melanoma and sarcoma treated by intravascular high-dose tumour necrosis factor alpha (TNFα). Int J Cancer 57:656–663, 1994.
51. Renard N, Nooijen PTGA, Schalkwijk L, et al. VWF release and platelet aggregation in human melanoma after perfusion with TNFα. J Pathol 176:279–287, 1995.
52. Watanabe N, Niitsu Y, Umeno H, et al. Toxic effect of TNF on tumor vasculature in mice. Cancer Res 49:2179–2183, 1988.
53. Sato N, Goto T, Haranaka K, et al. Actions of TNF on cultured vascular endothelial cells: Morphological modulation, growth inhibition and cytotoxicity. J Natl Cancer Inst 76:1113–1121, 1986.
54. Bloksma N, van de Wiel PA, Kuper CF, Hofhuis FMA. Multiple facets of induction of tumor necrosis. Ann Inst Pasteur/Immunol 139:294–299, 1988.
55. Nawroth P, Handley D, Matsueda G, et al. TNF/cachectin-induced intravascular fibrin formation in Meth-A fibrosarcomas. J Exp Med 168:637–647, 1988.
56. Manusama ER, Stavast J, Marquet RL, Eggermont AMM. Total body irradiation (TBI) attenuates antitumor effects of TNFα in isolated limb perfusions (ILP) in the rat (abstr). Eur J Surg Res 27(Suppl 1):110, 1995.
57. Prograbniak HW, Witt CJ, Terrill R, et al. Isolated lung perfusion with tumor necrosis factor: A swine model in preparation of human trials. Ann Thorac Surg 57:1477–1483, 1994.
58. Fraker DL, Alexander HR, Thom AK. Use of tumor necrosis factor in isolated hepatic perfusion. Circ Shock 44:45–50, 1994.
59. Vries de MR, Borel Rinkes IHM, Wiggers T, Jonker AM, Weijers-Hille MJ, Eggermont AMM. Hyperthermic isolated hepatic perfusion with TNFα with and without melphalan in pigs (abstr). Eur J Surg Res 27(Suppl 1):81, 1995.
60. Veen van de AH, Manusama ER, Kampen van CA, Durante NMC, Marquet RL, Eggermont AMM. Eur J Surg Oncol 20:404–405, 1994.

14. Soft tissue sarcomas in children

Alberto S. Pappo and Charles B. Pratt

Introduction

Soft tissue sarcomas of children and adolescents continue to present problems with pathologic diagnosis, staging, and treatment. In this chapter we review some of these difficulties and discuss recent clinical and laboratory findings associated with rhabdomyosarcoma and non-rhabdomyosarcomatous soft tissue sarcomas (NRSTS).

Rhabdomyosarcoma

Epidemiology and genetics

As reported by the Surveillance Epidemiology and End Results (SEER) section of the National Cancer Institute, the incidence of soft tissue sarcomas has remained remarkably constant over the last 13 years. In contrast, the incidence of other sarcomas, particularly Kaposi sarcoma, dramatically increased over the same period. The upsurge in Kaposi sarcoma is believed to be secondary to the AIDS epidemic [1].

In a study of international population- and hospital-based registries for the years 1970–1979, Stiller and Parkin found that pediatric soft tissue sarcomas accounted for 4–8% of all pediatric cancers [2]. Rhabdomyosarcoma, the most common sarcoma, comprised 60–70% of the cases, with an age-standardized annual incidence rate of 4–7 patients per million children. One third of the cases occurred between the ages of 5 and 9 years, and there was a slight male predominance overall.

Genetic predisposition and environmental factors may influence the development of pediatric soft tissue sarcomas. Hartley et al. [3] estimated the frequency of neoplastic disease in 151 families of children aged less than 15 years who had soft tissue sarcomas. Fifty families had histories consistent with a genetic predisposition for cancer, 15 of which had either a classic Li-Fraumeni syndrome or a pattern consistent with this syndrome. Diller et al. [4] screened 33 patients with rhabdomyosarcoma for mutations in the *p53* gene.

J. Verweij, H.M. Pinedo, and H.D. Suit (eds). SOFT TISSUE SARCOMAS: PRESENT ACHIEVEMENTS AND FUTURE PROSPECTS.

Heterozygous constitutional mutations in *p53* were detected in 3 of 13 children younger than 3 years. In contrast, none of the samples from the 20 children over the age of 3 years demonstrated these abnormalities. These findings suggest that the mutant *p53* carrier state contributes to the early development of malignancies. Grufferman et al. [5] conducted a case-controlled study of 351 children who were enrolled in the Intergroup Rhabdomyosarcoma Studies (IRS). Their findings suggested that parental use of recreational drugs increases the risk of rhabdomyosarcoma in their offspring.

Classification and prognosis

The conventional pathologic classification system proposed by Horn and Enterline correlates with survival in most cases of rhabdomyosarcoma but fails to independently predict outcome when matched for other prognostic factors, such as tumor site, age, and clinical group. To improve the classification of rhabdomyosarcoma, the IRS pathology committee conducted a comparative trial assessing the reproducibility and prognostic significance of four pathologic classification systems [6]. Sixteen internationally recognized pathologists reviewed 800 samples from patients with rhabdomyosarcoma who were enrolled in IRS-II. This panel of experts then devised a modified classification system that recognizes three major histologic subgroups of rhabdomyosarcoma: embryonal, alveolar, and undifferentiated tumors.

Among the samples presented to the panel, those of the botryoid and spindle cell variants of embryonal rhabdomyosarcoma were associated with an excellent survival. Other tumors with embryonal histology correlated with an intermediate prognosis, and patients with alveolar or undifferentiated tumors tended to fare poorly. In other studies, alveolar rhabdomyosarcomas, characterized by t(2;13)(q35;q14), frequently were found on the trunk of adolescents, who also tended to have disseminated disease, often involving the bone marrow, and poor responses to conventional therapy [7]. Alveolar rhabdomyosarcoma with t(1;13)(p36;q14) were rarer, often occurring in the extremities of younger patients [8].

The solid alveolar variant of rhabdomyosarcoma has recently been recognized. This variant lacks typical alveolar spaces and can be confused with embryonal rhabdomyosarcoma and extraosseous Ewing's sarcoma [9]. Characteristic of other alveolar rhabdomyosarcomas solid variant tumors are clinically aggressive and possess t(2;13)(q35;q14).

The rare pleomorphic subtype was excluded from the modified classification scheme. In a separate study, the IRS reviewed the clinocopathologic features of 110 pleomorphic (anaplastic) rhabdomyosarcomas [10], all of which microscopically demonstrated a clear transition between the anaplastic and alveolar or embryonal components. Although prominent anaplasia was associated with a poor outcome, the IRS concluded that the pleomorphic variant should no longer be considered to be a separate entity.

Similar to the association between histologic subtype and outcome, the

DNA content of rhabdomyosarcoma cells may have important prognostic significance. Among 34 children with inoperable embryonal rhabdomyosarcoma who were enrolled in IRS-III, hyperdiploidy conferred an excellent clinical outcome, and patients with diploid tumors fared poorly. The estimated 5-year progression-free survival rates were 91% versus 17%, respectively [11]. Other European studies have confirmed the association between DNA content and outcome [12,13]. These observations suggest that ploidy should be prospectively evaluated to ascertain its prognostic merit and to assess its inclusion in the pretreatment evaluation and risk stratification of children with rhabdomyosarcoma.

Molecular pathology, pathogenesis, and diagnosis

Rhabdomyosarcoma and fetal skeletal muscle share patterns of muscle-specific gene expression, including the MyoD family of genes [14,15]. These genes orchestrate the genetic events leading to the transcription of DNA sequences that encode muscle-specific genes [14–16]. Paradoxically, rhabdomyosarcoma cells cannot differentiate into myotubes, suggesting that rhabdomyoblasts may be deficient in a factor responsible for proper MyoD function or may contain an inhibitor of its function [17].

Altered expression of the retinoblastoma gene (*Rb*) has been documented in adult sarcomas; however, this gene was functionally and structurally normal in samples form 11 rhabdomyosarcoma cell lines and 18 primary tumors. These findings suggest that abnormalities in *Rb* or its product do not significantly contribute to the pathogenesis of pediatric rhabdomyosarcoma [18].

Embryonal rhabdomyosarcomas lack tumor-specific translocations but show consistent loss of heterozygosity at chromosome 11p15.5, suggesting that loss of a tumor-suppressor gene may play a role in their pathogenesis [19]. In contrast, alveolar rhabdomyosarcomas are characterized by t(2;13)(q35;q14) and, less commonly, t(1;13)(p36;q14) [7,8,19,20]. The t(2;13) results in the fusion of the *PAX3* gene, a presumed transcription factor expressed during early embryogenesis that is located on chromosome 2 band q35 with *FKHR*, a novel member of the forkhead family of transcription factors located on chromosome 13 at band q14 [20,21]. In the t(1;13), the intact binding domain of *PAX7*, located on chromosome 1p36, is fused to a truncated *FKHR* gene on chromosome 13 [8].

Although the precise contributions of PAX3-FKHR and PAX7-FKHR to tumorigenesis are unclear, these chimeric molecules may regulate a common set of genes that are primarily involved in the pathogenesis of alveolar rhabdomyosarcoma. Fredericks et al. proposed that the PAX3-FKHR fusion protein is an aberrant transcription factor that regulates PAX3 targets [22]. Epstein et al. have recently shown that PAX3 may inhibit terminal differentiation of limb myoblasts and that the PAX3-FKHR transcript is a more potent inhibitor of myogenic differentiation [23].

The identification of PAX3-FKHR and PAX7-FKHR fusion products has led to the development of several diagnostic assays. Downing et al. [24] have developed an enzyme-linked immunosorbent assay–based reverse transcriptase polymerase chain reaction (RT-PCR) assay in which samples may be tested simultaneously for Ewing's sarcoma (EWS-FLI1 transcript) and alveolar rhabdomyosarcoma (*PAX3-FKHR* transcript). In addition, fluorescence in situ hybridization (FISH) has also been used to identify the t(2;13) in interphase or metaphase nuclei [25]. These sensitive techniques contribute to the rapid and accurate diagnosis of alveolar rhabdomyosarcoma in samples from primary and metastatic sites (i.e., bone marrow) and are useful in monitoring occult residual disease.

Monoclonal antibodies that recognize muscle-associated proteins are helpful when diagnosing soft tissue sarcomas. For example, monoclonal antibodies to MyoD that are suitable for use with fresh-frozen and paraffin-embedded tissue should facilitate the differential diagnosis of small round cell tumors of childhood [9]. In addition, a monoclonal antibody to human dystrophin reacted against 8 of 9 samples of rhabdomyosarcoma but failed to recognize any of those from 14 other tumors. These findings illustrate the potential usefulness of antidystrophin in diagnosing rhabdomyosarcoma [26].

Clinical studies

Orbital rhabdomyosarcoma. Rousseau reported the results of 31 children with nonmetastatic orbital rhabdomyosarcomas who were enrolled in the Malignant Mesenchymal Study 84 (MMT 84) [27]. This protocol used a primary chemotherapy approach with vincristine, actinomycin, and ifosfamide ± cisplatin and doxorubicin. Radiotherapy was reserved for patients who failed to achieve a complete response after chemotherapy. The 4-year event-free survival and overall survival were 62% and 86%, respectively. Local recurrences arose in 11 patients, 10 of whom were not irradiated. Six patients were subsequently salvaged with irradiation, chemotherapy, and/or surgery. Radiation was avoided in 12 patients.

Neonatal soft tissue sarcomas. The mean age at presentation was 19 days for 14 neonates with rhabdomyosarcoma enrolled in the Intergroup Rhabdomyosarcoma Studies I–IV [28]. Male sex (1.8:1), embryonal histology (64%), and unresectable tumors (50%) predominated. Half of the tumors were located caudally (in the sacrococcygeal region, buttock, perirectal area, bladder, or vagina). Overall survival at 3 years was 49%. Patients with caudal tumors fared better than those with tumors in noncaudal sites (89% vs. 14%).

Dillon et al. [29] described 32 neonates with soft tissue sarcomas who were seen at 11 Children's Cancer Group (CCG) institutions over a 22-year period. Congenital fibrosarcoma was the most common tumor (n = 12), followed by rhabdomyosarcoma (n = 11) and other nonrhabdomyosarcoma soft tissue sarcomas (n = 9). At the time of the report, all patients with fibrosarcoma were alive. In contrast, only two children diagnosed with rhabdomyosarcoma and five with nonrhabdomyosarcomatous lesions were free of disease. These findings suggest that pathology, extent of disease, and resectability are important predictors of outcome in neonates with soft tissue sarcomas.

Pelvic rhabdomyosarcoma. Twenty-seven children with vaginal (n = 24) or vulvar (n = 3) rhabdomyosarcoma were treated in IRS-III [30]. The children with vulvar primary tumors presented with clinical group I (n = 2) or II disease (n = 1). These patients remain disease-free after treatment with vincristine, actinomycin ± cisplatin, doxorubicin, cyclophosphamide ± radiotherapy.

Twenty of 24 vaginal tumors treated in IRS-III were unresectable. Chemotherapy for this subgroup consisted of vincristine, actinomycin, cyclophosphamide, doxorubicin, and cisplatin. Second-look surgery, as mandated by the protocol, was performed at week 20 in 16 patients. Definitive surgical procedures were performed in seven patients, six of whom showed no histologic evidence of viable tumor. At 66–107 months after diagnosis, 17 of the 20 patients with unresectable vaginal tumors were alive and disease-free [31].

At 1.5–6 years after diagnosis, 9 of 14 children with uterine rhabdomyosarcoma treated in the IRS-III and -IV pilot protocols were free of tumor [131]. Four patients died of sepsis or chemotherapy-related toxicity, and only one developed tumor progression.

Using data from 292 children who were enrolled in the IRS I–III studies, Hays reviewed the advances in the clinical management of bladder/prostate rhabdomyosarcoma [32]. The percentage of patients with intact functional bladders at 3 years was 22% for IRS-I, 25% for IRS-II, and 60% for IRS-III. The marked improvement of bladder preservation rates in IRS-III was attributed to the fixed timing of radiotherapy (at week 6) and the addition of doxorubicin and cisplatin to standard vincristine, actinomycin, cyclophosphamide (VAC) chemotherapy.

Partial cystectomy was performed in 40 patients with rhabdomyosarcoma of the bladder and/or prostate during the course of the three IRS studies. The overall survival rate for these patients was 80%. Among the 32 survivors, one has required a secondary cystectomy, whereas 75% of the remaining cases had no bladder-related symptoms or demonstrable functional difficulties. In addition, prostatectomy without cystectomy was performed in 15 patients, 6 of whom have relapsed.

Paratesticular. In IRS-III, 121 patients with nonmetastatic paratesticular rhabdomyosarcoma underwent pathologic and clinical evaluation of their retroperitoneal lymph nodes [33]. Conflicting data were obtained on 14 of the 110 patients who were evaluated by both methods. Computed tomography scans yielded false-negative results in 13 cases and false-positive findings in 1 case. Retroperitoneal node relapse was rare, occurring in only two patients. The overall probability of survival at 5 years was 91% for the entire group. Patients with clinically negative nodes fared better than those with clinically positive nodes (5-year survivals, 96% and 69%, respectively, $p < 0.001$). Children younger than 10 years of age had a significantly better 5-year survival (97%) than did patients 10 years of age or older (85%, $p = 0.003$). Because retroperitoneal node dissection or biopsy of clinically negative nodes is not routinely recommended, patients in IRS-IV are being monitored closely for evidence of retroperitoneal involvement.

In another study, the IRS examined the clinicopathologic characteristics of children with the spindle cell variant of paratesticular rhabdomyosarcoma and found that these patients often have localized disease, a low incidence of nodal metastases, and an excellent outcome [34].

Second-look biopsies. The authors of the MMT 84 study assessed the predictive value of second-look biopsies after three or six courses of chemotherapy in children with nonmetastatic soft tissue sarcomas [35]. Despite negative biopsy specimens in 51 of 52 patients with rhabdomyosarcoma, 27 children (51%) had local recurrence of their tumor. The local failure rate for nonbiopsied patients was similar (48%). The outcome for children with recurrent disease was poor regardless of the biopsy results, suggesting that this procedure has limited prognostic and therapeutic value.

Radiotherapy. Investigators at St. Jude Children's Hospital used low-dose irradiation (40 Gy) to treat residual microscopic tumor following chemotherapy in 28 clinical group III patients with rhabdomyosarcoma. The local control rate (78%) was similar to that achieved in clinical group II patients. This result suggests that patients with microscopic residual tumor after induction chemotherapy and/or surgery for unresectable disease may safely be treated with lower radiation doses [36].

Local tumor control rates in the German CWS-86 trial improved dramatically for patients with rhabdomyosarcoma who had macroscopic tumor at the time of initiation of radiotherapy when compared with the results obtained in the previous CWS-81 study (95% vs. 30%, $p < 0.001$). In addition, the total dose required to control disease in children with clinical remission was reduced to from 44.4 Gy to 34.4 Gy. These encouraging results were attributed to earlier preoperative hyperfractionated radiotherapy (week 7–10 vs. 16–20) that was concomitantly administered with chemotherapy [37].

An IRS pilot study investigated the feasibility and toxicity of hyperfractionated radiotherapy (1.1 Gy fractions bid, total dose of 59.4 Gy) in 284 evaluable children with clinical group III and IV rhabdomyosarcoma. Severe or life-threatening toxicity (mostly hematopoietic), attributed to the combined chemotherapy and radiotherapy, was seen in 75% of group III and 65% of group IV cases. Toxicity was greatest for patients with parameningeal and genitourinary/pelvis primary tumors, and occurred mostly at the end of radiation therapy. Hyperfractionated radiotherapy proved to be feasible in these group of patients and led to toxicity similar to that seen in IRS-III with conventional radiation. The current IRS-IV study will prospectively compare conventional versus hyperfractionated radiotherapy in patients with inoperable or metastatic tumors [38].

Clinical trials

Outcome data were recently reported for IRS-II (1978–1984) and IRS-III (1984–1991), which accrued 999 and 1062 eligible patients, respectively [39,40]. Distributions by clinical groups I–IV were 13%, 17%, 53%, and 17% for IRS-II and 20%, 19%, 47%, and 14% for IRS-III. For both studies primary tumors were most commonly located in the head-and-neck region (including orbit and parameningeal), followed by genitourinary and extremity sites. Embryonal tumors predominated (about 50%), and alveolar histology was seen in approximately 20% of cases. In IRS-II, treatment was assigned according to clinical group and tumor site. In IRS-III, patients were stratified into eight different treatment subgroups according to clinical group, primary site, and histologic subtype (Table 1). The relevant treatment comparison groups of IRS-II and IRS-III, as well as the outcome of specific patient subgroups, is depicted in Table 1.

The International Society of Pediatric Oncology (SIOP) MMT89 study accrued 362 nonmetastatic rhabdomyosarcoma patients and evaluated therapy stratified according to primary tumor site and stage [41]. Chemotherapy for completely resected stage I patients consisted of vincristine and actinomycin. Ifosfamide was added to vincristine and actinomycin for the remaining patients, who received up to six courses of chemotherapy. All patients older than 3 years who had primary parameningeal tumors received adjuvant radiotherapy. Radiation was given to other patients based on the response of their tumors to chemotherapy. At 3 years, the overall survival and event-free survival were 78% and 62%, respectively. Local relapse remained the most frequent adverse event, occurring in 28% of patients with incompletely excised tumors.

In MMT 89, 75 children with metastatic soft tissue sarcomas were treated over a 3-year period. Fifty of these patients had rhabdomyosarcoma and received multiagent chemotherapy comprised of carboplatin, epirubicin, vincristine, ifosfamide, etoposide, and actinomycin. The estimated 4-year overall survival was 20%. Multivariate analysis revealed that extent of tumor and metastases to bone and bone marrow significantly influenced outcome. None of the children with all three risk features survived, whereas 60% of those who had none of these indicators were free of tumor at the time of the report [42].

A complete response rate of 50% was documented in 164 patients with metastatic rhabdomyosarcoma who were enrolled in four different European studies from 1975 through 1988. The probabilities of overall and disease-free survival were 18 and 15%, respectively. Excluding those lesions of the bladder and prostate, patients with genitourinary tumors had the most favorable outcome [43].

Table 1. Therapy and outcome according to specific patient subgroups in IRS-II and IRS-III

	IRS-II		IRS-III		
Risk subgroup	Treatment	5-yr survival (%)	Treatment	5-yr survival (%)	Comments
Group I (favorable histology)	VA × 1 yr VAC × 2 yr	84 85	VA × 1 yr	93	Alkylating agents and anthracyclines can be safely deleted without compromising outcome.
Group II (favorable histology)	VA + RT × 1 yr VAC + RT × 1 yr	88 79	VA + RT × 1 yr VAAdr + RT × 1 yr	54 89	Based on IRS-III results, the role of doxorubicin in this group of patients needs to be further clarified.
Groups I and II (unfavorable histology)	VA ± C ± RT × 1–2 yr	71	VAdrC-VA + CDDP + RT × 1 yr	80	Intensified therapy improved outcome in IRS-III when compared with IRS-II.
Group II (paratesticular)	VA + RT × 1 yr VAC + RT × 1 yr	 81	VA + RT × 1 yr	81	Reduced therapy with VA is safe and effective for this group of patients; thus alkylators can be safely deleted.
Groups II and III (orbit and head)	VA ± C ± Adr + RT × 1–2 yr	91	VA + RT × 1 yr	91	VA in IRS-III yielded equivalent results to VA in IRS-II; thus cyclophosphamide can be deleted from this regimen.

Group III (special pelvic sites)	VAC ± RT ± S × 2 yr	72	VAdrC-VA + CDDP ± A + VP16 ± RT ± × 2 yr	83	Intensive therapy, introduction of early radiotherapy, and second-look operations contributed to improved outcome when compared with IRS-II.
Group III (excluding special pelvic sites and other selected sites)	VAC + RT × 2 yr		VA + RT × 2 yr	70	Overall outcome for group III patients was significantly better in IRS-III than in IRS-II (5-year survival 65% vs. 59% p = 0.03).
	VAdrC-VAC	59	VAdrC-VA + CDDP + RT × 2yr	63	
			VAdrC-VA + CDDP + VP16 + RT × 2 yr	64	
Group IV	VAC + RT × 2 yr	24	VA + RT × 2 yr	27	No significant differences between studies or among regimens have been noted since the inception of I RS-I.
	VadrC-VAC + RT × 2 yr	26	VAdrC-VA + CDDP + RT × 2 yr	31	
			VAdrC-VA + CDDP + VP16 + RT × 2 yr	29	
Overall results		63		71	

V = vincristine; A = dactinomycin; C = cyclophosphamide; Adr = Adriamycin; VP = etoposide; CDDP = cisplatin; RT = radiotherapy; S = surgery.

Patients who present with advanced-stage rhabdomyosarcoma or develop recurrent disease continue to have a poor prognosis, and this situation has prompted the development of novel therapeutic strategies. Marrow ablation and subsequent autologous transplantation has been evaluated as treatment for rhabdomyosarcoma. Other approaches rely on the innovative application of modalities known to be active against rhabdomyosarcoma, and include dose intensification and the introduction of new treatment schedules or combinations of agents. In addition, analogues of effective drugs and novel agents identified in xenograft systems may expand the repertoire of drugs used to treat childhood rhabdomyosarcoma.

Autologous bone marrow transplantation for the treatment of childhood rhabdomyosarcoma has not dramatically improved response or survival. Horowitz et al. used total-body irradiation and autologous bone marrow support as consolidation treatment in 25 children with high-risk rhabdomyosarcoma [44]. In their experience, this strategy failed to significantly improve outcome, with a 6-year survival of 30%. Philip recently summarized the results from the European Bone Marrow Transplant Registry of 179 rhabdomyosarcoma patients who received autografts [45]. The 5-year survival rates ranged from 17% to 28%. Outcome was dependent on the clinical status of the patient at the time of transplantation. Dumontet et al. transplanted 22 patients with advanced soft tissue sarcomas (including 11 rhabdomyosarcomas) using melphalan-, ifosfamide-, or cyclophosphamide-containing regimens with a response rate of 66%. Survival for the entire group at 5 years was only 32% [46]. Using a regimen of escalating doses of carboplatin (1800–2100 mg/m^2) and etoposide (1200–1500 mg/m^2) followed by autologous bone marrow transplantation, Santana et al. [47] treated 30 children with relapsed pediatric solid tumors (including three sarcomas). Responses were seen in 44% of patients, primarily among those with neuroblastoma and Hodgkin's disease.

In a phase II 'up-front window study,' investigators at St. Jude Children's Research Hospital documented the significant clinical activity of ifosfamide (86% PR rate) in 22 previously untreated patients with advanced-stage rhabdomyosarcoma [48]. The activity of this agent in combination with etoposide and actinomycin is currently being tested and compared with cyclophosphamide in the IRS-IV study.

The CCG conducted a phase II trial of carboplatin (560 mg/m^2) for relapsed solid tumors. Thrombocytopenia and neutropenia were the most commonly noted toxicities. Ototoxicity, electrolyte abnormalities, nephrotoxicity, and nausea and vomiting were infrequent. Only 7% of patients with soft tissue sarcomas had a clinical response [49].

Phillips et al. treated 23 patients who had relapsed soft tissue sarcomas with a rapid schedule of intravenous etoposide (100 mg/m^2 daily for 3 days weekly over 3 weeks) and observed a response rate of 42% among 19 children with rhabdomyosarcoma. Grade 3–4 neutropenia and thrombocytopenia were observed in 38% and 10% of the courses, respectively [50]. These results are especially encouraging in light of the fact that the single-agent activity of etoposide in a previous CCG study was only 16% [51].

The combination of ifosfamide, carboplatin, and etoposide (ICE) has been used by investigators at St. Jude Children's Research Hospital [52], the Pediatric Oncology Group (POG) [53], and the CCG [54] to treat patients with recurrent solid tumors. Encouraging responses (overall CR + PR = 46%) have been noted in patients with sarcomas (45%), Wilms' tumor (67%), neuroblastoma (44%), and non-Hodgkin's lymphoma (80%) [54]. Dose intensification of ifosfamide has recently become possible with the use of granulocyte-macrophage–colony-stimulating factor (GM-CSF) [55]. Amelioration of myelosupression has also been reported following GM-CSF and PIXY 321 administration [56,57].

Preclinical studies of the camptothecin analogue CPT-11 in the xenograft model demonstrate complete tumor regression without evidence of tumor regrowth in 5 of 6 rhabdomyosarcoma lines [58]. Further, CPT-11 retained significant activity against sublines selected for resistance to vincristine, melphalan, and topotecan. In a similar experiment, the highest dose level of the bis-naphtalimide antitumor agent, DMP-840, led to complete regression of 5 of 6 rhabdomyosarcoma xenografts [59].

Complications of therapy

In a pilot study of 194 children with group III rhabdomyosarcoma, the introduction of ifosfamide was associated with renal tubular dysfunction in 14% of cases [60]. Preexisting renal abnormalities, age younger than 3 years, and doses $>72\,g/m^2$ significantly increased the risk of renal dysfunction. In another series [61], ifosfamide nephrotoxicity was dose dependent and increased after nephrectomy or administration of cisplatin. Ashraf et al. found evidence of renal dysfunction in 19 of 20 patients with sarcomas who received ifosfamide who were comprehensively studied [62].

Preliminary analysis of data from the IRS-III revealed 5 cases of secondary acute myelogenous leukemia (AML) among 1062 eligible patients [63]. Patients who received cyclophosphamide and epipodophylotoxins had a sevenfold greater risk of developing this complication compared with patients who received cyclophosphamide alone.

Of 109 children with bladder and prostate rhabdomyosarcoma who were treated in IRS studies I and II, 54 retained their bladders. Normal bladder function was reported in 73% of these patients. The most common complications included urinary incontinence, urinary frequency, and nocturia. Significant growth abnormalities were present in 10% of patients [64].

Eighteen children with paratesticular rhabdomyosarcoma were treated with chemotherapy ± surgery at St. Jude Children's Research Hospital. Two patients died of postoperative or therapy-related complications, and five had long-term nonfatal complications (including hypogonadism, inguinal neuralgia, lymphedema, and bile duct obstruction). Compared with their pretreatment measures, 13 children were in a lower percentile of height-for-age and/or had decreased height standard deviation scores [65].

In IRS-IV, seven patients with rhabdomyosarcoma who received multiagent chemotherapy, including high-dose cyclophosphamide, developed venoocclusive disease of the liver. Six of the seven recovered and two continued to receive cyclophosphamide without recurrence of this complication [66].

Nonrhabdomyosarcomatous soft tissue sarcomas (NRSTS)

NRSTS are a rare and heterogenous group of tumors that account for 3% of childhood malignancies. The natural history and response to therapy of these tumors has been well studied in adults. However, the frequency and clinical behavior of NRSTS in the pediatric population remains largely unknown.

Pathology

Histologic grading has a profound effect on clinical outcome in adults with soft tissue sarcomas. In 1986, the POG conducted a prospective study in which children with grossly resected NRSTS (clinical groups I and II) were randomized to no further therapy ± radiation or adjuvant chemotherapy (with vincristine, actinomycin, doxorubicin, and cyclophosphamide) ± radiation [67]. Tumors were graded according to a modified classification scheme that was based on percent of tumor necrosis, histologic subtype, and mitotic count (Table 2). At 3 years, 92% of patients with grade 1–2 lesions were disease-free, compared with 75% of those with grade 3 lesions ($p = 0.018$). Nine of 11 relapses occurred in the lung. These findings confirm that tumor grade has prognostic significance in clinical group I and II pediatric NRSTS, and this feature may help refine risk-directed therapy [67–69].

In a similar report, McCoy et al. reported their experience with 35 patients with NRSTS. The most common histologies were synovial sarcoma, desmoid tumors, and liposarcoma. Histologic grade and tumor size influenced disease-free survival [70].

Synovial sarcoma was the predominant histologic type among 28 patients younger than 16 years of age with NRSTS seen at the Royal Marsden Hospital. Younger patients fared better than their adult counterparts (82% 5-year survival vs. 63%, $p < 0.05$), but the patterns of local and distant recurrence were not significantly different [71]. Another recent report described the clinical features and outcome of 37 children with synovial sarcoma who were treated at St. Jude Children's Research Hospital over a 30-year period. Clinical group (I and II vs. III and IV), tumor invasiveness (T1 vs. T2), and histologic grade (grade 2 vs. 3) independently predicted clinical outcome [72].

Synovial sarcoma, neurogenic tumors, and malignant fibrous histiocytoma

Table 2. Pediatric Oncology Group NRSTS grading system

Grade 1 lesions
Myxoid and well-differentiated liposarcoma
Deep-seated dermatofibrosarcoma protuberans
Well-differentiated or infantile hemangiopericytoma (≤4 years old)
Well-differentiated or infantile fibrosarcoma (≤4 years old)
Well-differentiated malignant peripheral nerve sheath tumor
Extraskeletal myxoid chondrosarcoma
Angiomatoid malignant fibrous histiocytoma
Grade 2 lesions
Soft tissue sarcomas not included in grades I and III, and in which there is <15% necrosis and the mitotic count is <5/10 high-powered fields
Tumor not markedly cellular and nuclear atypia not marked
Grade 3 lesions
Pleomorphic or round cell liposarcoma
Mesenchymal chondrosarcoma
Extraskeletal osteosarcoma
Triton tumor
Alveolar soft part sarcoma
Any other sarcoma with >15% necrosis or >5 mitosis/10 high-powered fields using a 40× objective

Data from Parham et al. [67].

Table 3. Chromosomal abnormalities of selected solid tumors and their corresponding genes

Histology	Chromosomal abnormality	Fusion transcript
Synovial sarcoma	t(X;18)(p11.2;q11.2)	*STY-SSX*
Clear cell sarcoma	t(12;22)(q13–14;q12–13)	*ATF1-EWS*
Myxoid liposarcoma	t(12;16)(q13;p11)	*FUS-CHOP*
Peripheral neuroepithelioma	t(11;22)(q21–24;q11–13)	*FLI1-EWS*
	t(21;22)(q22;q12)	*ERG-EWS*
Desmoplastic small cell tumor	t(11;22)(p13;q11.2–21)	*WT1-EWS*

Data from Sreekantaiah et al. [75], Rabbits [76], and Shipley et al. [77].

were the most common histologies among 154 children treated for NRSTS at St. Jude Hospital. In over two thirds of cases, tumors arose in the trunk and lower extremities. Prognostic factors included tumor size, invasiveness, histologic grade, and clinical group [73]. These findings suggest that these pretreatment features can help identify patients who have an increased risk of treatment failure and should be addressed in the planning and design of future trials.

LaQuaglia reviewed the clinical outcome of 18 pediatric patients with liposarcoma who were treated at the Memorial Sloan-Kettering Cancer Center [74]. The myxoid histologic subtype predominated (13 cases), and only one tumor was categorized as high grade. All but 1 of 11 patients who had complete surgical resection are alive; in contrast, all four patients with gross residual tumor died of disease progression.

Many NRSTS have nonrandom chromosomal translocations that result in the fusion of disparate genes, thereby creating a chimeric fusion transcript. These transcripts can be detected by polymerase chain reaction–based assays and/or FISH, which enable improved diagnosis of these rare neoplasms. Table 3 shows chromosomal abnormalities in selected pediatric neoplasms [75–77].

Acknowledgments

This research was supported in part by grants CA 21765 and CA 23099 from The National Cancer Institute and by the American Lebanese Syrian Associated Charities (ALSAC). We wish to thank Amy Frazier for editorial assistance.

References

1. Ross JA, Severson RK, Davis S, et al. Trends in the incidence of soft tissue sarcomas in the United States from 1973 through 1987. Cancer 72:486–490, 1993.
2. Stiller CA, Parkin DM. International variations in the incidence of childhood soft tissue sarcomas. Paediatr Perinat Epidemiol 8:107–119, 1994.
3. Hartley AL, Birch JM, Blair V, et al. Patterns of cancer in the families of children with soft tissue sarcoma. Cancer 72:923–930, 1993.
4. Diller L, Sexsmith E, Gottlieb A, et al. Germline p53 mutations are frequently detected in young children with rhabdomyosarcoma. J Clin Invest 95:1606–1611, 1995.
5. Grufferman S, Schwartz AG, Ruymann FB, et al. Parent's use of cocaine and marijuana and increased risk of rhabdomyosarcoma in their children. Cancer Causes Control 4:217–224, 1993.
6. Asmar L, Geham EA, Newton WA, et al. Agreement among and within groups of pathologists in the classification of rhabdomyosarcoma and related childhood sarcomas. Report of an international study of four pathology classifications. Cancer 74:2579–2588, 1994.
7. Douglass EC, Shapiro DN, Valentine M, et al. Alveolar rhabdomyosarcoma with the t(2;13): Cytogenetic findings and clinicopathologic correlations. Med Pediatr Oncol 21:83–87, 1993.
8. Davis RJ, D'Cruz CM, Lovell MA, et al. Fusion of PAX7 to FKHR by the variant t(1;13)(p36;q14) translocation in alveolar rhabdomyosarcoma. Cancer Res 54:2869–2872, 1994.
9. Tsokos M. The diagnosis and classification of childhood rhabdomyosarcoma. Semin Diag Pathol 11:26–38, 1994.
10. Kodet R, Newton WA Jr., Hamoudi AB, et al. Childhood rhabdomyosarcoma with anaplastic (pleomorphic) features. A report of the Intergroup Rhabdomyosarcoma Study. Am J Surg Pathol 17:443–453, 1993.
11. Pappo AS, Crist WM, Kuttesch J, et al. Tumor-cell DNA content predicts outcome in children and adolescents with clinical group III embryonal rhabdomyosarcoma. The Intergroup Rhabdomyosarcoma Study Committee of the Children's Cancer Group and the Pediatric Oncology Group. J Clin Oncol 11:1901–1905, 1993.
12. Niggli FK, Powell JE, Parkes SE, et al. DNA ploidy and proliferative activity (S-phase) in childhood soft-tissue sarcomas: Their value as prognostic indicators. Br J Cancer 69:1106–1110, 1994.
13. Mathieu MC, Niggli F, Viehl P. Prognostic value of flow cytometric DNA ploidy in childhood rhabdomyosarcomas enrolled in SIOP-MMT89 Study. Med Pediatr Oncol 23:223, 1994.

14. Weintraub H. The MyoD family and myogenesis: Redundancy, networks, and thresholds. Cell 75:1241–1244, 1993.
15. Parham DM. The molecular biology of childhood rhabdomyosarcoma. Semin Diagn Pathol 11:39–46, 1994.
16. Buckingham M. Molecular biology of muscle development. Cell 78:15–21, 1994.
17. Tapscott SJ, Thayer MJ, Weintraub H. Deficiency in rhabdomyosarcomas of a factor required for MyoD activity and myogenesis. Science 259:1450–1453, 1993.
18. De Chiara A, T'Ang A, Triche TJ. Expression of the retinoblastoma susceptibility gene in childhood rhabdomyosarcomas. J Natl Cancer Inst 85:152–157, 1993.
19. Scrable HJ, Witte DP, Shimada H. Molecular differential pathology of rhabdomyosarcoma. Genes Chromosom Cancer 1:23–35, 1989.
20. Shapiro DN, Sublett JE, Li B, et al. Fusion of PAX3 to a member of the forkhead family of transcription factors in human alveolar rhabdomyosarcoma. Cancer Res 53:5108–5112, 1993.
21. Barr FG, Galili N, Holick J, et al. Rearrangement of the PAX3 paired box gene in the paediatric solid tumour alveolar rhabdomyosarcoma. Nat Genet 3:113–117, 1993.
22. Fredericks WJ, Galili N, Mukhopadhyay S, et al. The PAX3-FKHR fusion protein created by the t(2;13) translocation in alveolar rhabdomyosarcoma is a more potent transcriptional activator than PAX3. Mol Cell Biol 15:1522–1535, 1995.
23. Epstein JA, Lam P, Jepeal L, et al. PAX3 inhibits myogenic differentiation of cultured myoblast cells. J Biol Chem 270:11719–11722, 1995.
24. Downing JR, Khandekar A, Shurtleff SA, et al. Multiplex RT-PCR assay for the differential diagnosis of alveolar rhabdomyosarcoma and Ewing's sarcoma. Am J Pathol 146:626–634, 1995.
25. Biegel JA, Nycum LM, Valentine V, et al. Detection of the t(2;13)(q35;q14) and PAX3-FKHR fusion in alveolar rhabdomyosarcoma by fluorescence in situ hybridization. Genes Chromosomes Cancer 12:186–192, 1995.
26. Pinto A, Paslawski D, Sarnat HB, et al. Immunohistochemical evaluation of dystrophin expression in small round cell tumors of childhood. Mod Pathol 6:679–683, 1993.
27. Rousseau P, Flamant F, Quintana E, et al. Primary chemotherapy in rhabdomyosarcomas and other malignant mesenchymal tumors of the orbit: Results of the International Society of Pediatric Oncology MMT 84 study. J Clin Oncol 12:516–521, 1994.
28. Lobe TE, Wiener ES, Hays DM, et al. Neonatal rhabdomyosarcoma: The IRS experience. J Pediatr Surg 29:1167–1170, 1994.
29. Dillon PW, Whalen TV, Azizkhan RG, et al. Neonatal soft tissue sarcomas: The influence of pathology on treatment and survival. Children's Cancer Group Surgical Committee J Pediatr Surg 30:1038–1041, 1995.
30. Andrassy RJ, Hays DM, Raney RB, et al. Conservative surgical management of vaginal and vulvar pediatric rhabdomyosarcoma: A report from the Intergroup Rhabdomyosarcoma Study III. J Pediatr Surg 30:1034–1037, 1995.
31. Corpron CA, Andrassy RJ, Hays DM, et al. Conservative management of uterine pediatric rhabdomyosarcoma: A report from the Intergroup Rhabdomyosarcoma Study III and IV pilot. J Pediatr Surg 30:942–944, 1995.
32. Hays DM. Bladder/prostate rhabdomyosarcoma: Results of the multi-institutional trials of the Intergroup Rhabdomyosarcoma Study. Semin Surg Oncol 9:520–523, 1993.
33. Wiener ES, Lawrence W, Hays D, et al. Retroperitoneal node biopsy in paratesticular rhabdomyosarcoma. J Pediatr Surg 29:171–177, 1994.
34. Leuschner I, Newton WA Jr., Schmidt D, et al. Spindle cell variants of embryonal rhabdomyosarcoma in the paratesticular region. A report of the Intergroup Rhabdomyosarcoma Study. Am J Surg Pathol 17:221–230, 1993.
35. Godzinski J, Flamant F, Rey A, et al. Value of postchemotherapy bioptical verification of complete clinical remission in previously incompletely resected (Stage I and II pT3) malignant mesenchymal tumors in children: International Society of Pediatric Oncology 1984 Malignant Mesenchymal Tumors Study. Med Pediatr Oncol 22:22–26, 1994.

36. Regine WF, Fontanesi J, Kumar P, et al. Local tumor control in rhabdomyosarcoma following low-dose irradiation: Comparison of group II and select group III patients. Int J Radiat Oncol Biol Phys 31:485–491, 1995.
37. Koscielniak E, Treuner J. Improvement of local tumor control in primary nonresectable rhabdomyosarcoma (RMS) in children by early, preoperative, hyperfractionated radiotherapy (RT) given simultaneous to chemotherapy (CT): Report of the German Cooperative Soft Tissue Sarcoma Studies CWS-81 and 86. Proc Am Soc Clin Oncol 13:415 (abstr 1416), 1994.
38. Donaldson SS, Asmar L, Breneman J, et al. Hyperfractionated radiation in children with rhabdomyosarcoma — Results of an Intergroup Rhabdomyosarcoma pilot study. Int J Radiat Oncol Biol Phys 32:903–911, 1995.
39. Maurer HM, Gehan EA, Beltangady M, et al. The Intergroup Rhabdomyosarcoma Study — II. Cancer 71:1904–1922, 1993.
40. Crist W, Gehan EA, Ragab AH, et al. The Intergroup Rhabdomyosarcoma Study. J Clin Oncol 13:610–630, 1995.
41. Stevens MCG, Oberlin O, Rey A, et al. Nonmetastatic rhabdomyosarcoma: Experience from the SIOP MMT89 study. Med Pediatr Oncol 23:171 (abstr 0–6), 1994.
42. Carli M, Pinkerton P, Frascella E, et al. Risk group analysis in metastatic soft tissue sarcomas (STS) in children. European Intergroup Study MMT89. Proc Am Soc Clin Oncol 14:449 (abstr 1438), 1995.
43. Koscielniak E, Rodary C, Flamant F, et al. Metastatic rhabdomyosarcoma and histologically similar tumors in childhood: A retrospective European multi-center analysis. Med Pediatr Oncol 20:209–214, 1992.
44. Horowitz ME, Kinsella TJ, Wexler LH, et al. Total-body irradiation and autologous bone marrow transplant in the treatment of high-risk Ewing's sarcoma and rhabdomyosarcoma. J Clin Oncol 11:1911–1918, 1993.
45. Philip T. High dose therapy and ABMT rescue in lymphoma and solid tumours. Eur J Cancer 31A:808–809, 1995.
46. Dumontet C, Biron P, Bouffet E, et al. High dose chemotherapy with ABMT in soft tissue sarcomas: A report of 22 cases. Bone Marrow Transplant 10:405–408, 1992.
47. Santana VM, Schell MJ, Williams R, et al. Escalating sequential high-dose carboplatin and etoposide with autologous marrow support in children with relapsed solid tumors. Bone Marrow Transplant 10:457–462, 1992.
48. Pappo AS, Etcubanas E, Santana VM, et al. A phase II trial of ifosfamide in previously untreated children and adolescents with unresectable rhabdomyosarcoma. Cancer 71:2119–2125, 1993.
49. Ettinger LJ, Gaynon PS, Krailo MD, et al. A phase II study of carboplatin in children with recurrent or progressive solid tumors. A report from The Childrens Cancer Group. Cancer 73:1297–1301, 1994.
50. Phillips MB, Flamant F, Sommelet-Olive D, et al. Phase II study of rapid-scheduled etoposide in paediatric soft tissue sarcomas. Eur J Cancer 31A:782–784, 1995.
51. Chard R Jr, Krivit W, Bleyer WA, et al. Phase II study of VP-16-213 in children with malignant disease: A Children's Cancer Study Group report. Cancer Treat Rep 63:1755–1759, 1979.
52. Marina NM, Rodman J, Shema SJ, et al. Phase I study of escalating targeted doses of carboplatin combined with ifosfamide and etoposide in children with relapsed solid tumors. J Clin Oncol 11:554–560, 1993.
53. Kung FH, Goorin AM, Harris MB, et al. Ifosfamide/carboplatin/etoposide (ICE) in children with recurrent/resistant malignant solid tumors. Proc Am Assoc Cancer Res 34:230 (abstr 1372), 1993.
54. Cairo MS. The use of ifosfamide, carboplatin, and etoposide in children with solid tumors. Semin Oncol 22:23–27, 1995.
55. Kung FH, Goorin AM, Harris MB, et al. Dose intensification in ICE therapy for recurrent malignant solid tumors of childhood. Proc Am Soc Clin Oncol 14:440 (abstr 1404), 1995.

56. Cairo MS, Weinthal JA, Garrison L, et al. Results of a phase I trial of PIXY321 following ifosfamide, carboplatin, and etoposide (ICE) chemotherapy in children with recurrent solid tumors (RST): Improved multi-lineage hematopoietic reconstitution. Proc Am Soc Clin Oncol 14:255 (abstr 693), 1995.
57. Marina M, Shema SJ, Bowman LC, et al. Failure of granulocyte-macrophage colony-stimulating factor to reduce febrile neutropenia in children with recurrent solid tumors treated with ifosfamide, carboplatin and etoposide chemotherapy. Med Pediatr Oncol 23:328–334, 1994.
58. Houghton PJ, Chesire PJ, Hallman CJ, et al. Therapeutic efficacy of the topoisomerase I inhibitor 7-ethyl-10-(4-[piperidino]-1-piperidino)-carbonyloxy-camptothecin against tumor xenografts: Lack of cross-resistance in vivo in tumors with acquired resistance to the topoisomerase I inhibitor 9-dimethylaminomethyl-10-hydroxycamptothecin. Cancer Res 53:2823–2829, 1993.
59. Houghton PJ, Cheshire PJ, Hallman JC III, et al. Evaluation of a novel bis-naphthalimide anticancer agent, DMP 840, against human xenografts derived from adult, juvenile and pediatric cancers. Cancer Chemother Pharmacol 33:265–272, 1994.
60. Raney B, Ensign LG, Foreman J, et al. Renal toxicity of ifosfamide in pilot regimens of the Intergroup Rhabdomyosarcoma Study for patients with gross residual tumor. Am J Pediatr Hematol Oncol 16:286–295, 1994.
61. Rossi R, Godde A, Kleinebrand A, et al. Unilateral nephrectomy and cisplatin as risk factors of ifosfamide-induced nephrotoxicity: Analysis of 120 patients. J Clin Oncol 12:159–165, 1994.
62. Ashraf MS, Brady J, Breatnach F, et al. Ifosfamide nephrotoxicity in paediatric cancer patients. Eur J Pediatr 153:90–94, 1994.
63. Heyn R, Khan F, Ensign LG, et al. Acute myeloid leukemia in patients treated for rhabdomyosarcoma with cyclophosphamide and low-dose etoposide on Intergroup Rhabdomyosarcoma Study III: An interim report. Med Pediatr Oncol 23:99–106, 1994.
64. Raney B Jr., Heyn R, Hays DM, et al. Sequelae of treatment of 109 patients followed for 5 to 15 years after diagnosis of sarcoma of bladder and prostate. A report from the Intergroup Rhabdomyosarcoma Study Committee Cancer 71:2387–2394, 1993.
65. Hughes LL, Baruzzi MJ, Ribeiro RC, et al. Paratesticular rhabdomyosarcoma: Delayed effects of multimodality therapy and implications for current management. Cancer 73:476–482, 1994.
66. Ortega JA, Donaldson S, Ivy SP, et al. Veno–oclusive disease (VOD) of the liver following vincristine-actinomycin D-cyclophosphamide (VAC) therapy for rhabdomyosarcoma (RMS): A report from the Intergroup Rhabdomyosarcoma Study (IRS) Group. Proc Am Soc Clin Oncol 14:44 (abstr 1401), 1995.
67. Parham DM, Webber BL, Jenkins JJ III, et al. Nonrhabdomyosarcomatous soft tissue sarcomas of childhood: Formulation of a simplified system for grading. Mod Pathol, 8:705–710, 1995.
68. Jenkins J, Parham DM, Webber BL, et al. Prognostic value of grading in pediatric non-rhabdomyosarcomatous soft tissue sarcomas. Mod Pathol 6:126A (abstr 736), 1993.
69. Maurer HM, Cantor A, Salzberg A, et al. Adjuvant chemotherapy vs. observation for localized non-rhabdomyosarcoma soft tissue sarcomas (NRSTS) in children. Med Pediatr Oncol 20:388 (abstr 71), 1992.
70. McCoy DM, Levine EA, Ferrer K, et al. Pediatric soft tissue sarcomas of nonmyogenic origin. J Surg Oncol 53:149–153, 1993.
71. Skene AI, Barr L, Robinson M, et al. Adult type (nonembryonal) soft tissue sarcomas in childhood. Med Pediatr Oncol 21:645–648, 1993.
72. Pappo AS, Fontanesi J, Luo X, et al. Synovial sarcoma in children and adolescents: The St Jude Children's Research Hospital experience. J Clin Oncol 12:2360–2366, 1994.
73. Rao BN. Nonrhabdomyosarcoma in children: Prognostic factors influencing survival. Semin Surg Oncol 9:524–531, 1993.
74. Laquaglia MP, Spiro SA, Ghavimi F, et al. Liposarcoma in patients younger than or equal to 22 years of age. Cancer 72:3114–3119, 1993.

75. Sreekantaiah C, Ladanyi M, Rodriguez E, et al. Chromosomal aberrations in soft tissue tumors. Relevance to diagnosis, classification, and molecular mechanisms. Am J Pathol 144:1121–1134, 1994.
76. Rabbitts TH. Chromosomal translocation in human cancer. Nature 372:143–149, 1994.
77. Shipley J, Crew J, Gusterson B. The molecular biology of soft tissue sarcomas. Eur J Cancer 29A:2054–2058, 1994.

Index